Enzymes in Farm Animal Nutrition, 3rd Edition

Enzymes in Farm Animal Nutrition, 3rd Edition

Edited by

Michael R. Bedford, AB Vista, UK

Gary G. Partridge (retired), Danisco Animal Nutrition, UK

Milan Hruby, ADM, USA

and

Carrie L. Walk, DSM, UK

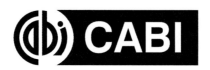

CABI is a trading name of CAB International

CABI
Nosworthy Way
Wallingford
Oxfordshire OX10 8DE
UK

CABI
WeWork
One Lincoln St
24th Floor
Boston, MA 02111
USA

Tel: +44 (0)1491 832111
Fax: +44 (0)1491 833508
E-mail: info@cabi.org
Website: www.cabi.org

Tel: +1 (617)682-9015
E-mail: cabi-nao@cabi.org

A catalogue record for this book is available from the British Library, London, UK.

Library of Congress Cataloging-in-Publication Data

Names: Bedford, Michael R. (Michael Richard), 1960- editor. | Partridge, Gary G., 1953- editor. | Hruby, Milan (Editor on animal nutrition) editor. | Walk, Carrie, editor.
Title: Enzymes in farm animal nutrition / edited by Michael R. Bedford, AB Vista, UK, Gary G. Partridge (retired), Danisco Animal Nutrition, UK, Milan Hruby, ADM, USA and Carrie Walk, DSM, UK.
Description: 3rd edition. | Oxfordshire, UK ; Boston, MA : CAB International, [2022] | Includes bibliographical references and index. | Summary: "This fully updated new edition provides a comprehensive guide to enzyme-supplemented animal feeds. It explores using enzymes in fish and shrimp diets, new understanding of how phytases function, and NSPase research. It also includes new chapters on enzyme combinations, antibiotic free diets and measuring response in feed trials"-- Provided by publisher.
Identifiers: LCCN 2021033216 (print) | LCCN 2021033217 (ebook) | ISBN 9781789241563 (hardback) | ISBN 9781789241570 (ebook) | ISBN 9781789241587 (epub)
Classification: LCC SF98.E58 E59 2022 (print) | LCC SF98.E58 (ebook) | DDC 636.08/52--dc23
LC record available at https://lccn.loc.gov/2021033216
LC ebook record available at https://lccn.loc.gov/2021033217

References to Internet websites (URLs) were accurate at the time of writing.

ISBN-13: 9781789241563 (hardback)
         9781789241570 (ePDF)
         9781789241587 (ePub)
DOI: 10.1079/9781789241563.0000

Commissioning Editor: Alex Lainsbury
Editorial Assistant: Emma McCann
Production Editor: Shankari Wilford

Typeset by SPi, Pondicherry, India
Printed and bound in the UK by Severn, Gloucester

Contents

_____

Contributors

Ajay Badhan, Lethbridge Research and Development Centre, 5403 1st Avenue South, Lethbridge, Alberta T1J 4B1, Canada. Email: ajay.badhan@agr.gc.ca

Karen A. Beauchemin, Lethbridge Research and Development Centre, PO Box 3000, 5403 1st Avenue South, Lethbridge, Alberta T1J 4B1, Canada. Email: karen.beauchemin@agr.gc.ca

Todd Becker, IFF, 925 Page Mill Road, Palo Alto, CA 94304, USA. Email: todd.becker@iff.com

Michael R. Bedford, AB Vista, 3 Woodstock Court, Blenheim Road, Marlborough, Wiltshire, SN8 4AA, UK. Email: mike.bedford@abvista.com

Kyle D. Brown, Department of Poultry Science, Texas A&M University, College Station, Texas, USA. Email: kyledeanbrown@yahoo.com

Aaron J. Cowieson, DSM Nutritional Products, Wurmisweg 576, 4303 Kaiseraugst, Switzerland. Email: aaron.cowieson@dsm.com

Douglas Dale, IFF, 925 Page Mill Road, Palo Alto, CA 94304, USA. Email: doug.dale@iff.com

Richard Ducatelle, Department of Pathology, Bacteriology and Avian Medicine, Faculty of Veterinary Medicine, Ghent University, Merelbeke, Belgium. Email: Richard.Ducatelle@UGent.be

Venessa Eeckhaut, Department of Pathology, Bacteriology and Avian Medicine, Faculty of Veterinary Medicine, Ghent University, Merelbeke, Belgium. Email: Venessa.Eeckhaut@UGent.be

Ceinwen Evans, Danisco Animal Nutrition, Danisco (UK) Ltd, PO Box 777, Marlborough, Wiltshire, SN8 1XN, UK. Email: ceinwen.evans@iff.com

Evy Goossens, Department of Pathology, Bacteriology and Avian Medicine, Faculty of Veterinary Medicine, Ghent University, Merelbeke, Belgium. Email: Evy.Goossens@UGent.be

Ralf Greiner, Federal Research Institute of Nutrition, and Food Institute of Food Technology and Bioprocess Engineering, Haid-und-Neu-Straße 9, 76131 Karlsruhe, Germany. Email: ralf.greiner@mri.bund.de

Laerke T. Haahr, Novozymes A/S, Biologiens Vej 2, 2800 Kgs., Lyngby, Denmark. Email: ltvh@novozymes.com

Adrian J. Hernández, Núcleo de Investigación en Producción Alimentaria, Depto de Ciencias Agropecuarias y Acuícolas, Facultad de Recursos Naturales, Universidad Católica de Temuco, Avda. Rudecindo Ortega, 02950, Temuco, Chile. Email: ajhernandez@uct.cl

Milan Hruby, ADM, 4666 Faries Parkway, Decatur, IL 62526, USA. Email: milan.hruby@ adm.com

Hamish Irving, Danisco Animal Nutrition, Genencor International BV, Willem Einthoven-straat 4, 2342 BG Oegstgeest, the Netherlands. Email: hamish.irving@iff.com

Ursula Konietzny, Walsdtrasse 5c, D-76706 Dettenheim, Germany. Email: uschi.greiner@ yahoo.de

Imke Kühn, AB Vista, AB Enzymes GmbH, Feldbergstrasse 78, D-64293 Darmstadt, Germany. Email: imke.kuhn@abvista.com

Jason T. Lee, CJ Bio America, 2001 Butterfield Rd, Downers Grove, IL 60515, USA. Email: jason.lee2@cj.net

Qingyun Li, Cargill Premix and Nutrition, 6571 State Route 503, Lewisburg, OH 45338, USA. Email: qli@provimi-na.com

Lorenzo Márquez, Grupo de Modelización Digestiva, Universidad de Almería, La Cañada de San Urbano, 04120 Almería, Spain. Email: marquez.lorenzo728@gmail.com

Sam Maurer, IFF, 925 Page Mill Road, Palo Alto, CA 94304, USA. Email: sam.maurer@iff.com

Daniel Menezes-Blackburn, Department of Soils, Water and Agricultural Engineering, Sultan Qaboos University, PO Box 34, Al-khod 123, Sultanate of Oman. Email: danielblac@squ.edu.om

Tim A. McAllister, Lethbridge Research and Development Centre, Lethbridge, Alberta, Canada. Email: tim.mcallister@agr.gc.ca

Gabriel A. Morales, Instituto de Investigaciones en Producción Animal – Consejo Nacional de Investigaciones Científicas y Técnicas (INPA-CONICET), Buenos Aires, Argentina; Departamento de Producción Animal, Facultad de Agronomía, Universidad de Buenos Aires, Av. San Martín 4453, Cap. Fed. C1417DSE, Buenos Aires, Argentina. Email: moralesg@agro.uba.ar

Edwin T. Moran Jr, Poultry Science Department, Auburn University, 260 Lem Morrison Drive, Auburn, AL 36849, USA. Email: moranet@auburn.edu

Francisco J. Moyano, Grupo de Modelización Digestiva, Universidad de Almería, La Cañada de San Urbano, 04120 Almería, Spain. Email: fjmoyano@ual.es

John F. Patience, Department of Animal Science, Iowa State University, 3026 Roxboro Drive, Ames, IA 50010, USA. Email: jfp@iastate.edu

Amy L. Petry, Texas Tech University, 203 Animal and Food Sciences Building, PO Box 42141, Lubbock, TX 79409, USA. Email: amy.petry@ttu.edu

Michael Reichman, IFF, 925 Page Mill Road, Palo Alto, CA 94304, USA. Email: michael. reichman@iff.com

Markus Rodehutscord, Department of Animal Nutrition, University of Hohenheim, Emil-Wolff-Strasse 10, D-70599 Stuttgart, Germany. Email: markus.rodehutscord@ uni-hohenheim.de

Christine Rosser, Lethbridge Research and Development Centre, PO Box 3000, 5403 1st Avenue South, Lethbridge, Alberta T1J 4B1, Canada. Email: clrosser.17@gmail.com

Noel Sheehan, AB Vista, Unit 6, Innovation & Technology Building, Tredomen Park, Hengoed, Ystrad Mynach, CF82 7FQ, UK. Email: noelsheehan@abvista.com

Lars K. Skov, Novozymes A/S, Biologiens Vej 2, 2800 Kgs., Lyngby, Denmark. Email: laks@ novozymes.com

Paul Steen, AB Vista, AB Agri Ltd, 3 Woodstock Court, Blenheim Road, Marlborough, Wiltshire, SN8 4AN, UK. Email: paul.steen@abvista.com

Vera Sommerfeld, Department of Animal Nutrition, University of Hohenheim, Emil-Wolff-Strasse 10, D-70599 Stuttgart, Germany. Email: v.sommerfeld@uni-hohenheim.de

Stephanie A. Terry, Lethbridge Research and Development Centre, PO Box 3000, 5403 1st Avenue South, Lethbridge, Alberta T1J 4B1, Canada. Email: stephanie.terry@agr.gc.ca

Filip Van Immerseel, Department of Pathology, Bacteriology and Avian Medicine, Faculty of Veterinary Medicine, Ghent University, Merelbeke, Belgium. Email: Filip.VanImmerseel@UGent.be

Jari Vehmaanperä, (retired) Roal Oy, Tykkimäentie 15b, 05200 Rajamäki, Finland. Email: jari.vehmaanpera@helsinki.fi

Carrie L. Walk, DSM Nutritional Products, 5 Delves Road, Heanor, Derbyshire, DE75 7SY, UK. Email: carrie.walk@dsm.com

1 The Feed Enzyme Market in 2020 and Beyond

Ceinwen Evans[1]* and Hamish Irving[2]

[1]*Danisco Animal Nutrition, Danisco (UK) Ltd, Marlborough, UK; [2]Danisco Animal Nutrition, Genencor International BV, Oegstgeest, the Netherlands*

1.1 Historic Use of Feed Enzymes

Commercial feed enzymes were first introduced in 1984 in Finland by Suomen Rehu and had the aim of significantly improving the nutritional quality of barley-based rations (Bedford and Partridge, 2001). The enzymes used were originally developed for the brewing industry and then leveraged into animal nutrition. Through their mode of action in targeting specific antinutrients present in key raw materials in the feed, enzymes help reduce antinutritional effects and improve feed efficiency by allowing the animals to extract more nutritional value from the feed ingredients. Their use has enabled producers to see direct and immediate economic returns through the ability to alter their feed formulations, reducing the use of expensive ingredients (e.g. fat, synthetic amino acids and inorganic phosphorus) while still meeting the animal's nutritional requirements. The use of enzymes in the feed also allows producers to have more flexibility in their feed formulations through inclusion of lower-quality raw materials or by-products in the diet when prices of the main grains are high, helping them to better manage feed cost volatility in their systems.

These immediate returns on investment for users helped adoption of feed enzymes as a new technology and has driven the growth of the market.

There are also additional benefits to the use of feed enzymes. The fact that the animal is able to extract more nutrients from the feed has the benefit of reducing the wastage from animal production systems; this is especially important in markets where land mass is an issue for disposal of waste or where there is strong environmental legislation. Through improved feed efficiency producers are also able to get animals to market weight quicker, using less feed. As feed is the greatest contributor to production costs (approximately 70%), any action that can bring down the price per tonne and the feed cost per animal in the system is of benefit for the profitability of the producer (Barletta, 2010).

1.2 Why Have Feed Enzymes Traditionally Been Used?

Historically, the use of feed enzymes has been with a nutritional focus in mind. The market to date has been dominated by

*Email: ceinwen.evans@iff.com

©CAB International 2022. *Enzymes in Farm Animal Nutrition, 3rd Edition* (M. Bedford *et al.* eds)
DOI: 10.1079/9781789241563.0001

enzyme activities targeting the main potential antinutrients found in livestock diets such as fibre, proteinaceous compounds (e.g. lectins, trypsin inhibitors) and phytate. Starch digestion can also be compromised and can potentially benefit from exogenous amylase addition.

1.2.1 Fibre-degrading enzymes

The first feed enzymes to be introduced were β-glucanases in the early 1980s for barley-based diets followed by xylanases in the late 1980s (Bedford and Partridge, 2001). These enzymes target β-glucans and arabinoxylans, which are soluble fibre fractions found in cereals and other raw materials present in the feed. Soluble fibre, if not dealt with, can lead to issues with viscosity, especially in poultry. Increasing levels of viscosity have a direct negative correlation with feed conversion and metabolizable energy. This is due to the viscous conditions in the gut hindering digestion of key nutrients and thereby decreasing bird growth. With the initial introduction of fibre-degrading enzymes, the visual effects of the enzyme could be seen within the production systems with reductions in sticky droppings, wet litter, dirty eggs and carcass downgrading issues such as breast blisters or carcass contamination.

While viscosity issues mainly affect poultry, other negative effects of fibre can affect performance of both poultry and swine. For example, in piglets the ability of fibre to increase the bulkiness of feed can negatively impact feed intakes during this critical phase and have detrimental effects on lifelong performance as a result. Clear benefits can also therefore be seen with use of xylanase for young pigs.

Initially these enzymes were targeted to those markets that were using viscous grains in their diets such as wheat, barley and rye. The nutritive value of these grains can be highly variable, introducing variability into the production system that can impact flock or herd uniformity, which is a big issue when animals are being grown to target weights for the market. Today most poultry

diets containing wheat, barley or other viscous grains would contain a xylanase and/or β-glucanase. Use of feed enzymes in piglet diets containing these grains is also high and adoption in grower-finisher diets is increasing.

1.2.2 Protein-degrading enzymes

Introduced soon after xylanase, proteases target the storage protein and proteinaceous antinutrients found in key feed ingredients such as soybean meal and other vegetable proteins. Key proteinaceous antinutrients present in legumes include trypsin inhibitors, which inhibit digestion by blocking the activity of trypsin. Through the use of exogenous proteases these inhibitors can be broken down and the protease can supplement the action of the endogenous proteases produced by the animal. Use of proteases also decreases nitrogen excretion, which can reduce ammonia production in animal houses and also has positive environmental impacts.

Protein digestibility of major protein sources is not complete, varying from 73.0 to 79.5% for meat and bone meal and canola meal to 91% for soybean meal (Rostagno et al., 2011). This means there is a large amount of undigested substrate to target with an exogenous protease. There are also potential gut health benefits through a reduction in undigested protein reaching the caeca of birds or hindguts of pigs, meaning less substrate available for potentially pathogenic protein-fermenting bacteria such as *Clostridium perfringens*.

1.2.3 Starch-degrading enzymes

As is the case with protein, starch digestibility is also not complete in the animal. For example, in poultry starch digestibility increases in the animal as endogenous amylase production increases during the early weeks of life, but while amylase production continues to scale up in the animal's gut, the overall digestion of starch tends to peak at about 85% (Noy and Sklan, 1995). This indicates that a high amount of substrate is still available for an exogenous amylase to target and enhance digestibility. Amylases are currently used in both monogastrics and ruminants, however application into ruminants is still in its infancy.

1.2.4   Phytate-degrading enzymes

Phytases dominate the current feed enzyme market and are ubiquitous in most poultry and pig feeds globally. They target the antinutrient phytate, which is the main storage form of phosphorus in plants. Phosphorus is crucial for good growth and bone development. Levels of phytate vary between raw materials and also between batches of raw material. Monogastric animals lack the enzyme activities needed to degrade phytate and therefore phosphorus in the form of phytate is largely unavailable to the animal. Prior to commercialization of phytases, in order to meet the animal's requirement for phosphorus, it was necessary to include inorganic forms of phosphorus in the diet. Such a diet would contain excess indigestible phosphorus and large amounts of phosphorus were excreted in the animal's manure. Environmental concerns due to pollution of natural waterways with phosphorus excreted by livestock led to the development and initial adoption of phytases in monogastric feeds in the 1990s. Widespread adoption followed once feed cost savings were achieved through application of phosphorus and calcium nutrient matrix values to the phytase and also through the reduced costs of disposing of the lower-phosphorus waste.

More recent research has demonstrated that the phytate molecule, targeted by phytases, not only makes phosphorus unavailable but is also a powerful antinutrient, impeding the digestion of amino acids and minerals, negatively impacting the effectiveness of the animal's endogenous protease and increasing endogenous losses from animals. The result of not dealing with phytate is therefore decreased nutrient digestion and feed efficiencies, impairing animal performance.

Since the initial introduction of phytase, ongoing investment in animal research by phytase suppliers and growing competition have led to the development of more efficient enzymes with significantly higher economic benefits for producers and lower costs of inclusion. With a deeper understanding of the negative effects of phytate and the benefits of phytase, there have been two major developments. Doses have increased beyond the traditional standard dose of 500 FTU/kg feed, especially in regions such as Asia where feeds can contain high levels of phytate-rich rice bran or other similar raw materials, the aim being to degrade the phytate as quickly as possible, reducing the antinutrient effects of phytate. Also, additional nutritional value is now assigned to the enzyme, with many suppliers having now introduced energy and amino acid values to the phytase nutrient matrix. This substantially increases the potential feed cost savings, leads to a higher optimal phytase dose and has therefore driven up the use of phytase.

1.2.5   Is more than one enzyme activity needed?

Most diets fed globally contain cereals and protein sources, with the dominant protein source being soybean meal. In cereals there is a close association between starch, protein and fibre-rich cell walls. For example, the endosperm of cereal grains is made up of a starch/protein matrix. Using enzymes to break down either the starch or the protein is therefore likely to also increase digestion of the other component. It is for this reason that when nutrient values are assigned to an enzyme product, they may include nutrients that are not the primary target of the enzyme. In the case of soybean products there is a large amount of protein present but also several antinutrients such as trypsin inhibitors and also non-starch polysaccharides. Some protein will be trapped due to the 'cage effect' of this fibre and therefore it is likely that a xylanase will complement the protease activity and provide additional benefits. When considering the feed enzymes to use it is important to look at the ingredients in the diet and the likely substrate levels that are present for the enzymes to act on. Enzymes can then be selected that are suitable for the main antinutritional substrates found in the diet.

1.3   Current Feed Enzyme Market Size

Recent market reports estimate the current size of the global feed enzyme market at US$1.2 billion. Projections for market growth differ, in the range of 5–10% compound annual growth rate (Marketsandmarkets.com, 2019; Mordor Intelligence, 2019). Market projections are typically prepared by analysts who look at data available in annual reports of publicly listed companies. As the largest feed enzyme suppliers are part of larger companies, there is little publicly available data on exactly how much revenue is generated with feed enzymes and how fast the market is growing. Factors that influence this growth rate include:

- Penetration of enzymes in the market. This typically increases as the level of sophistication of production systems increases.
- Enzyme inclusion levels (dosing). This typically increases as operations become more skilled in the use of enzymes.
- Emissions from animal production. Regulatory and consumer pressures to reduce emissions are expected to increase (FAO, 2019).
- Animal protein production output. Animal protein production is forecast to increase over the next decade.

While the exact magnitude of expected growth is unclear, analysts agree that the market and demand for feed enzymes will continue to increase. The key drivers for growth are a growing global population combined with a rise in the share of people in developing countries who can afford animal protein, despite a growing number of Western consumers who are reducing their meat consumption. Per capita meat consumption is forecast to increase in all regions, with Asia expected to see the largest growth. Meat consumption in China and South-East Asia is projected to increase by 2028 to 5 and 4 kg/capita, respectively, with the main increases coming from poultry and pork meat (OECD/FAO, 2019). In mature markets, meat consumption is also expected to grow, albeit at a lower rate, despite the growing trends for meat replacement.

Market needs to reduce feed costs and emissions in animal production will drive growth of feed enzymes, even in mature markets. Global livestock production is projected to expand by 13% by 2028, with an equivalent growth in feed production. The majority of livestock production growth will come from further intensification of production, by both increased outputs per animal through increased slaughter weights as well as increasing the number of animals through shortening time to market (OECD/FAO, 2019). To achieve these production improvements, efficiency of feed utilization will be a key parameter and feed enzymes are proven to contribute to this. An additional likely consequence of an increased human population and growing demand for animal protein is that there may be more episodes of increased competition for major grains between food, fuel and feed, driving up the costs of grains, incentivizing animal producers to use lower-quality ingredients in animal diets. This is likely to increase target substrates for feed enzymes.

1.4   Who's Who in the Feed Enzyme Market?

The number of players in the feed enzyme market continues to increase, as does the trend for mergers and acquisitions within the industry. In key growth markets such as India and China, there are increasing numbers of local companies producing the main classes of feed enzymes. As the experience of these producers and the quality of their products increase, some of these local products are starting to enter other global markets. Globally some of the main players who currently continue to dominate the industry are Danisco Animal Nutrition, Novozymes/DSM, BASF, Adisseo/Bluestar, Huvepharma and AB Vista.

Danisco Animal Nutrition (Leiden, the Netherlands) is a unit within the Health and Biosciences division of IFF (Wilmington, USA). Danisco Animal Nutrition (formerly known as Finnfeeds International Ltd) pioneered the development of feed enzymes in the 1980s. Their enzyme products include the phytases Axtra® PHY and Phyzyme® XP, and a range of single- and multi-activity carbohydrase/protease-based products – Danisco® Xylanase, Axtra® XB, Axtra® XAP and Axtra® PRO. The portfolio also includes products for swine and poultry that combine enzymes with probiotic technologies to maximize gut health and nutrient digestibility under the Syncra® brand. DuPont also sells natural betaine into the feed additive sector.

Novozymes (Denmark) and DSM (the Netherlands) formed a strategic alliance in 2001. DSM is responsible for the sales, marketing and distribution of Novozymes' feed enzymes. Novozymes is responsible for product development and R&D. The alliance covers pigs, poultry, ruminants and pet feed. Their portfolio of feed enzyme products currently includes a phytase, Ronozyme® HiPhos, and a range of single- and multi-activity carbohydrase/protease-based products including Ronozyme® ProAct, Ronozyme® WX, Roxazyme® G2, Ronozyme® RumiStar™ and Ronozyme® MultiGrain. The portfolio also includes a muramidase with the trade name Balancius®, which is an enzyme designed to digest bacterial waste within the gut of birds to help maximize digestion. DSM also sells other additive types including carotenoids, eubiotics and vitamins.

BASF's feed enzyme portfolio includes Natuphos®, which was the first commercial feed phytase, Natuphos® E (phytase) and Natugrain® (carbohydrase). Their portfolio also includes glycinates, carotenoids, organic acids, vitamins and clay products.

Adisseo (France) was acquired by Bluestar group (China) in 2006. Bluestar Adisseo (France) specializes in animal nutrition, providing amino acids, vitamins and enzymes to the animal feed industry. Their feed enzyme portfolio currently includes Rovabio® Excel (carbohydrase), Rovabio®

Advance (carbohydrase) and Rovabio® Advance PHY (carbohydrase and phytase).

Huvepharma (Bulgaria) is a company focused on human and veterinary pharmaceuticals. Their products include coccidiostats, enzymes, vaccines and other veterinary products. The Huvepharma feed enzyme portfolio includes Hostazym® C and Hostazym® X (carbohydrases) and OptiPhos® (phytase) that they acquired from Enzyvia LLC in 2013.

AB Vista is the feed additives business owned by AB Agri (UK). Their enzyme portfolio includes Quantum® Blue (phytase), Finase® EC (phytase), Econase® XT (carbohydrase) and Signis® (a combination of a xylanase and xylo-oligomers). Their portfolio also includes betaine and live yeast.

1.5 Regulation of Feed Enzymes

Most markets around the world have regulations in place to govern the placement of feed enzymes on to the market. Those producing feed enzymes or placing them on to the market must provide proof that the enzyme is safe and efficacious for the target species. Proof of product quality such as consistency and stability must also be demonstrated. Approval times vary by market and can range from 3 months to over 2 years depending on the level of detail needed in the regulatory dossier. The most highly regulated markets include the EU, the USA and Brazil, but the trend is for increased levels of regulation globally.

To gain approval to sell in the EU, enzymes must gain approval under Regulation EC 1831/2003. A full dossier detailing the identity, characterization and conditions of use for the enzyme must be provided to the European Food Safety Authority (EFSA). The source of most feed enzymes remains microorganisms and therefore full details on the characterization of the production organism are also required. Safety of the enzyme must be demonstrated via a full toxicity test, and tolerance studies must also be provided looking at the target species. Enzyme products, due to their proteinaceous nature, are presumed to be respiratory sensitizers and particle size data are used to assess the likelihood of exposure and risk to the users. As well as assessing safety, the EU dossier also requires proof of efficacy for the intended use. Studies must demonstrate significant effects at the lowest recommended dose in three studies per major target species conducted according to common feed manufacturing, animal husbandry and farming practices in the EU. Approval of the dossier by EFSA once it is prepared and submitted takes approximately 2 years (EFSA, 2019).

In the USA any product intended for use as an animal food ingredient is considered a food and the Food and Drug Administration's (FDA) Center for Veterinary Medicine (CVM) is responsible for the regulation of animal food products. Producers are able to submit a self Generally Recognized as Safe (GRAS) notification. This requires a similar safety assessment to the EU approval but requires only one proof-of-efficacy study. To achieve self GRAS, the information should be assessed by a group of experts known as a GRAS panel (FDA, 2020).

In other markets around the world there is a trend for increasing regulations. For example, in China and Canada if the enzyme production host is genetically modified then it is necessary to register the enzyme production host. Only once these are approved and on the positive list can one pursue a product registration. This process can be lengthy and up to 48 months in China. In Brazil regulations have also recently been reviewed and increased, with a new requirement introduced that every product presentation (liquid, granule, powder) and every product concentration needs its own efficacy study for each animal category.

1.6   How are Enzymes Used in Feed?

There are two main methods of using feed enzymes. The first is to assign and apply a nutrient matrix to the feed enzymes to account for the nutrients released by the enzyme. Matrix values for carbohydrases and proteases typically include energy, protein and amino acids. When first launched the matrix values assigned to phytases were for calcium and phosphorus only. However, as more is now understood about the negative effects of phytate, most producers also recommend energy, amino acids and other minerals to be assigned. The matrix values are usually generated using animal studies which have looked at digestibility improvements that can be gained through use of the enzymes. The benefit of assigning matrix values is that it results in reductions in feed costs while animal performance (growth, feed efficiency, egg production, etc.) is maintained. The matrix values can be used either to replace expensive ingredients in the formulation (e.g. fat or synthetic amino acids) or to relax constraints on the inclusion of lower-cost, poorer-quality ingredients. This is the preferred method of application as the cost savings achieved through the use of the enzyme(s) are immediately apparent to the user and will usually more than cover the cost of the enzyme addition.

The second method of using feed enzymes is to add the enzyme to the standard feed with no reformulation. The enzyme(s) will still release nutrients and improve efficiency of feed utilization resulting in improved animal performance. The economic benefits of this method of application are typically realized at the end of the production cycle, either in heavier slaughter weights or more production cycles per unit of time. Users can alternatively get the benefit of both application methods by applying a discount to the matrix provided by the enzyme suppliers at the same time as realizing some performance benefits.

There are several considerations for the physical product form. Enzymes are protein products which need to have sufficient shelf life to cover transportation, storage time and storage conditions, whether that is in pure form, in premix or in feed. They must also be robust enough to withstand feed processing conditions.

Enzymes can be added as liquid or dry product forms into the feed. Liquid product forms are usually non-thermostable and therefore have to be added to the feed via a post-pelleting liquid application (PPLA) system. Although PPLA systems are relatively complex they have several advantages. First, PPLA enables enzyme application to feed produced under harsh processing conditions. Such processing conditions can be used for several reasons, for example as a strategy to minimize *Salmonella* spp. contamination. Second, PPLA offers dosing flexibility where enzyme dose (especially phytase) can be varied from batch to batch, something which could be harder if the alternative is enzyme inclusion via the premix. Ideally, liquid enzymes would be sufficiently thermostable to allow them to be dosed directly into the feed mixer pre-pelleting, just like liquid amino acids are today. This would combine dosing flexibility and automation with a much simpler and cheaper dosing system than PPLA.

Dry product forms can be either thermostable or non-thermostable. The advantage of dry thermostable product is that it can be dosed either directly into the feed mixer or included in the premix, thus simplifying operations versus PPLA. As the majority of monogastric feed is pelleted, the majority of feed enzymes used today are dry thermostable products. Dry non-thermostable product is typically used in mash feed, which is not pelleted.

Finally, some thought should be given to safety and ease of handling. Some enzyme suppliers have started to offer high-concentration dry powder forms which are often highly dusty. To avoid worker exposure, which could lead to allergic reactions, proper containment procedures need to be put in place when handling high-concentration enzyme powders. Enzymes in granular form or in liquid form have a far lower worker safety exposure risk and are easier to handle safely.

Taking all these elements into consideration, the user should select the product and product form that best suits their operations.

1.7 The Changing World of Animal Production – An Opportunity for Feed Enzymes?

The animal production industry is currently undergoing a period of change. Globally there is a drive to reduce or remove antibiotics from animal production, mainly due to concerns over antibiotic resistance and possible implications for animal health. The use of antibiotics in animal production has been long established practice and their removal has big implications for producers. Without the antibiotic line of defence, animal production becomes more complex with unpredictable disease challenges on the rise. As a result, the importance of maintaining good gut health is receiving more focus and the necessity of feeding not just the animal but also its gut microbiome is clear.

While ensuring that the animal has all the nutrients needed to reach its full growth potential is a top priority, it is also important to either limit the amount of undigested nutrients or control the types of undigested nutrients that reach the terminal ileum or hindgut, so as not to provide substrates upon which non-beneficial bacterial populations can feed and thrive. Feed enzymes have a major contribution to make in this area as they are known to improve digestibility and limit the amounts of undigested nutrients in the lower gastrointestinal tract. For example, proteases and also carbohydrases and phytases will reduce the amount of undigested protein reaching the hindgut where it would be utilized by protein fermenters such as *C. perfringens* which can cause disease issues if their population gets out of control. Xylanase has also been shown to produce oligomers that are most suitable as a substrate for beneficial bacterial populations. Further research is currently under way across the industry to build on these known proven effects. A fuller understanding of which substrates can be utilized by the microbial populations in the gut and how to increase those of benefit will be key. In addition, a greater understanding will be necessary of how the nutritional changes and reductions in antinutritional effects achieved with enzymes influence other factors such as immune responses and gut function.

Due to the many issues that removing antibiotics may cause, it is probable that multiple technologies will be needed to replace them. As a result, we will likely be seeing more technology combinations in the marketplace, as well as novel enzyme activities that have a primary mode of action more related to gut health effects rather than nutritional effects per se. Recent years have also seen veterinary pharmaceutical companies moving into the feed additive space as they look for ways to replace the lost revenue streams from the removal of antibiotics from livestock diets.

Another trend starting to influence animal production is the growing concern over climate change and sustainability with a spotlight being shone on the animal production industry. Feeding a fast-growing human population is likely to lead to more intensification of the livestock industry. As farms become larger, concerns over emissions will continue to grow. Enzymes, through influencing the substrates available for bacterial fermentation, will likely have value in this application.

The current feed enzyme market is dominated by products aimed at monogastrics (pigs and poultry). Opportunities for market growth also exist in the ruminant and aquaculture industries. The challenge for the ruminant space is having enzymes that can either act in or survive the rumen. For aquaculture feeds it is likely that the successful enzymes will need to have different biochemical properties from those used for pigs and poultry, such as optimum temperature and pH as well as salt tolerance in the case of saltwater fish.

While to date the nutritional cost savings seen with enzymes has driven their market adoption, in the future a better understanding of their full mode of action may bring new value propositions. This is being reflected in the research approaches being adopted by major feed enzyme companies. All major enzyme producers are expanding their research disciplines to understand how enzymes can continue to improve via: (i) nutrition (where enzymes are traditionally key); (ii) the microbiome; and (iii) gut/immune function. It is in the latter two categories where the effects of enzymes are gradually becoming clearer from recent research. Factors such as diet, digestion and absorption, gastrointestinal tract microbiota and mucosa, welfare and performance, and immune status all need consideration. These show the agreement within the feed enzyme industry for a need to understand, at a much deeper level, the benefits that enzymes can bring. The ultimate aim is to help animal and feed producers navigate the options that are put to them and to demonstrate the importance of enzyme technology in the fast-changing world of animal production.

References

Barletta, A. (2010) Introduction: current market and expected developments. In: Bedford, M.R. and Partridge, G.G. (eds) *Enzymes in Farm Animal Nutrition*, 2nd edn. CAB International, Wallingford, UK, pp. 1–11.

Bedford, M.R. and Partridge, G.G. (2001) Preface. In: Bedford, M.R. and Partridge, G.G. (eds) *Enzymes in Farm Animal Nutrition*, 1st edn. CAB International, Wallingford, UK, p. ix.

EFSA (2019) Feed additive applications: regulations and guidance. European Food Safety Authority, Parma, Italy. Available at: https://www.efsa.europa.eu/en/applications/feedadditives/regulationsandguidance (accessed 22 January 2020).

FAO (2019) Five practical actions towards low-carbon livestock. Food and Agriculture Organization of the United Nations, Rome. Available at: http://www.fao.org/3/ca7089en/CA7089EN.pdf (accessed 22 January 2020).

FDA (2020) Generally Recognized as Safe (GRAS) Notification Program. US Food and Drug Administration, Silver Spring, Maryland. Available at: https://www.fda.gov/animal-veterinary/animal-food-feeds/generally-recognized-safe-gras-notification-program (accessed 22 January 2020).

Marketsandmarkets.com (2019) Feed Enzymes Market by Type (Phytase, Carbohydrase, and Protease), Livestock (Poultry, Swine, Ruminants, and Aquatic Animals), Source (Microorganism, Plant, and Animal), Form (Dry and Liquid), and Region – Global Forecast to 2025. MarketsandMarkets™ Research Pvt Ltd, Pune, India. Available at: https://www.marketsandmarkets.com/Market-Reports/feed-enzyme-market-1157.html (accessed 22 January 2020).

Mordor Intelligence (2019) Global feed enzymes market share, size-growth, trends and forecasts (2020–2025). Mordor Intelligence, Hyderabad, India. Available at: https://www.mordorintelligence.com/industry-reports/global-animal-feed-enzymes-market-industry (accessed 22 January 2020).

Noy, Y. and Sklan, D. (1995) Digestion and absorption in the young chick. *Poultry Science* 74, 366–373.

OECD/FAO (2019) *OECD-FAO Agricultural Outlook 2019–2028*. OECD Publishing, Paris/Food and Agriculture Organization of the United Nations, Rome. https://doi.org/10.1787/agr_outlook-2019-en

Rostagno, H.S., Albino, L.F.T., Donzele, J.L., Gomes, P.C., de Oliveira, R.F., *et al.* (2011) *Brazilian Tables for Poultry and Swine*, 3rd edn. Universidade Federal de Viçosa, Departamento de Zootecnia, Viçosa, Brazil.

2 Feed Enzymes: Enzymology, Biochemistry, and Production on an Industrial Scale

Jari Vehmaanperä*

Roal Oy, Rajamäki, Finland

2.1 Introduction

Fibre-degrading enzymes or non-starch polysaccharidases (NSPases) were first launched as feed additives for poultry in the 1980s followed by the introduction of phytase early in the 1990s for the main monogastric farm animals, poultry and pigs (Barletta, 2010; Bedford and Partridge, 2010). Since then the feed enzyme market has grown to about a quarter of the total industrial enzymes segment, comparable in size to detergent enzymes (Garske *et al.*, 2017). Phytase has achieved high inclusion rates (70–80%) in all diets for swine and poultry (Lei *et al.*, 2013) but because of price erosion, the value of the market is now probably equal or less than feed NSPases, i.e. xylanases and β-glucanases. In addition to these two segments, some other enzyme classes are sold to niche applications. Feed enzymes present a rather small number of enzyme classes within the hydrolase group and mainly originate from microbial sources. The enzyme products are manufactured in large-scale bioreactors by a few established companies, although during the last few years novel Chinese suppliers have started to enter global markets, particularly with competitive

phytase products. To meet the needs of the markets, enzymes should be produced at an affordable cost, safely, with secure supply and exhibit advanced characteristics like thermostability. To meet these needs, the feed enzyme industry has explored the biodiversity in nature in search for optimal enzyme backbones and engineered them further *in vitro* (Shivange and Schwaneberg, 2017) and has also developed advanced product formulations (Meesters, 2010). Genetically modified organisms (GMOs) are widely used for production and these microbes are cultivated under contained conditions. The enzyme semifinals recovered after submerged fermentation in bioreactors are essentially enzyme monocomponents, which are processed and blended with other ingredients to make the final product. The manufacturing process and the products themselves both require regulatory approval.

Traditionally, enzymes have been classified biochemically according to the IUB (International Union of Biochemistry) Enzyme Nomenclature into seven main classes, each having a unique code starting with 'EC' (Enzyme Commission) and followed by four numbers separated by a period for further

*Email: jari.vehmaanpera@helsinki.fi

©CAB International 2022. *Enzymes in Farm Animal Nutrition, 3rd Edition* (M. Bedford *et al.* eds)
DOI: 10.1079/9781789241563.0002

refinement (Bairoch, 2000; McDonald *et al.*, 2009; Tipton, 2018). The IUB classification is based on the reaction type and the substrate specificity, rather than, e.g., the structure of the enzyme polypeptide. Phytases and NSPases belong to the main class of hydrolases (EC 3) which indicates either addition or removal of water in the reaction. In addition, carbohydrate-active enzymes, i.e. NSPases, are structurally classified based on their amino acid sequence or fold similarities according to the CAZy database (Carbohydrate-Active enZYmes; http://www.cazy.org, accessed 10 September 2021), which reflects better their phylogenetic relationships (Henrissat and Davies, 1997; Lombard *et al.*, 2014).

The required biochemical characteristics of feed enzymes include high specific activity at body temperature, optimal pH profile, pepsin resistance and preferably high thermostability. High specific activity, i.e. activity per milligram of enzyme protein, is essential for the economics of enzyme manufacturing, enabling supply of highly concentrated products and supporting affordable cost of dosing in feed for the customer. The pH in the crop and stomach (proventriculus and gizzard) in poultry varies in the range pH 4.5–6.5 and 1.9–4.5, respectively (Svihus, 2010); accordingly, a pH of 5.0 and 3.0, respectively, has been chosen in some *in vitro* simulation studies (Menezes-Blackburn *et al.*, 2015). For pigs, stomach pH values between pH 3.0 and 5.0 have been reported, pH 4.0 being a representative average (Svihus, 2010). Because of the high standards of hygiene in feed manufacture, most feed enzymes need to survive high temperatures during feed processing, e.g. 90–95°C for a retention time of 10–90 s in the conditioner, while having high activity at the animal's body temperature (Doyle and Erickson, 2006; Gilbert and Cooney, 2010). Thus the molecules need to retain flexibility near the active site while being rigid enough for high thermal resistance (Shivange and Schwaneberg, 2017). Fortuitously, better intrinsic thermal tolerance of the enzyme molecule often correlates to improved protease resistance, better storage stability and general robustness of the enzyme.

2.2 Phytase

2.2.1 The market and the substrate

The current feed enzyme market is worth close to US$1 billion in sales and phytase accounts for about half of this (Greiner and Konietzny, 2012; Arbige *et al.*, 2019; Herrmann *et al.*, 2019). Feed grains like maize and wheat store the phosphorus in seeds as phytate, a mixed salt of phytic acid (phytin) which can account for up to 80% of the seed phosphorus. Phytic acid is chemically described as a sixfold dihydrogenphosphate ester of inositol, also called *myo*-inositol hexakisphosphate ($InsP_6$ or IP_6) or inositol polyphosphate (Fig. 2.1) (Bohn *et al.*, 2008). At acidic pH (e.g. stomach) phytic acid is soluble as phytate (Cheryan, 1980). Monogastric farm animals such as swine, chicken and turkey are not able to release the phytate-phosphorus in the feed in their stomach and as a result undigested phosphorus is released in the excreta with a risk of pollution to the environment due to phosphorus run-off. Inorganic phosphorus, which is a finite resource in nature (Gilbert, 2009), needs normally to be added to the feed to meet the requirements of the animal (Greiner and Konietzny, 2010; Humer *et al.*, 2015).

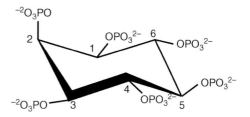

Fig. 2.1. Schematic presentation of phytic acid (*myo*-inositol(1,2,3,4,5,6)hexakisphosphate). Presented in the 'turtle' configuration as in Bohn *et al.* (2008) and Agranoff (2009). The four limbs and tail of the turtle are coplanar and represent the five equatorial hydroxyl groups. The turtle's head is erect and represents the axial hydroxyl group at the position 2. Looking down at the turtle from above, the numbering of the turtle begins at the right paw and continues past the head to the other limbs, thus numbering the inositol in the counterclockwise (D) direction (Bohn *et al.*, 2008). (Author's own figure.)

Phytate at low pH is negatively charged and acts as a strong chelator of cations, in particular zinc, iron, calcium and magnesium, and trace elements and proteins, making phytate also an antinutrient (Woyengo and Nyachoti, 2013; Dersjant-Li *et al.*, 2014). The chelating capability of the different inositol phosphate isomers (InsPs) is reduced rapidly when more phosphates are removed (Herrmann *et al.*, 2019) but, for example, InsP$_3$ still binds *in vitro* more than 80% of soluble zinc at pH 6 and above (Xu *et al.*, 1992) and InsPs above InsP$_2$ inhibit pepsin (Yu *et al.*, 2012). High doses of phytase (so-called 'superdosing') >1500 FTU/kg feed as compared with the more standard doses of 500–1000 FTU/kg (Bedford and Partridge, 2010) are reported to rapidly degrade the phytate to lower InsPs, removing or reducing its antinutritive effects in broilers and pigs (Goodband *et al.*, 2013; Santos *et al.*, 2014; Walk *et al.*, 2014; Kühn *et al.*, 2016). Furthermore, it has been proposed that *myo*-inositol (MI), the dephosphorylated backbone sugar-alcohol of phytic acid, would act as a semi-essential substrate or a prebiotic with clear benefits in the diet (Agranoff, 2009; Cowieson *et al.*, 2013; Sommerfeld *et al.*, 2018; Gonzalez-Uarquin *et al.*, 2020).

2.2.2   The enzyme

As biocatalysts, phytases are a group of phosphatases able to initiate the sequential release of phytate phosphate groups from phytate. Phytases in nature are grouped in four categories: histidine acid phytases (HAPhy), β-propeller phytases (BPPhy), cysteine phytases (CPhy) and purple acid phytases (PAPhy) (Greiner and Konietzny, 2010). All commercial phytases belong to the histidine acid phosphatases (HAPs) and are from microbial sources, belonging to branch 2 of the histidine phosphatase superfamily (Rigden, 2008). They share conserved active-site sequence motifs (RH-GXRXP and HD) and two structural domains (α-domain and α/β-domain) (Shivange and Schwaneberg, 2017). Recently, a different family of bacterial Minpp histidine

phosphatases, distinct from HAP phytases but belonging to the same branch 2, having an HAE motif instead of the HD, has been identified (Stentz *et al.*, 2014). Based on the carbon position on the phytate molecule at which the dephosphorylation preferably starts, the phytases are further classified as 3-phytases (EC 3.1.3.8) or 6-phytases (EC 3.1.3.26) (Table 2.1). Five of the phosphates in phytate are in an equatorial position, but the 2-phosphate is in an axial position, which makes it difficult for phytases to cleave. Thus, a complete dephosphorylation requires non-specific phosphatases (Fig. 2.1) (Wyss *et al.*, 1999; Hirvonen *et al.*, 2019).

The first commercially available phytase was a 3-phytase from *Aspergillus ficuum* (*niger*) launched by DSM in 1991 (Ullah and Dischinger, 1993; van Hartingsveldt *et al.*, 1993; Haefner *et al.*, 2005), later followed by other fungal phytases, including the consensus phytase based on the sequences of 13 fungal phytases (Lehmann *et al.*, 2000) and a 6-phytase from *Peniophora lycii* (Lassen *et al.*, 2001) (Table 2.1). The discovery that *Escherichia coli* and other enterobacterial 6-phytases have several-fold higher specific activities than the known fungal phytases (e.g. the *E. coli* phytase is reported to have an activity of approximately 800 U/mg protein as compared with approximately 100 U/mg for *A. niger* phytase (Wyss *et al.*, 1999)) and additionally possess other favourable characteristics like pepsin resistance (Rodriguez *et al.*, 1999) has resulted in many of the first-generation fungal phytases being replaced by their second-generation bacterial counterparts during the last 20 years (Table 2.1) (Greiner *et al.*, 1993; Garrett *et al.*, 2004; Pontoppidan *et al.*, 2012; Shivange *et al.*, 2012; Dersjant-Li *et al.*, 2014, 2020; Adedokun *et al.*, 2015; De Cuyper *et al.*, 2020). The first production hosts for the bacterial phytases were the yeasts *Pichia pastoris* and *Schizosaccharomyces pombe*. This was possibly because glycosylation has been speculated to improve thermostability (Rodriguez *et al.*, 2000). However, since the first reports of successful fungal expression (Löbel *et al.*, 2008), standard industrial hosts like *Trichoderma* and *Aspergillus* have also been widely used (Table 2.1).

Table 2.1. The main commercially available monocomponent GMO phytases recently submitted to EFSA or otherwise considered relevant.

Company	Trade name	Production organism	Source	Phytase class	Reference
Adisseo	Rovabio Advance PHY	Schizosaccharomyces pombe	Escherichia coli	6-phytase	Lawlor et al. (2019); ADISSEO France S.A.S. (2020)[a]
Adisseo	Rovabio PHY	Penicillium funiculosum	P. funiculosum	3-phytase	EFSA (2007b)
Andrés Pintaluba S.A.	Apsa Phytafeed	Pichia pastoris (Komagataella pastoris)	Not disclosed	6-phytase	Andrés Pintaluba S.A. (2019); EFSA FEEDAP Panel (2019)
BASF	Natuphos E	Aspergillus niger	Hybrid of Hafnia/Yersinia/Buttiauxella	6-phytase	EFSA FEEDAP Panel (2017b)
BASF	Natuphos	A. niger	Aspergillus ficuum	3-phytase	Wyss et al. (1999); EFSA (2006b)
DuPont Animal Nutrition	Axtra PHY Gold	Trichoderma reesei	Biosynthetic bacterial 6-phytase	6-phytase	Dersjant-Li et al. (2020); Ladics et al. (2020)
DuPont Animal Nutrition	Axtra PHY	T. reesei	Buttiauxella sp.	6-phytase	Kumar et al. (2012); Adedokun et al. (2015); EFSA FEEDAP Panel (2016a)
DuPont Animal Nutrition	Phyzyme XP	S. pombe	E. coli	6-phytase	EFSA (2006d)
Huvepharma	OptiPhos Plus	P. pastoris (Komagataella. phaffii)	E. coli, new generation	6-phytase	De Cuyper et al. (2020); EFSA FEEDAP Panel (2020)
Huvepharma	OptiPhos	P. pastoris (K. pastoris)	E. coli	6-phytase	EFSA FEEDAP Panel (2011); She et al. (2018)
Kaesler Nutrition	Enzy Phostar	P. pastoris (K. pastoris)	E. coli, synthetic	6-phytase	EFSA FEEDAP Panel (2015b)
Novozymes/DSM	Ronozyme HiPhos	Aspergillus oryzae	Citrobacter braakii	6-phytase	Lichtenberg et al. (2011); EFSA FEEDAP Panel (2012a); Pontoppidan et al. (2012)
Novozymes/DSM	Ronozyme P, NP	A. oryzae	Peniophora lycii	6-phytase	Lassen et al. (2001); EFSA (2008c); EFSA FEEDAP Panel (2010)
Novozymes/DSM	Phytase SP 1002	Hansenula polymorpha	Consensus fungal phytase	3-phytase	Lehmann et al. (2002); Esteve-Garcia et al. (2005); EFSA (2006c)
Novus Int.	Cibenza Phytaverse	Pseudomonas fluorescent	E. coli, modified	6-phytase	Almeida et al. (2017); Solomon (2017)
Roal/AB Vista	Quantum Blue	T. reesei	E. coli, enhanced	6-phytase	EFSA FEEDAP Panel (2013c)
Roal/AB Vista	Finase EC	T. reesei	E. coli	6-phytase	EFSA FEEDAP Panel (2009b)

EFSA, European Food Safety Authority.
[a]It is assumed that the 6-phytase described in the multicomponent product Rovabio Max (Lawlor et al., 2019) is the same molecule marketed as the Rovabio Advance 6-phytase.

During the last 10 years there has been an entry of second-generation Chinese 6-phytase products in the global market. These appear to be unmodified or thermostable variants of the *E. coli* phytase produced in *P. pastoris*: Beijing Smile Smizyme (Malloy *et al.*, 2017; She *et al.*, 2017), Guandong VTR Microtech (De Jong *et al.*, 2016) and Wuhan Sunhy SunPhase (Deniz *et al.*, 2013) being examples of some of the brands.

Because of the conditions under which animal feed is manufactured, phytases need to survive heat treatment steps during feed preparation. Intrinsically thermostable molecules have an advantage for high recovery, but this can be compensated by advanced granule formulations and coating for less thermostable phytases (Sands, 2007; De Jong *et al.*, 2016). However, formulation adds costs and therefore a search for more intrinsically thermostable phytases than the original *A. niger* phytase started early. The *Aspergillus fumigatus* phytase (Wyss *et al.*, 1998) and the consensus approach (Lehmann *et al.*, 2002) were the first advances in this direction and other phytase sequences were used as part of the first steps towards more thermostable variants. Since then impressive improvements in heat stability have been obtained using advanced evolution technologies like site-saturation mutagenesis for improving bacterial mesophilic phytases, without e.g. compromising the specific activity at body temperature (Garrett *et al.*, 2004; Herrmann *et al.*, 2019).

Preferably, the ideal phytase has high affinity (low K_M) to phytate and an ability to rapidly remove all the phosphates down to *myo*-inositol monophosphate. The phytase should maintain high activity at about pH 2.5 since the low pH of the stomach favours soluble and unchelated phytate and the gastric region is the only site in the animal where feed phytase can act because the pH in the remainder of the intestine is above 6. Until now the evolution work has focused on the activity on $InsP_6$ as the substrate, but obviously the kinetics and affinity of phytases differ on the lower InsPs which affect hydrolysis rates and the profile of the end products.

The biochemical characteristics of commercial phytases have been excellently summarized in more detail in the other publications (e.g. Lei *et al.*, 2013; Dersjant-Li *et al.*, 2014; Shivange and Schwaneberg, 2017).

2.3 Non-Starch Polysaccharide-Degrading Enzymes (NSPases)

2.3.1 The market and the substrate

NSPases contribute about half or more of the value of the feed enzyme market, xylanases having a significantly larger share than β-glucanases, while mannanases are used in some minor special applications (Paloheimo *et al.*, 2010). Wheat and barley, after maize, are the most commonly used energy sources in feeds for swine and poultry, particularly in Europe and outside the USA (Amerah, 2015; Ravn *et al.*, 2016). The non-starch polysaccharides (NSPs) in cereals range between 10 and 30%, are indigestible by monogastric animals and also have antinutritional effects (Choct, 1997, 2015). NSPs fall chemically into three categories: (i) cellulose; (ii) non-cellulosic polymers (including e.g. arabinoxylans and mixed β-glucans; Figs 2.2 and 2.3); and (iii) pectic polysaccharides. Cereal grains

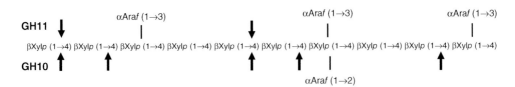

Fig. 2.2. Schematic presentation of the arabinoxylan structural units. βXyl*p*, D-xylopyranose; αAra*f*, L-arabinofuranosidase. The putative cleavage patterns of the GH11 and GH10 families are shown. (Adapted from Biely *et al.*, 1997; Choct, 1997.)

βGlup (1→4) β

(1→3) βGlup (1→4) βGlup (1→4) βGlup (1→4) βGlup

(1→3) βGlup (1→4) βGlup (1→4) βGlup

(1→3) βGlup (1→4) βGlup (1→4) βGlup (1→4) βGlup

Fig. 2.3. Schematic presentation of barley mixed-linked β-(1→3),(1→4)-D-glucan structure. βGlup, D-glucopyranose. (Adapted from Choct, 1997.)

contain predominantly arabinoxylans and mixed β-glucans (i.e. non-cellulosic polymers) and cellulose, but very little pectins (Choct, 1997). The NSPs in wheat, barley, rye, triticale and oats often create viscous digesta because a large portion of it is soluble, high-molecular-weight NSPs, whereas maize, sorghum and rice contain little soluble NSPs and are categorized as non-viscous (Choct, 2015). Wheat soluble NSPs consist mainly of arabinoxylan whereas in barley this is β-glucan.

The main chain of xylan is composed of 1,4-β-linked D-xylopyranose units (Aspinall, 1959; Wilkie, 1979) and in arabinoxylan (AX) the backbone is frequently substituted with L-arabinose residues through the xylosyl O-2 and O-3 atoms (Choct, 1997) (Fig. 2.2). Since xylose and arabinose are both pentose sugars, arabinoxylans are often called pentosans. The insoluble or water-unextractable arabinoxylans (WU-AX) are anchored to the cell walls or to other AX, whereas the unbound AX is soluble or water extractable (WE-AX) and can form highly viscous solutions (Choct, 1997; Moers et al., 2005).

Cereal soluble β-glucans consist of a linear glucose chain joined by mixed linkages of β-1,4- and β-1,3-glucosidic bonds. In barley, the β-glucans contain approximately 70% β-1,4 linkages and 30% β-1,3 linkages, in which segments of two or three 1,4 linkages are separated by a single 1,3 linkage (Fig. 2.3) (Choct, 1997). Although these β-glucans have the same β-1,4 bond as in cellulose, the β-1,3 linkages break up the uniform structure of the β-D-glucan molecule and make it soluble and flexible. The ratio of pentosan (xylan) to β-glucan varies from about 1.3 for barley to more than 10 for wheat and triticale (Henry, 1985).

Viscosity reduction, cell wall degradation and prebiotic effects have been proposed to account for the positive effect of NSPases on the nutritional value of feed. The soluble NSPs in the viscous cereals

hold significant amounts of water and cause increased intestinal viscosity when they are present in the feed (Choct and Annison, 1992; Bedford and Schulze, 1998). This is believed to contribute to the antinutritional effects in the animal by limiting the absorption of nutrients, which may result in reduced feed conversion ratio (FCR) and weight gain as well as wet droppings in poultry. Use of NSPases in the feed reduces the viscosity and improves animal performance. However, NSPases also upgrade the 'non-viscous' cereals like maize or sorghum (Choct, 2006) and it is assumed that release of valuable nutrients from the endosperm and aleurone layer improves the feed quality of these grains.

During the last few years more evidence has accumulated to suggest that oligosaccharides derived from the feed hemicelluloses due to the action of NSPases have a prebiotic effect and this is suggested to be one cause of the benefits of added xylanases and β-glucanases in feed (Bedford, 2018). These oligosaccharides have between three and ten sugar residues and would stimulate the gut microbiome to synthesize short-chain fatty acids (SCFAs) such as butyric acid which act as signals in the animal in multiple ways, improving its performance (Craig et al., 2020).

2.3.2 NSPase enzymes

Several enzyme activities are able to act on the xylans and β-glucans in feeds, and unlike phytase, the same enzyme backbones have frequently been cross-leveraged into adjacent industries like textile, detergent, biomass conversion, paper and pulp, and baking. All NSPases used in feed applications are endo-acting enzymes (Table 2.2), cutting in the middle of the polymer chain and therefore rapidly reducing viscosity;

Table 2.2. Selected commercial NSP feed enzyme products (NSPases). The table is based on the products for which documentation has recently been submitted to EFSA or which otherwise are considered relevant. For the GMO strains not all the donor organisms are included, as these are not disclosed in the public domain. Common names for the enzyme activities are used as follows. Xylanase: endo-1,4-β-xylanase (EC 3.2.1.8); β-glucanase: endo-1,3(4)-β-glucanase (EC 3.2.1.6); cellulase: endo-1,4-β-glucanase (EC 3.2.1.4); β-mannanase: endo-1,4-β-mannanase (EC 3.2.1.78).

Company	Trade name	Declared activity	Production organism	Gene source/other comments	Reference
Adisseo	Rovabio Advance	Xylanase	*Talaromyces versatilis* sp. nov. (formerly *Penicillium funiculosum*)	Self-cloned regulator modifications (*xlnR*[+])	Cozannet *et al.* (2017); Llanos *et al.* (2019)
Adisseo	Rovabio Excel	Xylanase β-Glucanase	*T. versatilis* sp. nov. (formerly *P. funiculosum*)	Non-GMO	Guais *et al.* (2008); EFSA FEEDAP Panel (2013a); Deshors *et al.* (2019)
Andrés Pintaluba S.A.	Endofeed DC	Xylanase β-Glucanase	*Aspergillus niger*	Non-GMO	EFSA FEEDAP Panel (2017c); Gifre *et al.* (2017)
BASF	Natugrain TS	Xylanase β-Glucanase	*A. niger*	Thermostable, both genes derived from *Talaromyces emersonii* (synonym *Rasamsonia emersonii*[a])	EFSA (2008b)
Belfeed DuPont Animal Nutrition	Belfeed B Axtra XB	Xylanase Xylanase β-Glucanase	*Bacillus subtilis* *Trichoderma reesei*	GMO Xylanase by a GMO host, β-glucanase by a non-GMO	EFSA FEEDAP Panel (2016b) EFSA FEEDAP Panel (2016a)
DuPont Animal Nutrition	Danisco Xylanase	Xylanase	*T. reesei*	Thermostable, Y5 mutant of the endogenous xylanase II (GH11)	Fenel *et al.* (2004); Jones (2010); Rasmussen (2010); Romero Millán *et al.* (2014)
Elanco	Hemicell HT	β-Mannanase	*Paenibacillus lentus* (formerly *Bacillus lentus*)	GMO	EFSA FEEDAP Panel (2018)
Huvepharma	Hostazym X	Xylanase	*Trichoderma citrinoviride*	Non-GMO	SCAN (2002); EFSA FEEDAP Panel (2017a); Gifre *et al.* (2017)
Novozymes/DSM	Bio-Feed Plus (Ronozyme W)	Xylanase Cellulase Multicomponent	*Humicola insolens*	Non-GMO	Cowan *et al.* (1996); SCAN (2002); Andersson *et al.* (2003); Choct *et al.* (2004)

Company	Product	Enzyme	Production organism	Notes	References
Novozymes/DSM	Bio-Feed Wheat (Ronozyme WX)	Xylanase	Aspergillus oryzae	Thermostable GH11 xylanase A Gene donor Thermomyces lanuginosus (formerly Humicola lanuginosa)	Schlacher et al. (1996); Bergman and Broadmeadow (1997); SCAN (2002); Andersson et al. (2003); Choct et al. (2004); Rasmussen (2010); EFSA FEEDAP Panel (2012b); Romero Millán et al. (2014); Ravn et al. (2016)
Novozymes/DSM	Bio-Feed Combi	Xylanase β-Glucanase	A. oryzae	Gene donors T. lanuginosus (xylanase) and Aspergillus aculeatus (β-glucanase)	EFSA FEEDAP Panel (2005)
Novozymes/DSM	Roxazyme G2	Xylanase Cellulase β-Glucanase	T. reesei (formerly Trichoderma longibrachiatum)	Non-GMO	EFSA FEEDAP Panel (2012c); Gifre et al. (2017)
Roal/AB Vista	Econase XT	Xylanase	T. reesei	Thermostable GH11 xylanase Gene from Nonomuraea flexuosa (formerly Actinomadura flexuosa)	Leskinen et al. (2005); EFSA (2008a); Rasmussen (2010); Maurer et al. (2013); Romero Millán et al. (2014)
Roal/AB Vista	Econase GT	β-Glucanase	T. reesei	Thermostable GMO, gene donor not dislosed	EFSA FEEDAP Panel (2013b); Olimpo (2015)
Roal/AB Vista	Econase Wheat Plus	Xylanase β-Glucanase	T. reesei	Two monocomponents blended, endogenous genes from T. reesei	EFSA (2005)

EFSA, European Food Safety Authority.
aType strain CBS 393.64 (Houbraken et al., 2014) anamorph Penicillium emersonii, synonym Geosmithia emersonii (Salar and Aneja, 2007).

only limited hydrolysis of the substrate is required for the benefits to accrue. The main enzyme activity hydrolysing xylan, the endo-1,4-β-xylanase catalysing the endohydrolysis of (1→4)-β-D-xylosidic linkages, is designated as EC 3.2.1.8 in the IUB system (Bairoch, 2000). For β-glucan, two EC classes in the commercial NSPase preparations are declared as the main activities: endo-1,4-β-glucanase or cellulase (EC 3.2.1.4) and endo-1,3(4)-β-glucanase or laminarinase (EC 3.2.1.6). The former hydrolyses 1,4-β linkages in glucans also containing 1,3-β linkages. The latter catalyses endohydrolysis of both 1,3-β and 1,4-β linkages in β-D-glucans when the glucose residue whose reducing group is involved in the linkage to be hydrolysed is itself substituted at C-3 (Fig. 2.3).

The products in the market can be divided into three categories, reflecting roughly the different levels of development of the products: (i) first-generation multi-enzyme preparations produced by classical (non-GMO) strains having both xylanase and cellulase activity (e.g. Adisseo Rovabio Excel); (ii) second-generation monocomponent preparations produced by a GMO containing a selected main activity, often from a thermostable source (e.g. Econase XT, Natugrain TS); and (iii) monocomponent of a protein engineered thermostable molecule (e.g. Danisco Xylanase) (Table 2.2). However, whereas with the phytases (Table 2.1) the engineered molecules are the rule, the NSPases, particularly xylanases, even when they are thermostable, are still unmodified molecules derived from nature. Practically all feed NSPases today are produced by standard fungal hosts, mainly by *Trichoderma* or *Aspergillus*, and the gene donors are also mostly fungal (Table 2.2).

Rasmussen (2010) compared several thermostable xylanase products, i.e. Danisco Xylanase (engineered *Trichoderma reesei* xylanase), Ronozyme WX (*Thermomyces lanuginosus* xylanase) and Econase XT (*Nonomuraea flexuosa* xylanase), with Porzyme 9302 (*Trichoderma* native xylanase; Paloheimo *et al.*, 2010) in a pelleting stability trial (Table 2.2). Econase XT was the most thermostable preparation, starting

to lose significant activity only at 100°C, followed by Ronozyme WX and Danisco Xylanase performing well up to 95°C, whereas the Porzyme preparation started to lose activity already at 90°C. Most of these products are intrinsically more thermostable molecules than the phytases on the market today. It is interesting to note that Econase XT is the only thermostable bacterial NSPase in this comparison and possibly in the feed enzyme market in general (Leskinen *et al.*, 2005).

As far as can be determined from the literature, the majority of the commercial monocomponent feed xylanases belong to glycoside hydrolase family GH11 (Schlacher *et al.*, 1996; Choct *et al.*, 2004; Fenel *et al.*, 2004; Paloheimo *et al.*, 2010; Deshors *et al.*, 2019); however, the sequence identity of the cloned *Talaromyces emersonii* xylanase of BASF Natugrain TS (Table 2.2; Tuohy *et al.*, 1994) and the *Aspergillus aculeatus* xylanase C (tested by Choct *et al.*, 2004) are not disclosed, and they may belong to family GH10 (Rantanen *et al.*, 2007; Schröder *et al.*, 2019). Family GH11 xylanases produce longer xylo-oligosaccharides (XOS) than GH10 xylanases which, unlike the GH11 xylanases, can attack the bond next to a branch and require only two unsubstituted xylopyranosyl units between the branches while GH11 require three (Fig. 2.2). GH10 xylanases can also hydrolyse short artificial substrates like aryl-β-D-cellobiosides, which could be a benefit in assays (Biely *et al.*, 1997). GH11 xylanases are known to differ from each other in their selectivity towards WU-AX and WE-AX, making some, like the *Bacillus subtilis* xylanase which preferentially hydrolyses WU-AX and leaves WE-AX and S-AX (solubilized arabinoxylans) largely untouched, suitable for baking applications (Moers *et al.*, 2005). In the study *A. aculeatus* GH10 had the lowest specific activity towards WU-AX whereas the GH11 *T. reesei* pI 9.0 (xylanase II) had intermediate selectivity (Moers *et al.*, 2003). Arabinofuranosidases (non-reducing end α-L-arabinofuranosidases; EC 3.2.1.55) (De La Mare *et al.*, 2013) and β-xylosidases (exo-1,4-β-D-xylosidases; EC 3.2.1.37) trim the arabinoxylo-oligosaccharides (AXOS) to release arabinose and xylose, respectively. Since these seldom are declared activities in commercial products but are usually present as background activities of the (mesophilic) production host, and are not necessarily surviving the heat treatments, the oligosaccharide profiles obtained with purified enzymes or non-heat-treated enzyme products may not correlate fully with the performance of the products undergoing heat processing prior to being fed to the animal.

Although the feed enzyme business started with NSPase products high in β-glucanase (cellulase) activity such as products from *T. reesei* in the 1980s (Bedford and Partridge, 2010), there has lately been less development in choice of these enzyme backbones towards intrinsically or engineered thermostable variants (Table 2.2). *T. reesei* produces two main endo-1,4-β-glucanases, EGI (Cel7B) and EGII (Cel5A), which belong to the families GH7 and GH5, respectively (Henrissat *et al.*, 1998; Martinez *et al.*, 2008), and are able to cleave β-1,4 linkages on cereal β-glucans (Roubroeks *et al.*, 2001; Ajithkumar *et al.*, 2006). Of the two, EGI has been marketed also as a monocomponent product for feed as Econase Wheat Plus (Paloheimo *et al.*, 2010). There is little information in the public domain on the enzyme identity of the other commercial β-glucanases (Table 2.2), but earlier studies have shown that *A. niger* and *A. aculeatus* preparations have multiple activities against lichenin and CMC (carboxymethyl cellulose), suggesting activity also towards cereal β-glucans (Vahjen and Simon, 1999), and the CAZy database lists several GH5 and GH7 endoglucanases for these species, as well as for *T. emersonii* (Table 2.2).

2.3.3 Carbohydrate-binding modules (CBMs)

Many, but not all, fungal cellulases and a few hemicellulases are two-modular enzymes consisting of a catalytic core and a carbohydrate-binding module (CBM) separated by a linker. Previously the CBMs on cellulases were called cellulose-binding domains (CBDs). The binding domains may be N- or C-terminal, or in some rare cases at both ends or in the middle of the protein, and they are also separately classified in the CAZy database. The CBMs are believed to increase the affinity of the enzyme to cellulose, particularly under low concentrations of the substrate (Várnai *et al.*, 2014). The significance of CBMs under the physiological conditions in animals has not been identified but many of the most used commercial β-glucanases have a backbone which carries a CBM.

The junction between the linker and the catalytic core is often sensitive to protease cleavage, which may not show in a standard enzyme assay but may affect performance in the animal. The routine enzyme assays often use soluble cellulose derivatives like CMC or HEC (hydroxyethyl cellulose) as the substrate, in which case the binding module does not have a role in the hydrolysis (Suurnäkki *et al.*, 2000; Voutilainen *et al.*, 2007; Szijártó *et al.*, 2008) and thus the assay likely bears little resemblance to the conditions under which the enzyme functions in the animal. If needed, the expected molecular weight of the relevant NSPase can be checked using SDS-PAGE analysis to ensure that the enzyme is intact.

2.3.4 Mannanases

β-Mannan is a plant sugar polymer consisting of a linear chain of β-1,4-mannose, which may be partially substituted with galactose, glucose or glucuronic acid units. Mannans are present in relatively high amounts in relatively infrequently used feed ingredients like palm kernel or copra and are also found in legumes like soybeans (Jackson, 2010). Special mannans are also found in yeast and fungal cell walls as α-1,6-mannan with α-1,2- and α-1,3-linked branches.

Endo-1,4-β-D-mannanases (EC 3.2.1.78) hydrolyse β-1,4-mannans in a random endo fashion similar to endoglucanases and endoxylanases. Wood hemicellulose includes β-mannans, and saprophytic fungi and bacteria that degrade lignocellulosic materials often have a β-mannanase as part of their cellulase–hemicellulase enzyme profile (Stålbrand *et al.*, 1995; Li *et al.*, 2014). β-Mannanases and their alkaline or thermostable variants have been used in other industries like detergents and oil, but in feed their application has been limited (Chauhan *et al.*, 2012; Soni and Kango, 2013). Elanco Animal Nutrition (previously Chemgen Corporation) markets Hemicell, a feed β-mannanase, that is derived from *Bacillus lentus* CMG1240 or ATCC55045 (EFSA, 2006a; Carr *et al.*, 2014), currently reidentified as *Paenibacillus lentus* (Li *et al.*, 2014). Commercial fungal mannanases belonging to glycoside hydrolase family GH5 from *T. reesei* and *A. niger* are also available and have been occasionally used as feed additives (Stålbrand *et al.*, 1995; Ademark *et al.*, 1998; Dhawan and Kaur, 2007; van Zyl *et al.*, 2010).

β-Mannanases have been suggested to prevent or reduce a feed-induced immune response (FIIR) in poultry fed β-mannan- or β-galactomannan-containing diets, thus lowering metabolizable energy loss (Arsenault *et al.*, 2017).

2.4 Other Feed Enzymes

2.4.1 Proteases

Proteases are widely used in the detergent, food processing and other industries (Arbige *et al.*, 2019). In laundry detergents they are essential for removing protein-containing soils. These proteases are endopeptidases having a broad substrate spectrum, wide pH profile and are robust to withstand detergent formulations and storage. The detergent proteases are invariably bacterial serine proteases of the family S8, called subtilisins and belonging to the IUPAC (International Union of Pure and Applied Chemistry) class EC 3.4.21.62 (Rawlings and Barrett, 1994; Maurer, 2004).

In feed, proteases are suggested to improve feed protein digestibility and increase the availability of amino acids (Glitsø *et al.*, 2012). The main feed proteases in the market (Table 2.3) are all produced in standard

Bacillus hosts and are apparently cross-leveraged to feed from other industries. The subtilisins or subtilases of the family S8 are non-specific peptidases with a preference to cut after hydrophobic residues, whereas the S1 trypsin or chymotrypsin-like proteases cleave amide substrates following Arg or Lys at P1 or following one of the hydrophobic amino acids at P1, respectively. Proteases of the V8 family (EC 3.4.21.19) have a preferential cleavage after Glu or Asp, and the M4 metalloproteases have a preference for cleavage of Xaa + Yaa, in which Xaa is a hydrophobic residue and Yaa is Leu, Phe, Ile or Val (Rawlings *et al.*, 2012).

2.5 Enzyme Production

2.5.1 General

Feed enzymes, like other industrial enzymes, are mainly produced by microbial hosts in submerged cultivations under contained conditions in large bioreactors or fermenters. The production strains represent highly developed proprietary strain lineages optimized over many years or even decades for high yield and safe production and are important assets to the manufacturing companies. The production hosts can be classically developed strains (non-GMO); in other words, they have been developed by generations of mutagenesis and selection and produce only enzymes native to the host. Their enzyme preparations are usually multicomponent, although the strain improvement programmes may have significantly changed the activity profile as compared with the original wild-type isolate (Garske *et al.*, 2017; Arbige *et al.*, 2019).

Typically, modern production strains are further improved by gene technology (i.e. they are GMOs), combining the technology benefits with the expression potential of the classically developed strains to drive maximal expression of the cloned gene. Use of genetic engineering allows exploration of the entire enzyme diversity in nature when screening for an ideal molecule with the optimal performance in the animal and,

Table 2.3. Selected commercial feed protease products. The table is based on the products for which documentation has been recently submitted to EFSA.

Company	Trade name	Declared activity	Production organism	Gene source/protease class	Reference
DuPont Animal Nutrition	Axtra Pro	Serine protease (EC 3.4.21.62)	*Bacillus subtilis*	Non-GMO or self-cloned, gene from *Bacillus* spp. Subtilisin S8	DuPont Animal Nutrition (2020); Watts *et al.* (2020)
Kemin	Kemzyme W[a]	Bacillolysin (EC 3.4.24.28)	*Bacillus amyloliquefaciens*	Non-GMO or self-cloned M4 metalloprotease Similar but not identical to thermolysin	Vasantha *et al.* (1984); EFSA (2007a)
Novozymes/DSM	Ronozyme ProAct	Serine protease (EC 3.4.21.-)	*Bacillus licheniformis*	Gene from *Nocardiopsis prasina* Trypsin-like S1 Thermostable	EFSA FEEDAP Panel (2009a); Farrell *et al.* (2012); Glitsø *et al.* (2012); Lee *et al.* (2020)
Novus	Cibenza EP150 (Versazyme)	Serine protease[b] (EC 3.4.21.19)	*B. licheniformis*	Non-GMO S1 β-glutamyl peptidase (V8)	EFSA FEEDAP Panel (2015a)

EFSA, European Food Safety Authority.

[a]The product is a blend of multiple monocomponents, but only the protease activity is listed here.

[b]The declared activity EC 3.4.21.19 refers to a minor serine protease activity (Svendsen and Breddam, 1992), but the keratinase activity associated with the Cibenza protease (e.g. DP100) products would fit more to the main *B. licheniformis* subtilisin S8 protease/EC 3.4.21.62 (Lin *et al.*, 1995; Wang *et al.*, 2011).

moreover, permits further *in vitro* improvements by protein engineering. Gene technology also allows tailoring the strains by deleting the genes encoding harmful side activities like proteases, which may affect product stability during cultivation and storage. Because gene technology usually maximizes the expression of the gene encoding the target enzyme to such an extent that it represents the bulk of the total secreted protein, the products are virtually monocomponents. Patents are used to protect the novel enzymes by claiming primarily their amino acid sequences but also other dependent fields, like the product and use in application.

The microbial genetically modified hosts used for production of feed enzymes consist of a few standard hosts which are also used in manufacturing of other industrial enzymes. Many of the current hosts were developed from strains originally used as classical strains for commercial production of amylases, proteases, pectinases or cellulases for various industries. The bacterial host species include proprietary strains of the *Bacillus* genus, like *B. subtilis*, *Bacillus licheniformis* or *Bacillus amyloliquefaciens*, whereas the eukaryotic cell factories comprise yeasts like *Schizosaccharomyces pombe* or *P. pastoris* or filamentous fungi such as *A. niger*, *Aspergillus oryzae*, *Humicola insolens*, *Myceliophthora thermophila* (Dyadic's C1 platform) and *T. reesei* (Paloheimo *et al.*, 2016; Garske *et al.*, 2017). These hosts have the potential to naturally secrete a large array of enzymes at high concentrations, are non-pathogenic and easy to cultivate at industrial scale.

2.5.2 Production process

Nearly all microbially produced industrial enzymes are secreted and commercial enzyme preparations are, in their simplest form, concentrated cell-free spent culture media. Modern feed enzymes are produced in large bioreactors with the production phase volumes ranging from about 40 to 400 m³ (or 100,000 gallons). The smaller sizes are most suitable for bacterial cultivations requiring vigorous mixing and efficient cooling, whereas larger volumes are used for slower-growing yeasts and fungi. These are aseptic and aerobic fermentations, where the temperature, pH, foaming, aeration and mixing are carefully monitored and controlled (Fig. 2.4). The production phase takes from 1 to 2 days with bacteria and up to 1 week or more with yeasts and fungi.

After the cultivation the cells are separated from the spent medium, and the liquid part containing the secreted enzymes is concentrated by removing water, often by ultrafiltration, to produce what is termed a 'semifinal'. Typically, no enzyme purification is needed but if so, this can be done by selective crystallization or precipitation or by chromatographic methods. Liquid products made to the specifications by mixing semifinals at desired ratios with diluents (water/buffers) are then stabilized by adding stabilizers such as sorbitol or glycerol, and preservatives, like sodium benzoate, and then packaged (Fig. 2.4) (Paloheimo *et al.*, 2016; Arbige *et al.*, 2019).

Dry feed enzyme products are manufactured to varying qualities. The desired

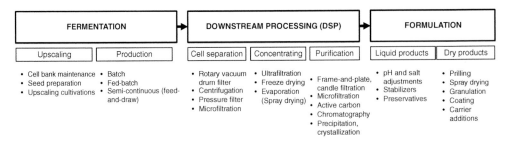

Fig. 2.4. Manufacturing process steps for feed enzyme products. The outline is representative for microbial submerged tank fermentations for secreted enzymes. (Author's own figure.)

characteristics are improved storage stability, low dusting potential, standard particle size and rapid release/dissolution. Furthermore, because enzymes are potential respiratory allergens, the exposure of users to the enzyme proteins is minimized by coating. Dry products include spray-dried powders and agglomerated granules manufactured by extrusion, high- and low-shear granulation and fluid bed techniques (Meesters, 2010), and may be coated or non-coated. In spray drying enzymes, the liquid or slurry is rapidly dried with the help of hot air by dispersing it through a nozzle or an atomizer. In combined or multistage drying, larger agglomerates can be produced. The dry semifinal is then mixed with a carrier to make the final product. In the extrusion technique the material is forced through a die and then cut into small pieces, which are further spheronized to granules. In high and low shear and in the fluid bed granulation, powder and liquid are mixed to build agglomerates of different size, porosity and density (Meesters, 2010). The hygienic requirements of feed pellets are typically met by a steam treatment which can reach temperatures in excess of 90°C (Gilbert and Cooney, 2010). To improve the recovery of particularly the intrinsically less thermostable enzymes, specific coating formulations have been developed with multiple layers of fat or wax or other moisture-resistant materials, like polyethylene glycol, which also improve storage stability (Haefner et al., 2005; Meesters, 2007; Jones, 2010). However, while providing thermostability the coating formulation needs to allow for rapid dissolution in the stomach of the animal to facilitate functionality.

2.6   Conclusions and Future Trends

Since the previous edition of this book in 2010, we have seen the introduction of the high-activity enterobacterial phytases and their protein engineered derivatives into the marketplace, replacing the first-generation fungal phytases (Table 2.1). This reflects the general trend in the industry where the native molecules are routinely further engineered and evolved to have optimal characteristics, like high thermostability. In the NSPase segment the development has been slower but there, too, we have seen the first-generation molecules gradually being replaced by intrinsically more thermostable counterparts (Table 2.2).

While the original benefit of the phytase releasing the phytate-phosphorus for the animal still holds, more evidence is accumulating that use of higher doses to remove the antinutritive effect of the high InsPs and to provide myo-inositol, which seems to have a special role, may bring significant additional benefits. With NSPases and particularly with the xylanases, the role of enzyme-generated oligosaccharides in contributing to the animal's gut health and consequent welfare is seen as increasingly important.

In manufacturing, technologies have been developed to provide thermostable coating formulations to compensate for the lower intrinsic thermostability of some molecules. As enzyme evolution techniques become more and more advanced, the targets of coating may shift more towards providing dust-free formulations to further minimize enzyme exposure of the workforce (Kuske et al., 2020).

Plant-based production systems for enzymes have received attention during recent years and producing transgenic feed enzymes in maize or other cereal seeds appears an attractive alternative. However, differences in post-translational modifications in plants may influence the molecule thermostability, the regulatory policies are still being established, prompt supply-on-demand would be challenging and finally the products need to have competitive prices as compared with microbially produced feed enzymes. Currently the industry is still at early stages (Brinch-Pedersen et al., 2006; Blavi et al., 2019; Broomhead et al., 2019).

References

Adedokun, S.A., Owusu-Asiedu, A., Ragland, D., Plumstead, P. and Adeola, O. (2015) The efficacy of a new 6-phytase obtained from *Buttiauxella* spp. expressed in *Trichoderma reesei* on digestibility of amino acids, energy, and nutrients in pigs fed a diet based on corn, soybean meal, wheat middlings, and corn distillers' dried grains with solubles. *Journal of Animal Science* 93, 168–175. doi: 10.2527/jas.2014-7912

Ademark, P., Varga, A., Medve, J., Harjunpää, V., Drakenberg, T., *et al.* (1998) Softwood hemicellulose-degrading enzymes from *Aspergillus niger*: purification and properties of a β-mannanase. *Journal of Biotechnology* 63, 199–210.

ADISSEO France S.A.S. (2020) Rovabio® Advance PHY Product Brochure. ADISSEO France S.A.S., Antony, France. Available at: https://www.adisseo.com/wp-content/uploads/2018/09/Rovabio-Ad-Phy-standard.pdf (accessed 7 May 2020).

Agranoff, B.W. (2009) Turtles all the way: reflections on *myo*-inositol. *The Journal of Biological Chemistry* 284, 21121–21126. doi: 10.1074/jbc.X109.004747

Ajithkumar, A., Andersson, R., Siika-Aho, M., Tenkanen, M. and Åman, P. (2006) Isolation of cellotriosyl blocks from barley β-glucan with endo-1,4-β-glucanase from *Trichoderma reesei*. *Carbohydrate Polymers* 64, 233–238. doi: 10.1016/j.carbpol.2005.11.033

Almeida, F.N., Vazquez-Añón, M. and Escobar, J. (2017) Dose-dependent effects of a microbial phytase on phosphorus digestibility of common feedstuffs in pigs. *Asian-Australasian Journal of Animal Sciences* 30, 985–993. doi: 10.5713/ajas.16.0894

Amerah, A.M. (2015) Interactions between wheat characteristics and feed enzyme supplementation in broiler diets. *Animal Feed Science and Technology* 199, 1–9. doi: 10.1016/j.anifeedsci.2014.09.012

Andersson, R., Eliasson, C., Selenare, M., Kamal-Eldin, A. and Åman, P. (2003) Effect of endo-xylanase-containing enzyme preparations and laccase on the solubility of rye bran arabinoxylan. *Journal of the Science of Food and Agriculture* 83, 617–623. doi: 10.1002/jsfa.1321

Andrés Pintaluba S.A. (2019) APSA PHYTAFEED® 20,000 L & APSA PHYTAFEED® 20,000 GR 6-phytase (ed.). EU Submission No. 1517480301188-2172. Andrés Pintaluba S.A., Reus, Spain, pp. 1–7.

Arbige, M.V., Shetty, J.K. and Chotani, G.K. (2019) Industrial enzymology: the next chapter. *Trends in Biotechnology* 37, 1355–1366. doi: 10.1016/j.tibtech.2019.09.010

Arsenault, R.J., Lee, J.T., Latham, R., Carter, B. and Kogut, M.H. (2017) Changes in immune and metabolic gut response in broilers fed β-mannanase in β-mannan-containing diets. *Poultry Science* 96, 4307–4316. doi: 10.3382/ps/pex246

Aspinall, G.O. (1959) Structural chemistry of the hemicelluloses. *Advances in Carbohydrate Chemistry* 14, 429–468.

Bairoch, A. (2000) The enzyme database in 2000. *Nucleic Acids Research* 28, 304–305.

Barletta, A. (2010) Introduction: current market and expected developments. In: Bedford, M.R. and Partridge, G.G. (eds) *Enzymes in Farm Animal Nutrition*, 2nd edn. CAB International, Wallingford, UK, pp. 1–11. doi: 10.1079/9781845936747.0001

Bedford, M.R. (2018) The evolution and application of enzymes in the animal feed industry: the role of data interpretation. *British Poultry Science* 59, 486–493. doi: 10.1080/00071668.2018.1484074

Bedford, M.R. and Partridge, G.G. (2010) Feed enzymes, the future: bright hope or regulatory minefield? In: Bedford, M.R. and Partridge, G.G. (eds) *Enzymes in Farm Animal Nutrition*, 2nd edn. CAB International, Wallingford, UK, pp. 304–311. doi: 10.1079/9781845936747.0001

Bedford, M.R. and Schulze, H. (1998) Exogenous enzymes for pigs and poultry. *Nutrition Research Reviews* 11, 91–114.

Bergman, A. and Broadmeadow, A. (1997) An overview of the safety evaluation of the *Thermomyces lanuginosus* xylanase enzyme (SP 628) and the *Aspergillus aculeatus* xylanase enzyme (SP 578). *Food Additives and Contaminants* 14, 389–398. doi: 10.1080/02652039709374542

Biely, P., Vranska, M., Tenkanen, M. and Kluepfel, D. (1997) Endo-beta-1,4-xylanase families: differences in catalytic properties. *Journal of Biotechnology* 57, 151–166.

Blavi, L., Muñoz, C.J., Broomhead, J.N. and Stein, H.H. (2019) Effects of a novel corn-expressed *E. coli* phytase on digestibility of calcium and phosphorous, growth performance, and bone ash in young growing pigs. *Journal of Animal Science* 97, 3390–3398. doi: 10.1093/jas/skz190

Bohn, L., Meyer, A.S. and Rasmussen, S.K. (2008) Phytate: impact on environment and human nutrition. A challenge for molecular breeding. *Journal of Zhejiang University SCIENCE B* 9, 165–191. doi: 10.1631/jzus.B0710640

Brinch-Pedersen, H., Hatzack, F., Stoger, E., Arcalis, E., Pontopidan, K. and Holm, P.B. (2006) Heat-stable phytases in transgenic wheat (*Triticum aestivum* L.): deposition pattern, thermostability, and phytate hydrolysis. *Journal of Agricultural and Food Chemistry* 54, 4624–4632. doi: 10.1021/jf0600152

Broomhead, J.N., Li, X. and Raab, R.M. (2019) Safety of corn-expressed carbohydrase when fed to broilers at a high dietary level. *Journal of Applied Poultry Research* 28, 631–637. doi: 10.3382/japr/pfz013

Carr, S., Allee, G., Rincker, P., Fry, R. and Boler, D.D. (2014) Effects of endo-1,4-β-D-mannanase enzyme (Hemicell HT 1.5×) on the growth performance of nursery pigs. *Professional Animal Scientist* 30, 393–399. doi: 10.15232/pas.2014-01326

Chauhan, P.S., Puri, N., Sharma, P. and Gupta, N. (2012) Mannanases: microbial sources, production, properties and potential biotechnological applications. *Applied Microbiology and Biotechnology* 93, 1817–1830. doi: 10.1007/s00253-012-3887-5

Cheryan, M. (1980) Phytic acid interactions in food systems. *Critical Reviews in Food Science and Nutrition* 13, 297–335. doi: 10.1080/10408398009527293

Choct, M. (1997) Feed non-starch polysaccharides: chemical structures and nutritional significance. *Feed Milling International (June)*, 13–26.

Choct, M. (2006) Enzymes for the feed industry: past, present and future. *World's Poultry Science Journal* 62, 5–16. doi: 10.1079/WPS200480

Choct, M. (2015) Feed non-starch polysaccharides for monogastric animals. *Animal Production Science* 55, 1360–1366. doi: 10.1071/AN15276

Choct, M. and Annison, G. (1992) Anti-nutritive effect of wheat pentosans in broiler chickens: roles of viscosity and gut microflora. *British Poultry Science* 33, 821–834. doi: 10.1080/00071669208417524

Choct, M., Kocher, A., Waters, D.L.E., Pettersson, D. and Ross, G. (2004) A comparison of three xylanases on the nutritive value of two wheats for broiler chickens. *British Journal of Nutrition* 92, 53–61. doi: 10.1079/BJN20041166

Cowan, W.D., Korsbak, A., Hastrup, T. and Rasmussen, P.B. (1996) Influence of added microbial enzymes on energy and protein availability of selected feed ingredients. *Animal Feed Science and Technology* 60, 311–319.

Cowieson, A.J., Ptak, A., Mackowiak, P., Sassek, M., Pruszynska-Oszmalek, E., *et al.* (2013) The effect of microbial phytase and *myo*-inositol on performance and blood biochemistry of broiler chickens fed wheat/corn-based diets. *Poultry Science* 92, 2124–2134. doi: 10.3382/ps.2013-03140

Cozannet, P., Kidd, M.T., Montanhini Neto, R. and Geraert, P.-A. (2017) Next-generation non-starch polysaccharide-degrading, multi-carbohydrase complex rich in xylanase and arabinofuranosidase to enhance broiler feed digestibility. *Poultry Science* 96, 2743–2750. doi: 10.3382/ps/pex084

Craig, A.D., Khattak, F., Hastie, P., Bedford, M.R. and Olukosi, O.A. (2020) Xylanase and xylo-oligosaccharide prebiotic improve the growth performance and concentration of potentially prebiotic oligosaccharides in the ileum of broiler chickens. *British Poultry Science* 61, 70–78. doi: 10.1080/00071668.2019.1673318

De Cuyper, C., Nollet, L., Aluwé, M., De Boever, J., Douidah, L., *et al.* (2020) Effect of supplementing phytase on piglet performance, nutrient digestibility and bone mineralisation. *Journal of Applied Animal Nutrition* 8, 3–10. doi: 10.3920/JAAN2019.0003

De Jong, J.A., DeRouchey, J.M., Tokach, M.D., Dritz, S.S., Goodband, R.D., *et al.* (2016) Stability of commercial phytase sources under different environmental conditions. *Journal of Animal Science* 94, 4259–4266. doi: 10.2527/jas2016-0742

De La Mare, M., Guais, O., Bonnin, E., Weber, J. and Francois, J.M. (2013) Molecular and biochemical characterization of three GH62 α-l-arabinofuranosidases from the soil deuteromycete *Penicillium funiculosum*. *Enzyme and Microbial Technology* 53, 351–358. doi: 10.1016/j.enzmictec.2013.07.008

Deniz, G., Gezen, S.S., Kara, C., Gencoglu, H., Meral, Y. and Baser, E. (2013) Evaluation of nutrient equivalency of microbial phytase in hens in late lay given maize–soybean or distiller's dried grains with solubles (DDGS) diets. *British Poultry Science* 54, 494–502. doi: 10.1080/00071668.2013.797954

Dersjant-Li, Y., Awati, A., Schulze, H. and Partridge, G. (2014) Phytase in non-ruminant animal nutrition: a critical review on phytase activities in the gastrointestinal tract and influencing factors. *Journal of the Science of Food and Agriculture* 95, 878–896. doi: 10.1002/jsfa.6998

Dersjant-Li, Y., Villca, B., Sewalt, V., De Kreij, A., Marchal, L., *et al.* (2020) Functionality of a next generation biosynthetic bacterial 6-phytase in enhancing phosphorus availability to weaned piglets fed a corn–soybean meal-based diet without added inorganic phosphate. *Animal Nutrition* 6, 24–30. doi: 10.1016/j.aninu.2019.11.003

Deshors, M., Guais, O., Neugnot-Roux, V., Cameleyre, X., Fillaudeau, L. and Francois, J.M. (2019) Combined *in situ* physical and *ex-situ* biochemical approaches to investigate *in vitro* deconstruction of destarched wheat bran by enzymes cocktail used in animal nutrition. *Frontiers in Bioengineering and Biotechnology* 7, 158. doi: 10.3389/fbioe.2019.00158

Dhawan, S. and Kaur, J. (2007) Microbial mannanases: an overview of production and applications. *Critical Reviews in Biotechnology* 27, 197–216. doi: 10.1080/07388550701775919

Doyle, M.P. and Erickson, M.C. (2006) Reducing the carriage of foodborne pathogens in livestock and poultry. *Poultry Science* 85, 960–973.

DuPont Animal Nutrition (2020) Axtra PRO Product Brochure. Available at: https://www.dupontnutritionand-biosciences.com/animal-nutrition/product-solutions/axtra-pro.html (accessed 20 February 2020).

EFSA (2005) Opinion of the Scientific Panel on Additives and Products or Substances used in Animal Feed on the safety of the enzyme preparation Econase Wheat Plus for use as feed additive for chickens for fattening. *The EFSA Journal* 231, 1–6.

EFSA (2006a) Opinion of the Scientific Panel on Additives and Products or Substances used in Animal Feed on the safety and efficacy of the enzymatic preparation Hemicell® Feed Enzyme (beta-D-mannanase) as a feed additive for chickens for fattening in accordance with Regulation (EC) No 1831/2003. *The EFSA Journal* 412, 1–12.

EFSA (2006b) Opinion of the Scientific Panel on Additives and Products or Substances used in Animal Feed and of the Scientific Panel on Genetically Modified Organisms on the safety and efficacy of the enzyme preparation Natuphos® (3-phytase) produced by *Aspergillus niger*. *The EFSA Journal* 369, 1–19.

EFSA (2006c) Opinion of the Scientific Panel on Additives and Products or Substances used in Animal Feed and of the Scientific Panel on Genetically Modified Organisms on the safety and efficacy of the enzyme preparation Phytase SP 1002 (3-phytase) for use as feed additive for piglets, pigs for fattening, sows, chickens for fattening, turkeys and laying hens. *The EFSA Journal* 333, 1–27.

EFSA (2006d) Opinion of the Scientific Panel on Additives and Products or Substances used in Animal Feed and of the Scientific Panel on Genetically Modified Organisms on the safety and efficacy of the enzymatic preparation Phyzyme XP (6-Phytase) for use as feed additive for chickens for fattening. *The EFSA Journal* 350, 1–14.

EFSA (2007a) Opinion of the Scientific Panel on Additives and Products or Substances used in Animal Feed on the safety of the enzyme preparation Kemzyme® W Dry for laying hens. *The EFSA Journal* 475, 1–4.

EFSA (2007b) Opinion of the Scientific Panel on Additives and Products or Substances used in Animal Feed and the Scientific Panel on Genetically Modified Organisms on the safety and efficacy of the enzyme preparation Rovabio™ PHY AP/LC (3-phytase) as feed additive for chickens for fattening, laying hens, piglets and pigs for fattening in accordance with Regulation (EC) No 1831/2003. *The EFSA Journal* 471, 1–29.

EFSA (2008a) Safety and efficacy of Econase XT P/L as feed additive for chickens for fattening, chickens reared for laying, turkeys for fattening, turkeys reared for breeding and piglets (weaned). *The EFSA Journal* 712, 1–19.

EFSA (2008b) Safety and efficacy of Natugrain® TS (endo-1,4-beta-xylanase and endo-1,4-beta-glucanase) as a feed additive for piglets (weaned), chickens for fattening, laying hens, turkeys for fattening and ducks. *The EFSA Journal* 914, 1–21.

EFSA (2008c) Safety and efficacy of the product Ronozyme® NP (6-phytase) for chickens for fattening. *The EFSA Journal* 871, 1–16.

EFSA FEEDAP Panel (2005) Opinion of the Scientific Panel on Additives and Products or Substances used in Animal Feed on the safety of the enzyme preparation Bio-Feed Combi for use as feed additive for chickens for fattening and piglets. *The EFSA Journal* 261, 1–6.

EFSA FEEDAP Panel (2009a) Safety and efficacy of Ronozyme® ProAct (serine protease) for use as feed additive for chickens for fattening. *The EFSA Journal* 1185, 1–15.

EFSA FEEDAP Panel (2009b) Scientific Opinion on the safety and efficacy of Finase® EC (6-phytase) as a feed additive for chickens for fattening and reared for laying, laying hens, turkeys for fattening and reared for breeding, ducks and other minor poultry species, piglets (weaned), pigs for fattening and sows. *EFSA Journal* 7, 1380. doi: 10.2903/j.efsa.2009.1380

EFSA FEEDAP Panel (2010) Scientific Opinion on Ronozyme® P (6-phytase) as feed additive for chickens and turkeys for fattening, laying hens, and piglets (weaned), pigs for fattening and sows (poultry and pigs). *EFSA Journal* 8, 1862. doi: 10.2903/j.efsa.2010.1862

EFSA FEEDAP Panel (2011) Scientific Opinion on the safety and efficacy of Optiphos® (6-phytase) as a feed additive for chickens and turkeys for fattening, chickens reared for laying, turkeys reared for breeding, laying hens, other birds for fattening and laying, weaned piglets, pigs for fattening and sows. *EFSA Journal* 9, 2414. doi: 10.2903/j.efsa.2011.2414

EFSA FEEDAP Panel (2012a) Scientific Opinion on the safety and efficacy of Ronozyme HiPhos GT (6-phytase) as feed additive for poultry and pigs. *EFSA Journal* 10, 2730. doi: 10.2903/j.efsa.2012.2730

EFSA FEEDAP Panel (2012b) Scientific Opinion on the safety and efficacy of Ronozyme WX (endo-1,4-beta-xylanase) as a feed additive for poultry, piglets (weaned) and pigs for fattening. *EFSA Journal* 10, 2790. doi: 10.2903/j.efsa.2012.2790

EFSA FEEDAP Panel (2012c) Scientific Opinion on the safety and efficacy of Roxazyme® G2 G/L (endo-1,4-beta-xylanase, endo-1,4-beta-glucanase and endo-1,(3)4-beta-glucanase) as a feed additive for poultry and piglets. *EFSA Journal* 10, 2930. doi: 10.2903/j.efsa.2012.2930

EFSA FEEDAP Panel (2013a) Scientific Opinion on Rovabio® Excel (endo-1,3(4)-beta-glucanase and endo-1,4-beta-xylanase) as a feed additive for chickens and turkeys for fattening, laying hens, piglets (weaned) and pigs for fattening, ducks, guinea fowls, quails, geese, pheasants and pigeons. *EFSA Journal* 11, e3321. doi: 10.2903/j.efsa.2013.3321

EFSA FEEDAP Panel (2013b) Scientific Opinion on the safety and efficacy of Econase® GT (endo-1,3(4)-beta-glucanase) as a feed additive for chickens for fattening and weaned piglets. *EFSA Journal* 11, 3432. doi: 10.2903/j.efsa.2013.3432

EFSA FEEDAP Panel (2013c) Scientific Opinion on the safety and efficacy of Quantum® Blue (6-phytase) as a feed additive for laying hens and minor laying poultry species. *EFSA Journal* 11, 3433. doi: 10.2903/j.efsa.2013.3433

EFSA FEEDAP Panel (2015a) Scientific Opinion on the safety and efficacy of Cibenza® EP150 (a preparation of *Bacillus licheniformis* (ATCC 53757) and its protease (EC 3.4.21.19)) as a feed additive for chickens for fattening, chickens reared for laying and minor avian species for fattening and to point of lay and ornamental birds. *EFSA Journal* 13, 4055. doi: 10.2903/j.efsa.2015.4055

EFSA FEEDAP Panel (2015b) Scientific Opinion on the safety and efficacy of ENZY PHOSTAR® (6-phytase) as a feed additive for avian and porcine species. *EFSA Journal* 13, 1–26 (e4159). doi: 10.2903/j.efsa.2015.4159

EFSA FEEDAP Panel (2016a) Safety and efficacy of Axtra® XB 201 (endo-1,4-beta-xylanase and endo-1,3(4)-beta-glucanase) as a feed additive for lactating sows and minor porcine species. *EFSA Journal* 14, 4350. doi: 10.2903/j.efsa.2016.4350

EFSA FEEDAP Panel (2016b) Safety and efficacy of Belfeed B MP/ML (endo-1,4-beta-xylanase) as feed additive for poultry, piglets (weaned) and pigs for fattening. *EFSA Journal* 14, 4562. doi: 10.2903/j.efsa.2016.4562

EFSA FEEDAP Panel (2017a) Safety and efficacy of HOSTAZYM® X (endo-1,4-β-xylanase) as a feed additive for chickens reared for laying and minor poultry species reared for laying. *EFSA Journal* 15, 4708. doi: 10.2903/j.efsa.2017.4708

EFSA FEEDAP Panel (2017b) Safety and efficacy of Natuphos® E (6-phytase) as a feed additive for avian and porcine species. *EFSA Journal* 15, 5024. doi: 10.2903/j.efsa.2017.5024

EFSA FEEDAP Panel (2017c) Safety of Endofeed® DC (endo-1,3(4)-β-glucanase and endo-1,4-β-xylanase) as a feed additive for chickens for fattening, laying hens, pigs for fattening and minor poultry and porcine species. *EFSA Journal* 15, 4706. doi: 10.2903/j.efsa.2017.4706

EFSA FEEDAP Panel (2018) Safety and efficacy of Hemicell® HT (endo-1,4-β-mannanase) as a feed additive for chickens for fattening, chickens reared for laying, turkey for fattening, turkeys reared for breeding, weaned piglets, pigs for fattening and minor poultry and porcine species. *EFSA Journal* 16, 5270. doi: 10.2903/j.efsa.2018.5270

EFSA FEEDAP Panel (2019) Safety and efficacy of APSA PHYTAFEED® 20,000 GR/L (6-phytase) as a feed additive for chickens for fattening, chickens reared for laying and minor growing poultry species. *EFSA Journal* 17, 5692. doi: 10.2903/j.efsa.2019.5692

EFSA FEEDAP Panel (2020) Safety and efficacy of OptiPhos® PLUS for poultry species for fattening, minor poultry species reared for breeding and ornamental birds. *EFSA Journal* 18, 6141. doi: 10.2903/j.efsa.2020.6141

Esteve-Garcia, E., Perez-Vendrell, A.M. and Broz, J. (2005) Phosphorus equivalence of a *Consensus* phytase produced by *Hansenula polymorpha* in diets for young turkeys. *Archives of Animal Nutrition* 59, 53–59. doi: 10.1080/17450390512331342386

Farrell, D., Webb, H., Johnston, M.A., Poulsen, T.A., O'Meara, F., *et al.* (2012) Towards fast determination of protein stability maps: experimental and theoretical analysis of mutants of a *Nocardiopsis prasina* serine protease. *Biochemistry* 51, 5339–5347. doi: 10.1021/bi201926f

Fenel, F., Leisola, M., Janis, J. and Turunen, O. (2004) A *de novo* designed N-terminal disulphide bridge stabilizes the *Trichoderma reesei* endo-1,4-beta-xylanase II. *Journal of Biotechnology* 108, 137–143.

Garrett, J.B., Kretz, K.A., O'Donoghue, E., Kerovuo, J., Kim, W., *et al.* (2004) Enhancing the thermal tolerance and gastric performance of a microbial phytase for use as a phosphate-mobilizing monogastric-feed supplement. *Applied and Environmental Microbiology* 70, 3041–3046.

Garske, A.L., Kapp, G. and McAuliffe, J.C. (2017) Industrial enzymes and biocatalysis. In: Kent, J.A., Bommaraju, T.V. and Barnicki, S.D. (eds) *Handbook of Industrial Chemistry and Biotechnology*, 13th edn. Springer, Cham, Switzerland, pp. 1571–1638. doi: 10.1007/978-3-319-52287-6

Gifre, L., Arís, A., Bach, À. and Garcia-Fruitós, E. (2017) Trends in recombinant protein use in animal production. *Microbial Cell Factories* 16, 40. doi: 10.1186/s12934-017-0654-4

Gilbert, C. and Cooney, G. (2010) Thermostability of feed enzymes and their practical application in the feed mill. In: Bedford, M.R. and Partridge, G.G. (eds) *Enzymes in Farm Animal Nutrition*, 2nd edn. CAB International, Wallingford, UK, pp. 249–259. doi: 10.1079/9781845936747.0001

Gilbert, N. (2009) The disappearing nutrient. *Nature* 461, 716–718.

Glitsø, V., Pontoppidan, K., Knap, I. and Ward, N. (2012) Development of a feed protease. *Industrial Biotechnology* 8, 172–175. doi: 10.1089/ind.2012.1531

Gonzalez-Uarquin, F., Rodehutscord, M. and Huber, K. (2020) *Myo*-inositol: its metabolism and potential implications for poultry nutrition – a review. *Poultry Science* 99, 893–905. doi: 10.1016/j.psj.2019.10.014

Goodband, R.D., Langbein, K.B., Tokach, M.D., DeRouchey, J.M. and Dritz, S.S. (2013) Influence of a super-dose of phytase (Optiphos) on finishing pig performance and carcass characteristics. *Kansas Agricultural Experiment Station Research Reports*, 116–120. doi: 10.4148/2378-5977.7049

Greiner, R. and Konietzny, U. (2010) Phytases: biochemistry, enzymology and characteristics relevant to animal feed use. In: Bedford, M.R. and Partridge, G.G. (eds) *Enzymes in Farm Animal Nutrition*, 2nd edn. CAB International, Wallingford, UK, pp. 96–128. doi: 10.1079/9781845936747.0001

Greiner, R. and Konietzny, U. (2012) Update on characteristics of commercial phytases. In: AB Vista (ed.) *Proceedings of IPS2 – The Second International Phytase Summit for Phytase Academics*. AB Vista, Marlborough, UK, pp. 96–107.

Greiner, R., Konietzny, U. and Jany, K.D. (1993) Purification and characterization of two phytases from *Escherichia coli*. *Archives of Biochemistry and Biophysics* 303, 107–113. doi: 10.1006/abbi.1993.1261

Guais, O., Borderies, G., Pichereaux, C., Maestracci, M., Neugnot, V., *et al.* (2008) Proteomics analysis of 'Rovabio™ Excel', a secreted protein cocktail from the filamentous fungus *Penicillium funiculosum* grown under industrial process fermentation. *Journal of Industrial Microbiology & Biotechnology* 35, 1659–1668. doi: 10.1007/s10295-008-0430-x

Haefner, S., Knietsch, A., Scholten, E., Braun, J., Lohscheidt, M. and Zelder, O. (2005) Biotechnological production and applications of phytases. *Applied Microbiology and Biotechnology* 68, 588–597. doi: 10.1007/s00253-005-0005-y

Henrissat, B. and Davies, G. (1997) Structural and sequence-based classification of glycoside hydrolases. *Current Opinion in Structural Biology* 7, 637–644.

Henrissat, B., Teeri, T.T. and Warren, R.A.J. (1998) A scheme for designating enzymes that hydrolyse the polysaccharides in the cell walls of plants. *FEBS Letters* 425, 352–354.

Henry, R.J. (1985) A comparison of the non-starch carbohydrates in cereal grains. *Journal of the Science of Food and Agriculture* 36, 1243–1253.

Herrmann, K.R., Ruff, A.J., Infanzón, B. and Schwaneberg, U. (2019) Engineered phytases for emerging biotechnological applications beyond animal feeding. *Applied Microbiology and Biotechnology* 103, 6435–6448. doi: 10.1007/s00253-019-09962-1

Hirvonen, J., Liljavirta, J., Saarinen, M.T., Lehtinen, M.J., Ahonen, I. and Nurminen, P. (2019) Effect of phytase on *in vitro* hydrolysis of phytate and the formation of *myo*-inositol phosphate esters in various feed materials. *Journal of Agricultural and Food Chemistry* 67, 11396–11402. doi: 10.1021/acs.jafc.9b03919

Houbraken, J., Vries, R.P. de and Samson, R.A. (2014) Modern taxonomy of biotechnologically important *Aspergillus* and *Penicillium* species. *Advances in Applied Microbiology* 86, 199–249. doi: 10.1016/B978-0-12-800262-9.00004-4

Humer, E., Schwarz, C. and Schedle, K. (2015) Phytate in pig and poultry nutrition. *Journal of Animal Physiology and Animal Nutrition* 99, 605–625. doi: 10.1111/jpn.12258

Jackson, M.E. (2010) Mannanase, alpha-galactosidase and pectinase. In: Bedford, M.R. and Partridge, G.G. (eds) *Enzymes in Farm Animal Nutrition*, 2nd edn. CAB International, Wallingford, UK, pp. 54–84. doi: 10.1079/9781845936747.0001

Jones, G. (2010) New thermostable enzyme helps meet demands for safer feed. *AllAboutFeed* 1, 8–9.

Kühn, I., Schollenberger, M. and Männer, K. (2016) Effect of dietary phytase level on intestinal phytate degradation and bone mineralization in growing pigs. *Journal of Animal Science* 94, 264–267. doi: 10.2527/jas2015-9771

Kumar, A., Bold, R.M. and Plumstead, P.W. (2012) Comparative efficacy of *Buttiauxella* and *E. coli* phytase on growth performance in broilers. *Poultry Science* 91(Suppl. 1), 90.

Kuske, M., Berndt, K., Spornraft-Ragaller, P., Neumeister, V., Raulf, M., *et al.* (2020) Occupational allergy to phytase. *Journal of the German Society of Dermatology* 18, 859–865. doi: 10.1111/ddg.14205

Ladics, G.S., Han, K.-H., Jang, M.S., Park, H., Marshall, V., *et al.* (2020) Safety evaluation of a novel variant of consensus bacterial phytase. *Toxicology Reports* 7, 844–851. doi: 10.1016/j.toxrep.2020.07.004

Lassen, S.F., Breinholt, J., Ostergaard, P.R., Brugger, R., Bischoff, A., *et al.* (2001) Expression, gene cloning, and characterization of five novel phytases from four basidiomycete fungi: *Peniophora lycii, Agrocybe pediades*, a *Ceriporia* sp., and *Trametes pubescens*. *Applied and Environmental Microbiology* 67, 4701–4707. doi: 10.1128/AEM.67.10.4701-4707.2001

Lawlor, P.G., Cozannet, P., Ryan, W.F. and Lynch, P.B. (2019) Effect of a combination phytase and carbohydrolase enzyme supplement on growth performance and bone mineralization of pigs from six weeks to slaughter at 105 kg. *Livestock Science* 223, 144–150. doi: 10.1016/j.livsci.2019.01.028

Lee, J.J., Kang, J., Park, S., Cho, J.H., Oh, S., *et al.* (2020) Effects of dietary protease on immune responses of weaned pigs. *Journal of Animal Science and Technology* 62, 174–179. doi: 10.5187/jast.2020.62.2.174

Lehmann, M., Kostrewa, D., Wyss, M., Brugger, R., D'Arcy, A., *et al.* (2000) From DNA sequence to improved functionality: using protein sequence comparisons to rapidly design a thermostable consensus phytase. *Protein Engineering* 13, 49–57. doi: 10.1093/protein/13.1.49

Lehmann, M., Loch, C., Middendorf, A., Studer, D., Lassen, S.F., *et al.* (2002) The consensus concept for thermostability engineering of proteins: further proof of concept. *Protein Engineering* 15, 403–411. doi: 10.1093/protein/15.5.403

Lei, X.G., Weaver, J.D., Mullaney, E., Ullah, A.H. and Azain, M.J. (2013) Phytase, a new life for an 'old' enzyme. *Annual Review of Animal Biosciences* 1, 283–309. doi: 10.1146/annurev-animal-031412-103717

Leskinen, S., Mäntylä, A., Fagerström, R., Vehmaanperä, J., Lantto, R., *et al.* (2005) Thermostable xylanases, Xyn10A and Xyn11A, from the actinomycete *Nonomuraea flexuosa*: isolation of the genes and characterization of recombinant Xyn11A polypeptides produced in *Trichoderma reesei*. *Applied Microbiology and Biotechnology* 67, 495–505. doi: 10.1007/s00253-004-1797-x

Li, Y.-F., Calley, J.N., Ebert, P.J. and Helmes, E.B. (2014) *Paenibacillus lentus* sp. nov., a β-mannanolytic bacterium isolated from mixed soil samples in a selective enrichment using guar gum as the sole carbon source. *International Journal of Systematic and Evolutionary Microbiology* 64, 1166–1172. doi: 10.1099/ijs.0.054726-0

Lichtenberg, J., Pedersen, P.B., Elvig-Joergensen, S.G., Skov, L.K., Olsen, C.L. and Glitsoe, L.V. (2011) Toxicological studies on a novel phytase expressed from synthetic genes in *Aspergillus oryzae*. *Regulatory Toxicology and Pharmacology* 60, 401–410. doi: 10.1016/j.yrtph.2011.05.010

Lin, X., Kelemen, D.W., Miller, E.S. and Shih, J.C. (1995) Nucleotide sequence and expression of *kerA*, the gene encoding a keratinolytic protease of *Bacillus licheniformis* PWD-1. *Applied and Environmental Microbiology* 61, 1469–1474.

Llanos, A., Déjean, S., Neugnot-Roux, V., François, J.M. and Parrou, J.-L. (2019) Carbon sources and XlnR-dependent transcriptional landscape of CAZymes in the industrial fungus *Talaromyces versatilis*: when exception seems to be the rule. *Microbial Cell Factories* 18, 14. doi: 10.1186/s12934-019-1062-8

Löbel, D., Schwarz, T., Paladino, S., Lingner, A., Leiss, G., *et al.* (2008) Overexpression of an *E. coli* phytase mutant in *Trichoderma reesei* and characterization of the enzyme. Presented at *9th European Conference on Fungal Genetics, Edinburgh, Scotland, 5–8 April 2008*, abstract/poster.

Lombard, V., Golaconda Ramulu, H., Drula, E., Coutinho, P.M. and Henrissat, B. (2014) The carbohydrate-active enzymes database (CAZy) in 2013. *Nucleic Acids Research* 42, D490–D495. doi: 10.1093/nar/gkt1178

Malloy, M.N., Stephens, A.G., Freeman, M.E., Jones, M.K., Faser, J.M., *et al.* (2017) Foot ash can replace tibia ash as a quantification method for bone mineralization in broilers at 21 and 42 days of age. *Journal of Applied Poultry Research* 26, 175–182. doi: 10.3382/japr/pfw060

Martinez, D., Berka, R.M., Henrissat, B., Saloheimo, M., Arvas, M., *et al.* (2008) Genome sequencing and analysis of the biomass-degrading fungus *Trichoderma reesei* (syn. *Hypocrea jecorina*). *Nature Biotechnology* 26, 553–560. doi: 10.1038/nbt1403

Maurer, K.H. (2004) Detergent proteases. *Current Opinion in Biotechnology* 15, 330–334. doi: 10.1016/j.copbio.2004.06.005

Maurer, K.-H., Elleuche, S. and Antranikian, G. (2013) Enzyme. In: Sahm, H., Antranikian, G., Stahmann, K.-P. and Takors, R. (eds) *Industrielle Mikrobiologie*. Springer, Berlin/Heidelberg, Germany, pp. 205–224. doi: 10.1007/978-3-8274-3040-3

McDonald, A.G., Boyce, S. and Tipton, K.F. (2009) ExplorEnz: the primary source of the IUBMB enzyme list. *Nucleic Acids Research* 37, D593–D597. doi: 10.1093/nar/gkn582

Meesters, G.M. (2007) Agglomeration of enzymes, micro-organisms and flavours. In: Salman, A.D., Hounslow, M. and Seville, J. (eds) *Handbook of Powder Technology*. Elsevier BV, Amsterdam, pp. 555–589.

Meesters, G.M. (2010) Encapsulation of enzymes and peptides. In: Zuidam, N. and Nedovic, V. (eds) *Encapsulation Technologies for Active Food Ingredients and Food Processing*. Springer, New York, pp. 253–268. doi: 10.1007/978-1-4419-1008-0_9

Menezes-Blackburn, D., Gabler, S. and Greiner, R. (2015) Performance of seven commercial phytases in an *in vitro* simulation of poultry digestive tract. *Journal of Agricultural and Food Chemistry* 63, 6142–6149. doi: 10.1021/acs.jafc.5b01996

Moers, K., Courtin, C.M., Brijs, K. and Delcour, J.A. (2003) A screening method for endo-beta-1,4-xylanase substrate selectivity. *Analytical Biochemistry* 319, 73–77. doi: 10.1016/S0003-2697(03)00161-1

Moers, K., Celus, I., Brijs, K., Courtin, C.M. and Delcour, J.A. (2005) Endoxylanase substrate selectivity determines degradation of wheat water-extractable and water-unextractable arabinoxylan. *Carbohydrate Research* 340, 1319–1327. doi: 10.1016/j.carres.2005.02.031

Olimpo, F.E. (2015) AB Vista: Spreading the superdosing gospel in Asia. Available at: http://www.efeedlink. com/contents/04-01-2015/f8df4be7-650b-43eb-8f60-4f6079118a7b-e321.html (accessed 16 September 2021).

Paloheimo, M., Piironen, J. and Vehmaanperä, J. (2010) Xylanases and cellulases as feed additives. In: Bedford, M.R. and Partridge, G.G. (eds) *Enzymes in Farm Animal Nutrition*, 2nd edn. CAB International, Wallingford, UK, pp. 12–53. doi: 10.1079/9781845936747.0001

Paloheimo, M., Haarmann, T., Mäkinen, S. and Vehmaanperä, J. (2016) Production of industrial enzymes in *Trichoderma reesei*. In: Schmoll, M. and Dattenböck, C. (eds) *Gene Expression Systems in Fungi: Advancements and Applications*. Springer, Cham, Switzerland, pp. 23–57. doi: 10.1007/978-3-319-27951-0

Pontoppidan, K., Glitsoe, V., Guggenbuhl, P., Quintana, A.P., Nunes, C.S., *et al.* (2012) *In vitro* and *in vivo* degradation of *myo*-inositol hexakisphosphate by a phytase from *Citrobacter braakii*. *Archives of Animal Nutrition* 66, 431–444. doi: 10.1080/1745039X.2012.735082

Rantanen, H., Virkki, L., Tuomainen, P., Kabel, M., Schols, H. and Tenkanen, M. (2007) Preparation of arabinoxylobiose from rye xylan using family 10 *Aspergillus aculeatus* endo-1,4-β-D-xylanase. *Carbohydrate Polymers* 68, 350–359. doi: 10.1016/j.carbpol.2006.11.022

Rasmussen, D.K. (2010) *Difference in Heat Stability of Phytase and Xylanase Products in Pig Feed*. Trial Report No. 875, Pig Research Centre, Danish Agriculture and Food Council, Copenhagen.

Ravn, J.L., Martens, H.J., Pettersson, D. and Pedersen, N.R. (2016) A commercial GH 11 xylanase mediates xylan solubilisation and degradation in wheat, rye and barley as demonstrated by microscopy techniques and wet chemistry methods. *Animal Feed Science and Technology* 219, 216–225. doi: 10.1016/j. anifeedsci.2016.06.020

Rawlings, N.D. and Barrett, A.J. (1994) Families of serine peptidases. *Methods in Enzymology* 244, 19–61.

Rawlings, N.D., Barrett, A.J. and Bateman, A. (2012) MEROPS: the database of proteolytic enzymes, their substrates and inhibitors. *Nucleic Acids Research* 40, D343–D350. doi: 10.1093/nar/gkr987

Rigden, D.J. (2008) The histidine phosphatase superfamily: structure and function. *The Biochemical Journal* 409, 333–348. doi: 10.1042/BJ20071097

Rodriguez, E., Porres, J.M., Han, Y. and Lei, X.G. (1999) Different sensitivity of recombinant *Aspergillus niger* phytase (r-PhyA) and *Escherichia coli* pH 2.5 acid phosphatase (r-AppA) to trypsin and pepsin *in vitro*. *Archives of Biochemistry and Biophysics* 365, 262–267. doi: 10.1006/abbi.1999.1184

Rodriguez, E., Wood, Z.A., Karplus, P.A. and Lei, X.G. (2000) Site-directed mutagenesis improves catalytic efficiency and thermostability of *Escherichia coli* pH 2.5 acid phosphatase/phytase expressed in *Pichia pastoris*. *Archives of Biochemistry and Biophysics* 382, 105–112. doi: 10.1006/abbi.2000.2021

Romero Millán, L.F., Yu, S., Walsh, M., Lantz, S., Mitchinson, C., *et al.* (2014) Methods and compositions to improve the nutritional value of lignocellulosic biomass. Patent Application WO2014202716.

Roubroeks, J., Anderson, R., Mastomaruo, R., Christensen, P.E. and Åman, P. (2001) Molecular weight, structure and shape of oat (1→3),(1→4)-beta-D-glucan fractions obtained by enzymatic degradation with (1→4)-beta-D-glucan 4-glucanohydrolase from *Trichoderma reesei*. *Carbohydrate Polymers* 46, 275–285.

Salar, R.K. and Aneja, K. (2007) Thermophilic fungi: taxonomy and biogeography. *Journal of Agricultural Technology* 3, 77–107.

Sands, J. (2007) The latest in phytase technology: minimising feed costs and improving the environment. Available at: http://animalnutrition.dupont.com/index.php?id=1391&tx_tcresourcelibrary_search%5Bresource% 5D=111&tx_tcresourcelibrary_search%5Bsecurity%5D=cf128e2b&tx_tcresourcelibrary_search%5

Baction%5D=forceDownload&tx_tcresourcelibrary_search%5Bcontroller%5D=Resource&cHash=
995489cb7b7ed816e5299b12e35b3328 (accessed 16 September 2021).

Santos, T.T., Walk, C.L., Wilcock, P., Cordero, G. and Chewning, J. (2014) Performance and bone characteristics of growing pigs fed diets marginally deficient in available phosphorus and a novel microbial phytase.
Canadian Journal of Animal Science 94, 493–497. doi: 10.4141/cjas2013-190

SCAN (2002) Opinion of the Scientific Committee on Animal Nutrition on the use of certain enzymes in animal feedingstuffs (adopted 4 June 1998, updated 16 October 2002). Scientific Committee on Animal
Nutrition (SCAN), European Commission. Available at: https://ec.europa.eu/food/system/files/2020-12/
sci-com_scan-old_report_out96.pdf (accessed 10 September 2021).

Schlacher, A., Holzmann, K., Hayn, M., Steiner, W. and Schwab, H. (1996) Cloning and characterization of
the gene for the thermostable xylanase XynA from *Thermomyces lanuginosus*. *Journal of Biotechnology*
49, 211–218. doi: 10.1016/0168-1656(96)01516-7

Schröder, S.P., De Boer, C., McGregor, N.G.S., Rowland, R.J., Moroz, O., *et al.* (2019) Dynamic and functional profiling of xylan-degrading enzymes in *Aspergillus* secretomes using activity-based probes. *ACS
Central Science* 5, 1067–1078. doi: 10.1021/acscentsci.9b00221

She, Y., Liu, Y., González-Vega, J.C. and Stein, H.H. (2017) Effects of graded levels of an *Escherichia coli*
phytase on growth performance, apparent total tract digestibility of phosphorus, and on bone parameters
of weanling pigs fed phosphorus-deficient corn–soybean meal based diets. *Animal Feed Science and
Technology* 232, 102–109. doi: 10.1016/j.anifeedsci.2017.08.005

She, Y., Sparks, J.C. and Stein, H.H. (2018) Effects of increasing concentrations of an *Escherichia coli* phytase
on the apparent ileal digestibility of amino acids and the apparent total tract digestibility of energy and
nutrients in corn–soybean meal diets fed to growing pigs. *Journal of Animal Science* 96, 2804–2816. doi:
10.1093/jas/sky152

Shivange, A.V. and Schwaneberg, U. (2017) Recent advances in directed phytase evolution and rational
phytase engineering. In: Alcalde, M. (ed.) *Directed Enzyme Evolution: Advances and Applications.*
Springer, Cham, Switzerland, pp. 145–172. doi: 10.1007/978-3-319-50413-1_6

Shivange, A.V., Serwe, A., Dennig, A., Roccatano, D., Haefner, S. and Schwaneberg, U. (2012) Directed
evolution of a highly active *Yersinia mollaretii* phytase. *Applied Microbiology and Biotechnology* 95,
405–418. doi: 10.1007/s00253-011-3756-7

Solomon, H.S. (2017) Evaluating two different doses and comparing a modified *E. coli* phytase to other heat
stable phytases by evaluating broiler performance and tibia ash. MSc thesis, University of Pretoria, Pretoria,
South Africa.

Sommerfeld, V., Künzel, S., Schollenberger, M., Kühn, I. and Rodehutscord, M. (2018) Influence of phytase or
myo-inositol supplements on performance and phytate degradation products in the crop, ileum, and
blood of broiler chickens. *Poultry Science* 97, 920–929. doi: 10.3382/ps/pex390

Soni, H. and Kango, N. (2013) Microbial mannanases: properties and applications. In: Shukla, P. and
Pletschke, B.I. (eds) *Advances in Enzyme Biotechnology.* Springer, New Delhi, pp. 41–56. doi:
10.1007/978-81-322-1094-8

Stålbrand, H., Saloheimo, A., Vehmaanperä, J., Henrissat, B. and Penttilä, M. (1995) Cloning and expression
in *Saccharomyces cerevisiae* of a *Trichoderma reesei* beta-mannanase gene containing a cellulose binding domain. *Applied and Environmental Microbiology* 61, 1090–1097.

Stentz, R., Osborne, S., Horn, N., Li, A.W., Hautefort, I., *et al.* (2014) A bacterial homolog of a eukaryotic
inositol phosphate signaling enzyme mediates cross-kingdom dialog in the mammalian gut. *Cell Reports*
6, 646–656. doi: 10.1016/j.celrep.2014.01.021

Suurnäkki, A., Tenkanen, M., Siika-Aho, M., Niku-Paavola, M.-L., Viikari, L. and Buchert, J. (2000) *Trichoderma
reesei* cellulases and their core domains in the hydrolysis and modification of chemical pulp. *Cellulose*
7, 189–209. doi: 10.1023/A:1009280109519

Svendsen, I. and Breddam, K. (1992) Isolation and amino acid sequence of a glutamic acid specific endopep-
tidase from *Bacillus licheniformis*. *European Journal of Biochemistry* 204, 165–171.

Svihus, B. (2010) Effect of digestive tract conditions, feed processing and ingredients on response to NSP enzymes. In: Bedford, M.R. and Partridge, G.G. (eds) *Enzymes in Farm Animal Nutrition*, 2nd edn. CAB
International, Wallingford, UK, pp. 129–159. doi: 10.1079/9781845936747.0001

Szijártó, N., Siika-Aho, M., Tenkanen, M., Alapuranen, M., Vehmaanperä, J., *et al.* (2008) Hydrolysis of
amorphous and crystalline cellulose by heterologously produced cellulases of *Melanocarpus albomyces*. *Journal of Biotechnology* 136, 140–147. doi: 10.1016/j.jbiotec.2008.05.010

Tipton, K. (2018) Translocases (EC 7): A new EC Class. Available at: https://iubmb.org/wp-content/uploads/
sites/10116/2018/10/Translocases-EC-7.pdf (accessed 6 September 2020).

Tuohy, M.G., Laffey, C.D. and Coughlan, M.P. (1994) Characterization of the individual components of the xylanolytic enzyme system of *Talaromyces emersonii*. *Bioresource Technology* 50, 37–42.

Ullah, A.H. and Dischinger, H.C. Jr. (1993) *Aspergillus ficuum* phytase: complete primary structure elucidation by chemical sequencing. *Biochemical and Biophysical Research Communications* 192, 747–753. doi: 10.1006/bbrc.1993.1477

Vahjen, W. and Simon, O. (1999) Biochemical characteristics of non starch polysaccharide hydrolyzing enzyme preparations designed as feed additives for poultry and piglet nutrition. *Archives of Animal Nutrition* 52, 1–14. doi: 10.1080/17450399909386147

van Hartingsveldt, W., van Zeijl, C.M., Harteveld, G.M., Gouka, R.J., Suykerbuyk, M.E., *et al.* (1993) Cloning, characterization and overexpression of the phytase-encoding gene (*phyA*) of *Aspergillus niger*. *Gene* 127, 87–94. doi: 10.1016/0378-1119(93)90620-I

van Zyl, W.H., Rose, S.H., Trollope, K. and Görgens, J.F. (2010) Fungal β-mannanases: mannan hydrolysis, heterologous production and biotechnological applications. *Process Biochemistry* 45, 1203–1213. doi: 10.1016/j.procbio.2010.05.011

Várnai, A., Mäkelä, M.R., Djajadi, D.T., Rahikainen, J., Hatakka, A. and Viikari, L. (2014) Carbohydrate-binding modules of fungal cellulases: occurrence in nature, function, and relevance in industrial biomass conversion. In: Sariaslani, S. and Gadd, G.M. (eds) *Advances in Applied Microbiology*, vol. 88, 1st edn. Academic Press, San Diego, California, pp. 103–165.

Vasantha, N., Thompson, L.D., Rhodes, C., Banner, C., Nagle, J. and Filpula, D. (1984) Genes for alkaline protease and neutral protease from *Bacillus amyloliquefaciens* contain a large open reading frame between the regions coding for signal sequence and mature protein. *Journal of Bacteriology* 159, 811–819.

Voutilainen, S.P., Boer, H., Linder, M.B., Puranen, T., Rouvinen, J., *et al.* (2007) Heterologous expression of *Melanocarpus albomyces* cellobiohydrolase Cel7B, and random mutagenesis to improve its thermostability. *Enzyme and Microbial Technology* 41, 234–243. doi: 10.1016/j.enzmictec.2007.01.015

Walk, C.L., Santos, T.T. and Bedford, M.R. (2014) Influence of superdoses of a novel microbial phytase on growth performance, tibia ash, and gizzard phytate and inositol in young broilers. *Poultry Science* 93, 1172–1177. doi: 10.3382/ps.2013-03571

Wang, D., Piao, X.S., Zeng, Z.K., Lu, T., Zhang, Q., *et al.* (2011) Effects of keratinase on performance, nutrient utilization, intestinal morphology, intestinal ecology and inflammatory response of weaned piglets fed diets with different levels of crude protein. *Asian-Australasian Journal of Animal Sciences* 24, 1718–1728. doi: 10.5713/ajas.2011.11132

Watts, E.S., Rose, S.P., Mackenzie, A.M. and Pirgozliev, V.R. (2020) The effects of supercritical carbon dioxide extraction and cold-pressed hexane extraction on the chemical composition and feeding value of rapeseed meal for broiler chickens. *Archives of Animal Nutrition* 74, 57–71. doi: 10.1080/1745039X.2019.1659702

Wilkie, K. (1979) The hemicelluloses of grasses and cereals. *Advances in Carbohydrate Chemistry* 36, 215–264.

Woyengo, T.A. and Nyachoti, C.M. (2013) Review: Anti-nutritional effects of phytic acid in diets for pigs and poultry – current knowledge and directions for future research. *Canadian Journal of Animal Science* 93, 9–21. doi: 10.4141/cjas2012-017

Wyss, M., Pasamontes, L., Rémy, R., Kohler, J., Kusznir, E., *et al.* (1998) Comparison of the thermostability properties of three acid phosphatases from molds: *Aspergillus fumigatus* phytase, *A. niger* phytase, and *A. niger* pH 2.5 acid phosphatase. *Applied and Environmental Microbiology* 64, 4446–4451.

Wyss, M., Brugger, R., Kronenberger, A., Rémy, R., Fimbel, R., *et al.* (1999) Biochemical characterization of fungal phytases (*myo*-inositol hexakisphosphate phosphohydrolases): catalytic properties. *Applied and Environmental Microbiology* 65, 367–373.

Xu, P., Price, J., Wise, A. and Aggett, P.J. (1992) Interaction of inositol phosphates with calcium, zinc, and histidine. *Journal of Inorganic Biochemistry* 47, 119–130.

Yu, S., Cowieson, A., Gilbert, C., Plumstead, P. and Dalsgaard, S. (2012) Interactions of phytate and *myo*-inositol phosphate esters (IP1–5) including IP5 isomers with dietary protein and iron and inhibition of pepsin. *Journal of Animal Science* 90, 1824–1832.

3   Xylanases and Cellulases: Relevance in Monogastric Nutrition – Pigs

John F. Patience[1]*, Qingyun Li[2] and Amy L. Petry[3]

[1]*Iowa State University, Ames, Iowa, USA;* [2]*Cargill Premix and Nutrition, Lewisburg, Ohio, USA;* [3]*Texas Tech University, Lubbock, Texas, USA*

3.1   Introduction

The United Nations has projected that the world population will reach 9.7 billion in 2050 and 10.9 billion in 2100 (United Nations, 2019). The challenge of expanding overall food production, combined with growing demand for animal protein, will test the capabilities of the world's agriculture sector to its limit. Two of the many challenges facing food production will be the development and implementation of technologies that support expanded and effective use of higher-fibre ingredients by monogastric farm species. Feed enzymes clearly present one opportunity to achieve success in this regard.

Maize, wheat and rice are the three main cereal grains grown around the world. In 2019/20, global maize consumption totalled 1134 million metric tonnes (MMT) compared with 734 MMT of wheat and 439 MMT of rice. In contrast, total barley consumption was only 27 MMT, total sorghum consumption was 4 MMT and total oats consumption was slightly more than 2 MMT (USDA, 2020). The dominance of maize reflects the already high and still increasing yield of the crop combined with the diversity of its uses for animal feed, human food and industrial purposes.

An increasing portion of the world's grain crop, especially maize, is being diverted from food and feed uses to fulfil industrial purposes, chief among them being the production of renewable fuels. For example, in the USA, ~38% of the maize crop is directed towards the production of ethanol alone (Mohanty and Swain, 2019). The consequences of the changing nature of global grain trade are: (i) greater competition for the source grains, which elevates prices and drives the need to find less expensive, alternative feed ingredients; and (ii) the utilization of industrial co-products, which are inherently of lower feeding value, notably due to higher fibre content.

Taking maize as an example, the unprocessed kernel contains 620 g starch/kg, 17 g cellulose/kg and 63 g total non-cellulosic polysaccharides (NCPs)/kg. In contrast, distillers' dried grains with solubles (DDGS), the principal co-product of ethanol production, contains only 60 g starch/kg, while cellulose and NCPs are increased in concentration to 67 and 215 g/kg, respectively. Thus, starch content is reduced by 90% while the amount of cellulose and NCPs is increased by 294 and

*Email: jfp@iastate.edu

©CAB International 2022. *Enzymes in Farm Animal Nutrition, 3rd Edition* (M. Bedford *et al.* eds)
DOI: 10.1079/9781789241563.0003

33

241%, respectively (Li, 2018). This single example illustrates the changing nature of pig diets as the industry moves to increased utilization of industrial co-products such as DDGS. Concurrent with this change is the need to utilize non-starch polysaccharides (NSPs), such as cellulose and xylans, more effectively. Enzymes represent one of the most probable technologies to achieve success in this regard.

The discovery, and first definition, of cellulose as $C_6H_{10}O_5$ is attributed to the French chemist Anselme Payen (Fisher, 1989). Cellulose is the most abundant organic polymer on earth and therefore also the most abundant polysaccharide, with global annual production of 1.5×10^{12} tonnes (Klemm *et al.*, 2005). About one-third of all plant material consists of cellulose, ranging from, on average, 90% of cotton, 59% of flax straw, 45% of wood, 42% of maize cobs, 36% of maize stalks, 34% of wheat straw to 3.5% of the barley kernel, 2.4% of the maize kernel and 1.6% of the wheat kernel. While its presence in plants is well known, there is less appreciation for the fact that algae, fungi and bacteria also produce cellulose. For example, it has been found that cellulose represents an essential structural component of bacterial biofilm formation (Thongsomboon *et al.*, 2018). While cellulose is widely distributed in nature, it poses significant challenges for animal nutritionists, especially those who specialize in swine, due to the pig's inability to digest or even ferment cellulose without the assistance of exogenous enzymes.

Xylans are the second most common polysaccharide and, like cellulose, are widely distributed in the plant kingdom. They fall within the category of matrix polysaccharides known as hemicellulose due to their random, amorphous structure. Xylans are composed of a primary chain of D-xylose residues, often with side chains of arabinose, mannose or glucose. In nature, xylans play an important role by increasing resistance to enzymes of plant cell walls. This poses a challenge to the effective use of exogenous xylanases in swine diets.

Presented with the problem of increasing global demand for animal protein and the need to expand and enhance the effective use of higher-fibre ingredients, enzymes represent a logical technological option. Their ability to assist the pig in digesting complex carbohydrates such as cellulose and xylans explains the current interest in their application in swine diets. However, a better understanding of the mode of action of enzymes is required in order to maximize their use. At the present time, the efficacy of xylanase when added to pig diets is highly variable and cellulases are only used as part of an enzyme 'cocktail'. This chapter presents current information on this topic, with particular emphasis on the underlying chemistry, physiology and immunology all considered in the context of improving diet digestibility, enhancing pig growth and improving pig health and liveability.

3.2 Substrates

Carbohydrases hydrolyse the NSP fraction of swine diets. NSPs are mainly found in the primary or secondary plant cell wall, are resistant to endogenous enzymes naturally secreted by the pig and may be fermented by the gastrointestinal (GI) microbiota. The concentration, type and source of NSPs within a diet are important considerations when adding carbohydrase(s) into the formulation matrix. The concentration of NSPs within a diet can vary considerably and is dependent on the ingredient composition of the diet. Cereal grains (e.g. maize, wheat, barley, etc.) have relatively low amounts of NSPs, oilseeds and legumes have low to moderate amounts of NSPs, and industrial cereal and oilseed co-products typically contain moderate to high amounts (Bach Knudsen, 1997). The types of NSPs also differ among feed ingredients; cereal grains and their co-products contain predominantly arabinoxylan and cellulose, and some contain β-glucans, while legumes and oilseeds are composed primarily of pectin, cellulose and xyloglucans. The structure of NSP types and location within the plant structure are important aspects to consider when selecting what type and concentration of carbohydrase(s) to supplement in the diet.

3.2.1 Cellulose in plants and plant products

Cellulose is a water-insoluble homopolysaccharide composed of glucose units that are linked by β-1,4-glycosidic bonds in a linear arrangement found in the cell walls of plants. The linearity and non-covalent bonds between glucose units allow the cellulose polymer to pack tightly to form an integral network of cellulose microfibres that in turn combine to form structural macrofibrils (Bach Knudsen, 2014). Hydroxyl groups among the glucose units form hydrogen bonds, giving cellulose its rigidity (Cummings and Stephen, 2007). More rigid cellulose, the result of more hydrogen bonding, is referred to as crystalline cellulose, and cellulose with fewer rigid portions is referred to as amorphous cellulose.

Amorphous cellulose is more susceptible to microbial enzymes and exogenous cellulases, while crystalline cellulose cannot be hydrolysed by cellulases under GI conditions and is considered unfermentable (Ciolacu et al., 2011). The pericarp contains about 25% of the total cellulose within a plant, another 20 to 30% is in the seedcoat, 9 to 12% in the aleurone layer and less than 1% in the endosperm layer (Bach Knudsen, 1997). The cellulose fraction of maize and maize co-product NSP ranges between 21 and 25 %, while wheat NSP has 8–18% cellulose and barley NSP is about 15% cellulose (Henry, 1988; Jaworski et al., 2015). The fermentability of cellulose in swine is very poor, but its degradation and fermentability may be improved by exogenous cellulases.

3.2.2 Xylans in plants and plant products

Xylans are the most abundant NCPs present on earth and can be found in all annual plants, the secondary cell walls of dicots and the cell walls of grasses. The general structure of xylan is a D-xylose backbone linked by β-1,4-glycosidic bonds in a linear or branched form with some fibres having side chains composed of arabinose, mannose or glucose monosaccharides (Cummings and Stephen, 2007). These hemicelluloses can be further classified into arabinoxylans, homoxylans, glucoxylans and glucuroarabinoxylans depending on their structure and side chain composition (Dodd and Cann, 2009). Arabinoxylan is the most complex and abundant xylan found in cereal grains, and it is the primary focus in this chapter.

The β-1,4-xylose backbone of arabinoxylan is highly substituted with arabinose side chains linked by α-1,2- or α-1,3-glycosidic bonds. In addition to arabinose, these side chains may also contain xylose, galactose and phenolic acid residues that may be esterified to lignin (Cummings and Stephen, 2007). The number and composition of L-arabinofuranosyl side chains and degree of lignin esterification can dictate the solubility and fermentability of arabinoxylan within the GI tract. Arabinoxylans that have an arabinose to xylose ratio in the range of 1:3 to 1:6 are considered insoluble and those with a ratio in the range of 1:1 to 1:2 are considered soluble in water (Bach Knudsen, 2014). The fermentability of arabinoxylan is not necessarily dependent on solubility. The degree of interaction with other plant components, along with the lignification of arabinoxylan, can be barriers to fermentation and hydrolysis by exogenous enzymes. The location of arabinoxylan within a grain can be an indicator of both structure and solubility. Non-lignified arabinoxylans are found in the aleurone layer, whereas arabinoxylans in the seedcoat and bran are generally more substituted with phenolic acids and are subject to lignification (Bach Knudsen, 1997).

Arabinoxylan is the most prominent hemicellulose in maize and maize co-products, and it comprises approximately 48.6% of the total NSP content in both maize and maize DDGS (Jaworski et al., 2015). The arabinoxylans found in maize and its co-products have low solubility due to high substitution of phenolic acids and increased amount of L-arabinofuranosyl side chains. Barley has between 4.5 and 8.0% arabinoxylan by weight, and the arabinoxylans in barley also have low solubility due to their complex structural interactions with other plant components (Henry, 1987; Bach Knudsen, 1997). In wheat, arabinoxylan can make up approximately 61% of the total NSP content, with about 30% of that being soluble in water (Bach Knudsen, 1997).

3.3 Enzymes

3.3.1 Enzyme classes

There are two major NSP enzyme classification systems. According to the IUB Enzyme Nomenclature (1992), NSP enzymes have been traditionally classified as glycosyl hydrolases (EC 3.2.1.x) based on reaction type and substrate specificity. For example, xylanases (EC 3.2.1.8) hydrolyse the endo-1,4-β-glycosidic linkages in xylan and cellulases (EC 3.2.1.x) catalyse the hydrolysis of cellulose or β-1,4-glucan. This classification system does not necessarily reflect the sequence and structural (three-dimensional crystal) features of the enzymes and does not take into account enzymes that can hydrolyse multiple substrates. More recently, another classification system based on amino acid sequence or fold similarities between enzymes became available (Henrissat, 1991). This classification has been greatly advanced with the increased analysis of gene sequences and definition of the three-dimensional structures of glycosyl hydrolases. There are currently 166 glycoside hydrolase (GH1–166) families listed in the database of Carbohydrate-Active enZYmes (CAZy; http://www.cazy.org, accessed 10 September 2021). Under this classification, GH families 5, 7, 8, 10, 11, 16, 43, 51 and 62 are associated with xylanases; GH families 5, 7, 8, 10, 11 and 43 contain a single xylanase catalytic domain; and GH families 16, 51 and 62 contain two enzyme catalytic domains (Collins *et al.*, 2005). Xylanase research has been primarily focused on GH10 and GH11.

3.3.2 Cellulases

Cellulases refer to a series of enzymes that hydrolyse cellulose or β-1,4-glucan to generate various lengths of oligosaccharides, including exoglucanases (cellobiohydralases; EC 3.2.1.91) and endoglucanases (EC 3.2.1.4). Complete depolymerization of cellulose to glucose requires endoglucanases, exoglucanases, cellodextrinases and β-glucosidases enzymes. Exoglucanases (1,4-β-D-glucan glucanohydrolases) act on 1,4-β-D-glucosidic linkages in the crystalline parts of cellulose and cellotetraose, liberating cellobiose from the non-reducing ends of the chains (Sadhu and Maiti, 2013). Endoglucanases (endo-1,4-β-D-glucan glucanohydrolases) cleave randomly at internal amorphous regions of the cellulose and cello-oligosaccharides. The enzymatic products of endoglucanase can be hydrolysed by exoglucanases to release reduced cello-oligosaccharides, cellobiose or glucose (Zhang and Zhang, 2013).

Cellobiases or β-glucosidases (EC 3.2.1.21) are often included in the cellulase complex because they cleave soluble cellodextrins and cellobiose to release glucose from the non-reducing end (Sadhu and Maiti, 2013). β-Glucanases (endo-1,3(4)-β-glucanases; EC 3.2.1.6) act on 1,3- or 1,4-β-glycosidic bonds of β-glucan. β-Glucanases are often mischaracterized as cellulases due to the structural similarity between β-glucan and cellulose (Adeola and Cowieson, 2011). β-Glucan is a major fibrous component in cereal grains often included in swine feed, such as barley and oats. Thus, the impact of β-glucanase supplementation in pig diets is also discussed in following sections of this chapter.

Commercially available cellulases for use in the diets of monogastric species are mainly produced by bacteria (e.g. *Bacillus subtilis*) and fungi (e.g. *Trichoderma* spp.), and have been widely reviewed (Sadhu and Maiti, 2013; Narsing Rao and Li, 2017).

3.3.3 Xylanases

The complete depolymerization of arabinoxylan requires a surfeit of enzymes: β-1,4-endoxylanases, β-xylosidases, α-arabinofuranosidases, α-arabinofuranohydrolases, α-glucuronidases, acetyl xylan esterases, and ferulic or coumaric acid esterases. Xylanases (endo-1,4-β-xylanases; EC 3.2.1.8) are often referred to as pentosanases and hemicellulases. Xylanases have been widely reviewed previously (Collins *et al.*, 2005; Bhardwaj *et al.*, 2019) and catalyse the hydrolysis of β-1,4-glycosidic bonds in xylan (or arabinoxylan in cereal grains) to release xylo-oligosaccharides (Dodd and Cann, 2009). Xylo-oligosaccharides are then broken down to produce xylose and other pentose monomers (e.g. arabinose) by β-D-xylosidases (EC 3.2.1.37), along with several accessory enzymes that attack side groups of xylan, including α-L-arabinofuranosidases (EC 3.2.1.55), α-glucuronidase (EC 3.2.1.139), acetyl xylan esterase (EC 3.1.1.72), ferulic acid esterase (EC 3.1.1.73) and p-coumaric esterase (EC 3.1.1.B10) (Collins et al., 2005; Bhardwaj et al., 2019). The affinity of β-xylosidases can be hindered if the oligomers are branched (Gamauf et al., 2007). Xylanases exist in many living organisms, such as bacteria, fungi, protozoa, algae, crustaceans, insects, snails and plant seeds (Sunna and Antranikian, 1997). Ferulic and coumaric acids esterified to arabinose within the side chains are hydrolysed by feruloyl esterases and coumaroyl esterases, respectively.

Commercial xylanases used in animal feed are produced mainly from bacteria (e.g. *Bacillus* spp.) and filamentous fungi (commonly *Aspergillus* and *Trichoderma* spp.), and have been well reviewed previously (Paloheimo et al., 2010; Bhardwaj et al., 2019).

3.4 Impact of Xylanase and Cellulase on Nutrient Digestion and Fermentation

The breakdown of NSPs by carbohydrases, in theory, should improve dry matter, fibre and energy digestibility and improve growth performance in pigs, especially feed efficiency; indeed, in many studies, improvements in digestibility are observed. In fact, a meta-analysis of studies using xylanase in growing-finishing pigs conducted by Torres-Pitarch et al. (2019) found that xylanase supplementation improved the apparent total tract digestibility of dry matter, crude protein and gross energy, irrespective of diet composition. The mean improvement was 1.2, 0.9 and 1.4%, respectively. However, pig studies that show an improvement in digestibility in tandem with improved performance are uncommon. While many researchers have postulated why this

response, or lack thereof, occurs, there is still a dearth of empirical understanding on why performance responses are not better aligned with improvements in digestibility. The key to improving xylanase efficacy to yield improvements in both digestibility and performance lies with the elucidation of the *in vivo* mode of action.

Over the years, the mechanism by which xylanase improves nutrient and energy digestibility has been extensively debated. There are four plausible mechanisms of action commonly discussed: (i) xylanase increases energy and fibre digestibility in the pig by hydrolysing arabinoxylan to release fragments that can be either absorbed or fermented (Adeola and Cowieson, 2011); (ii) xylanase degrades the physical structure of the endosperm walls, releasing trapped nutrients, which results in improved fibre, energy and/or nutrient digestibility – the so-called 'encapsulation theory' (De Lange et al., 2010); (iii) xylanase mitigates various physiochemical properties associated with NSPs that can negatively impact the digestibility of nutrients and energy (De Vries et al., 2012); and (iv) xylanase reduces endogenous losses associated with the sloughing of epithelial cells and the erosion of mucin (Adeola and Cowieson, 2011). It is plausible that each of these modes of action is true but are situationally dependent on supplementation conditions. Among the digestibility responses reported, researchers have commonly associated their results with fibre solubility, substrate type, metabolic efficiencies of release products, production stage of the animal, length of supplementation, enzyme source and xylanase concentration. It is likely that a combination of these factors impairs or improves xylanase efficacy.

Historically, one expectation of supplementing xylanase is the hydrolysis of arabinoxylan in the small intestine to promote intestinal absorption of monosaccharides, rather than microbial fermentation. Energy derived from carbohydrate fermentation is metabolically less efficient when compared with direct absorption and utilization of monosaccharides, at least for hexoses. In the pig, pentoses (e.g. xylose and arabinose) are metabolically less efficient than hexoses, but it is not clear whether their energetic efficiency would be greater if they would be absorbed as such or fermented to short-chain fatty acids (SCFAs) (Huntley and Patience, 2018; Abelilla and Stein, 2019a).

There are few *in vivo* data that have quantified the actual extent of monosaccharide release. *In vitro* data would suggest that it is quite marginal, particularly with insoluble fibre (Dale *et al.*, 2019). Limited monosaccharide release, or inefficiency of pentose utilization for energy, could partially explain why apparent ileal digestibility of energy responses are less common than apparent total tract digestibility (Torres-Pitarch *et al.*, 2019). Likewise, if fibre hydrolysis in the small intestine is minimal, it may not be detected by commonly used methods of determining nutrient digestibility (Patience and Petry, 2019); however, fibre in the ileal effluent could be a more fermentable substrate for the hindgut microbiota.

Diet and ingredient composition may also impact the effectiveness and consistency of xylanase in the pig. The fermentability of NSPs differs among dietary ingredients and is related to the physiochemical properties and structure of the fibre (Anguita *et al.*, 2006). The physiochemical properties of arabinoxylan, particularly solubility, have been suggested to impact hydrolysis by xylanase (Stein, 2019). Soluble arabinoxylans are less lignified, have greater branching and a lower arabinose to xylose ratio (Oakenfull, 2000). These properties allow for greater water infiltration into the arabinoxylan matrix, subsequently increasing surface area and improving fermentation. It appears that digestibility is improved when xylanase is supplemented with substrates containing more soluble arabinoxylan, such as wheat and barley (Yin *et al.*, 2001; Abelilla and Stein, 2019b), but responses have also been observed when supplemented in diets containing insoluble arabinoxylan, such as maize (Petry *et al.*, 2019a).

Soluble arabinoxylans can also increase digestive viscosity by forming gels.

Viscous fibres impair nutrient digestibility by preventing interaction of nutrients with the brush border and decrease lipid emulsification (Dikeman and Fahey, 2006). In poultry diets, the cornerstone of xylanase supplementation is mitigation of the viscous nature of soluble arabinoxylans, thus improving nutrient and energy digestibility. However, the digestive anatomy and physiology differ greatly between pigs and poultry. In pigs, digesta viscosity seems to not interfere with nutrient digestibility to the same degree as in poultry (Duarte *et al.*, 2019). This may explain why xylanase efficacy is more consistent in poultry.

Considerable value has been placed on the ability of xylanase to degrade the physical structure of fibre cell walls, releasing trapped nutrients that were originally inaccessible to the pig. There is some *in vitro* microscopic evidence of this reported in the literature (Tervilä-Wilo *et al.*, 1996; Jha *et al.*, 2015; Ravn *et al.*, 2016), but by and large, this has been associated with improved digestibility of other dietary components, such as starch, phosphorus, calcium and various amino acids. Indeed, the value of xylanase is increased, if this is the case, but *in vivo* evidence is needed to confirm this mode of action.

In pigs, cellulase is most commonly supplemented as part of an enzyme blend. Research evaluating cellulase alone is scarce and partitioning the impact of cellulase on digestibility from enzyme blend research is unachievable. The lack of singular cellulase supplementation is likely due to the limited number of lignocellulose-degrading enzymes that are not produced as accessory enzymes. Theoretically, cellulase supplementation should increase insoluble fibre digestibility and improve energy utilization. This would be particularly beneficial if hydrolysis occurred in the small intestine and released glucose, but in-depth studies evaluating cellulase are unavailable. Improvements in energy digestibility have been reported with cellulase supplementation, but like many studies with carbohydrases, the experimental conditions and results vary considerably. Currently, cellulase activity is inconsistent and small relative to the amount of cellulose within typical diets, and the production of singular lignocellulose enzymes with consistent activity is rare or in the research and development stage (Wang *et al.*, 2012).

3.5 Impact of Xylanase and Cellulase on Animal Health

The effect of cellulases, β-glucanases and xylanases on animal health may occur mainly through modification of fibre structure and production of various chain lengths of oligosaccharides in the small and large intestine. These molecules may modulate intestinal microbiota as well as regulate intestinal function and immune status, either via direct interaction with epithelial cells and immune cells or via indirect interaction with microbes and microbial fermentation products (Courtin *et al.*, 2008; Samuelsen *et al.*, 2011; Chen *et al.*, 2012; Kiarie *et al.*, 2013; Mendis *et al.*, 2016). Very limited research has directly quantified oligosaccharides derived from fibre degradation under the influence of cellulase and xylanase in the intestinal tract of swine, either *in vivo* or *in vitro*. Lærke *et al.* (2015) reported that supplementing xylanase in wheat or rye diets increased the amount of arabinoxylo-oligosaccharides in both the dry matter and the liquid phase of the ileal digesta in growing pigs. Similarly, low-molecular-weight arabinoxylan in ileal digesta of grow-finish pigs was increased by xylanases (Pedersen *et al.*, 2015), demonstrating the efficacy of xylanases in swine feed.

3.5.1 Effects on intestinal function and immune status

The impact of carbohydrase supplementation on gut barrier function as well as intestinal and systemic immune status in pigs is largely unknown. Recently, Li *et al.* (2018a) reported that the addition of a carbohydrase blend (xylanase, β-glucanase and cellulase) in weaned pig diets reduced urinary lactulose:mannitol and increased ileal claudin-3

(*CLDN3*) mRNA abundance, indicating improved small intestinal barrier integrity. This is consistent with Tiwari *et al.* (2018) who observed increased protein concentration of claudin, occludin and ZO-1 in the jejunum by xylanase supplementation in nursery diets. Li *et al.* (2018b) also showed reduced markers of gut (ileal secretory IgA levels and *IL-22* mRNA) and systemic (plasma TNF-α, IL-1β and IL-8) inflammation by the carbohydrase blend, coinciding with improved growth performance (Li *et al.*, 2018a). These provide evidence that the mechanism of action whereby carbohydrases enhance growth in weaned pigs is probably due in part to improving gut barrier function and downregulating inflammation; this, in turn, decreases the amount of energy and nutrients used for maintenance of the immune system. The modulation of gut barrier and immune status may partly explain why the addition of xylanase in grow-finish diets improves survivability and the portion of pigs placed in a barn that are able to achieve market weight (Boyd *et al.*, 2019). The economic implications of reduced mortality are substantial and easily dwarf modest improvements in growth rate or feed efficiency.

Pigs fed diets supplemented with both xylanase and the enzyme blend, but not individual enzymes, had greater colonic occludin (*OCLN*) and *CLDN3* mRNA, as well as lower levels of plasma IL-1β and TNF-α, compared with those receiving the control diet without enzymes (Li *et al.*, 2018b). This suggests synergistic effects of different enzymes or improved efficacy of enzymes with increased activities in reducing markers of inflammation. In contrast, Vila *et al.* (2018) reported that a carbohydrase blend (xylanase, β-glucanase, mannanase and galactosidase) increased IL-1β and decreased IL-11 (an anti-inflammatory cytokine) in the ileum of growing pigs, regardless of diet type, suggesting elevated immune activation in the intestine. The reason for this discrepancy between studies is unclear, but it may be attributed to differences in supplemental enzyme activities, thus resulting in different levels of fibre hydrolysis products in the intestine.

Mucins, major components of the intestinal mucus layer, are important for maintaining gut barrier function and may inhibit bacterial translocation across the gut (Usui *et al.*, 1999). Limited research has evaluated the effect of cellulases and xylanases on intestinal mucins in swine. Vila *et al.* (2018) reported that a multi-carbohydrase reduced ileal *MUC2* mRNA of growing pigs fed diets with 40% DDGS compared with those without carbohydrases; this appeared to agree with the increase in IL-1β and decrease in IL-11 discussed above. In contrast, a xylanase and β-glucanase blend did not change the mRNA abundance of *MUC4* and *MUC20* in growing pigs fed diets with 30% DDGS (Agyekum *et al.*, 2015).

Carbohydrases may regulate intestinal microbial populations in one of two ways: (i) reduction of undigested nutrients; and (ii) provision of prebiotic short-chain oligosaccharides (Bedford and Cowieson, 2012; Kiarie *et al.*, 2013). Modulation of the gut microbiota and associated changes in volatile fatty acids (VFAs) (e.g. acetate and butyrate) may partially contribute to changes in gut barrier integrity and the immune response of host animals (Peng *et al.*, 2009). This is supported by Tiwari *et al.* (2018) who reported that xylanases increased acetate, propionate and total VFAs *in vitro*, concurrent with improved intestinal barrier integrity *in vivo* in pigs. Milo *et al.* (2002) also showed that VFA (acetate, propionate and butyrate) supplementation increased ileal IL-1β and IL-6 concentration in pigs. The effect of carbohydrases on intestinal microbiota is discussed in detail in a following section.

3.5.2 Effects on enteric bacterial challenges

Because carbohydrases can indirectly modulate intestinal microbiota via the production of fermentable oligosaccharides and/or the reduction of other fermentable substrates flowing into the hindgut, they may exert some benefits by controlling enteric bacterial challenges such as enterotoxigenic *Escherichia coli* (ETEC) (Bedford and Cowieson, 2012; Kiarie *et al.*, 2013). For example, NSP hydrolysis products of certain feed ingredients (e.g. soybean meal, wheat middlings) generated by a carbohydrase blend with cellulase, xylanase, glucanase and other enzyme activities mitigated an ETEC infection by improving fluid balance in an *in situ* model (Kiarie *et al.*, 2008, 2010). Follow-up *in vivo* studies by the same researchers showed that weaned pigs fed diets containing NSP hydrolysis products had reduced faecal scores and serum haptoglobin as well as increased ileal mucosal adherent lactobacilli counts 48 h after a K88 ETEC challenge (Kiarie *et al.*, 2009a,b). These results suggest that enzyme hydrolysis products may mitigate or help control an ETEC infection in pigs. The *in vivo* studies, however, did not include a non-challenged control treatment or report the incidence of diarrhoea post-challenge to demonstrate the severity of the challenge; this made it difficult to fully understand the true protective effect of those enzyme hydrolysis products (Kiarie *et al.*, 2009a,b). In contrast, a recent study by Li *et al.* (2019) showed that an F18 ETEC challenge increased the incidence of diarrhoea, elevated markers of impaired gut barrier function and inflammation, and reduced growth performance of weaned pigs compared with a sham inoculum of phosphate-buffered saline. In the same study, the supplementation of multiple carbohydrases (xylanase, β-glucanase and pectinase) in a soluble fibre diet with sugarbeet pulp decreased markers of an inflammatory response (serum haptoglobin and ileal *TNF-α* mRNA) and increased markers of gut barrier integrity (*OCLN* and *ZO-1* mRNA). This appeared to contribute to improved pig growth compared with the ETEC-challenged control (Li *et al.*, 2019). The reduced immune activation and enhanced gut barrier integrity seemed to be associated with decreases in *Escherichia/Shigella* and increases in *Lactobacillus*, which may be a result of oligosaccharides released by enzyme supplementation (Chen *et al.*, 2012; González-Ortiz *et al.*, 2014). Increases in acetate and total VFAs as well as lower colonic pH observed in the same study may also play a partial role in enhancing gut barrier integrity, because acetate can be consumed by butyrogenic bacteria via a cross-feeding mechanism to produce butyrate (Peng *et al.*, 2009; Rios-Covian *et al.*, 2015). In addition to ETEC, xylanase supplementation in a non-extruded wheat diet also improved growth performance of pigs challenged with a virulent strain of *Brachyspira hyodysenteriae* (Durmic *et al.*, 1997).

Therefore, xylanases alone or in combination with cellulase, β-glucanase and/or other enzymes are promising in improving gut barrier function, resistance to enteric bacterial challenges and thus overall health of pigs. More studies are warranted to fully understand the modes of action through which these enzymes modulate animal health and to be able to successfully apply these enzyme technologies in commercial swine production.

3.6 Impact of Xylanase on Growth Performance

There is a very large number of publications addressing the impact of xylanase on growth performance. Unfortunately, the same cannot be said of cellulase; it is generally studied as a component of a multi-enzyme complex, rendering it impossible to separate the effect of cellulase from other individual carbohydrases present in the diet.

Recently, Torres-Pitarch *et al.* (2019) undertook a meta-analysis of publications evaluating the effect of carbohydrases on growth performance and nutrient digestibility in growing pigs. They identified 302 total publications dealing with growing pigs, of which only 67 met all of their selection criteria; these papers reported a total of 139 comparisons. Interestingly, the most common studies evaluated enzyme complexes, followed by xylanase, xylanase plus β-glucanase and mannanase. There were no reports of studies on cellulase alone but cellulase was included in many of the enzyme complexes that were investigated. Furthermore, most of the studies involved maize followed by wheat and then barley. A total of 120 studies investigated the impact of enzymes on growth performance; 38 of these

studies reported a positive impact, 78 showed no benefit and four saw a negative effect on feed efficiency. Their data revealed a clear effect of substrate. For example, xylanase improved average daily gain in maize and maize co-product diets, while multi-enzyme complexes improved both average daily gain and feed efficiency in diets based on maize, wheat, barley and co-products.

Adeola and Cowieson (2011) also surveyed published studies on the effect of carbohydrases on growth performance in swine. They reported that xylanase was the most common enzyme studied but concluded that carbohydrases had no consistent effect on growth performance. Zeng *et al.* (2018) completed a meta-analysis of 101 studies. Perhaps because this was a more recent analysis of the published literature and thus would represent advances in enzyme technology as well as our ability to utilize them more effectively, their conclusions differed from those of Adeola and Cowieson (2011). They reported that carbohydrases or proteases increased rate of gain by 3.0% in wheat-based diets, 2.1% in maize-based diets and 1.5% in barley-based diets. In turn, feed conversion efficiency was improved by 2.8, 1.6 and 2.7% in wheat-, maize- and barley-based diets, respectively.

It is puzzling how enzymes can be quite effective at improving energy and nutrient digestibility but, as Torres-Pitarch *et al.* (2019) point out, this is not always reflected in an increase in feed efficiency or growth rate. A number of possibilities exist to explain what appears to be an inconsistency in these data. First, the correlation between dietary energy intake and feed efficiency is highly variable; in some cases, it has been determined to be less than 0.15 (Oresanya *et al.*, 2008) and in other cases, highly correlated (Beaulieu *et al.*, 2009). This can be explained by the large number of factors that affect feed efficiency. Second, the improvement in digestibility may be of a magnitude too small to be measured in terms of feed efficiency. For example, in the Beaulieu *et al.* (2009) study cited above, each 1% increase in dietary energy concentration resulted in a 0.7% improvement in the gain:feed ratio. Therefore, if an enzyme improved energy digestibility by 1 to 3%, the expected improvement in feed efficiency would be well below the level of precision of many growth studies. However, this explanation is overly simplistic, because enzymes typically impact more than simply improving the digestibility of gross energy (Adeola and Cowieson, 2011; Bedford, 2019). Third, it is difficult, but certainly not impossible, to conduct a digestibility study with a high degree of precision and accuracy coincident with measurement of growth performance. This helps to explain why most studies separate the two, thus introducing problems associated with experiment-to-experiment variability. Fourth, as illustrated very well by the reviews of Adeola and Cowieson (2011) and Torres-Pitarch *et al.* (2019), the response to enzymes is in itself variable, especially in the growing pig. It can be influenced by the nature of the substrates present in the diet, the quantity and quality of the enzyme employed, the age and sex of the pig, the formulation of the experimental diet and the length of time the pig is exposed to the enzyme (Adeola and Cowieson, 2011; Petry *et al.*, 2019b).

Looking at various individual research reports on the topic of substrate, growth rate and feed efficiency on maize or maize DDGS diets were improved by xylanase (Lan *et al.*, 2017) in some instances, but sometimes only rate of gain benefited (Tsai *et al.*, 2017). Yet others reported no effect at all (Jones *et al.*, 2010, 2015). Similar observations have been reported using wheat as the basal ingredient. Owusu-Asiedu *et al.* (2010) reported that xylanase in combination with β-glucanase improved feed efficiency but provided no benefit in terms of rate of gain. Zijlstra *et al.* (2004) used diets based on wheat and canola meal; in nursery pigs, graded levels of a blend of xylanase and β-glucanase improved feed intake and feed efficiency, but not rate of gain. Omogbenigun *et al.* (2004) used a very different approach. They used three different enzyme preparations, but all contained eight or more enzymes. They reported that all of the enzyme combinations improved rate and efficiency of gain.

3.6.1 Impact of xylanases and cellulases in liquid feeding systems

Xylanase and other carbohydrases have sometimes been added to liquid feeding systems in order to enhance the breakdown of complex carbohydrates in the diet, thus maximizing digestion of dietary contents and thereby leading to improved growth performance. However, there are limited data on this topic. Choct *et al.* (2004) evaluated liquid feed provided to newly weaned piglets fed diets based on wheat; they reported that enzyme supplementation improved average daily gain by 15% ($P = 0.045$) but had no effect on feed conversion. Interestingly, steeping the liquid mixture for 15 h had the same impact as adding enzyme with only 1 h steeping. Indeed, there was no benefit from enzyme addition when 15 h steeping was applied. De Lange and Zhu (2012) reported that the addition of xylanase and β-glucanase to a liquid diet containing 30% maize DDGS improved average daily gain by almost 9% ($P = 0.007$) and feed:gain by 3% ($P = 0.022$). Moran *et al.* (2016) investigated the addition of xylanase to dry or liquid diets containing 30% wheat middlings or DDGS fed to growing pigs. They reported no improvement in any growth performance parameter.

3.7 Potential Modes of Action for Microbiome Modulation by Xylanase

The GI tract is home to a diverse microbiota that contributes to the nutrition, health and performance of pigs. Recently, due to the increased availability of culture-independent next-generation sequencing technologies (e.g. 16S rDNA sequencing) and the shift towards reducing reliance on antibiotics, research on the role of the microbiome in swine nutrition has intensified. A significant portion of this research has been directed at evaluating the ability of feed additives, such as carbohydrases, to modulate the microbiota. In fact, the interplay between the intestinal microbiota and phenotypic responses to carbohydrases was considered well before the wide adoption of culture-independent sequencing technologies (Bedford and Cowieson, 2012).

Diet composition directly impacts the substrates available for the gut microbiota. It is widely acknowledged that dietary fibre is the predominant colonic substrate and a potent microbiota modulator that can reduce pathogenic microbes, alter and increase the diversity of microbial communities, and improve the proliferation of 'beneficial' microbes (Isaacson and Kim, 2012; Fouhse et al., 2016). Carbohydrases have the unique ability to modulate GI microbial ecology through various mechanisms of altering dietary fibre. Carbohydrases have demonstrated positive effects in controlling infectious diseases such as post-weaning colibacillosis (Li et al., 2019), and there is a potential role for their use in non-antibiotic feeding systems as a potent gut microbiota stimulator. Due to the infancy of 16S rDNA research, this section does not review specific changes in microbiota composition, or the impact of cellulase on the microbiome due to a dearth of studies. Rather, it focuses on the potential modes of action for microbiome modulation by xylanase.

There are three commonly proposed mechanisms for GI microbial modulation by xylanase: (i) xylanase reduces undigested substrates in ileal digesta, thereby altering the composition of substrates entering the large intestine; (ii) xylanase alters the physiochemical properties of arabinoxylan and thus modifies substrate availability for gut microbiota; and (iii) the in situ production by xylanase of arabinoxylo-oligosaccharides, which have prebiotic-like effects (Bedford and Cowieson, 2012; Kiarie et al., 2013). These modes of action are likely occurring in tandem with each other and could potentially increase production of potent signalling SCFAs such as butyrate, reduce luminal pH, increase energy to the pig through improved fermentation, modulate the immune system, reduce pathogen adhesion to host cells and alter the brain–microbiome axis (Isaacson and Kim, 2012; Bourassa et al., 2016; Fouhse et al., 2016). But there are inconsistences in the

conditions in which these responses occur. Moreover, xylanase efficacy in modulating the GI microbiota, regardless of mode of action, is almost certainly dependent on diet composition.

As previously discussed, xylanase can alter the structural and physicochemical properties of arabinoxylan and, in turn, alter the substrates available to the microbiota. Substrates that were once available to the microbiota may now be utilized by the pig in the small intestine. In terms of dietary energy, this is beneficial to the pig, but it also increases the proportion of energetically less favourable substrates presented to the microbiota, such as proteins, and endogenous losses. This can result in an increase in production of branched-chain fatty acids and protein fermentation products, and reduce microbial diversity (Kim et al., 2017). However, in some instances, xylanase can improve the ileal digestibility of other dietary components, through the cell wall nutrient releasing mechanism, and reduce protein and starch fermentation. Likewise, through this mechanism, xylanase may reduce substrate competition between host and ileal microbiota and reduce the potential of pathogenic bacteria colonizing the ileum through microbial starvation (Bedford and Cowieson, 2012).

The solubility, viscosity and fermentability of fibre can impact the GI microbiota. Soluble NSPs are fermented more proximally (e.g. the ileum) and insoluble fibres are partially fermented in the distal colon, where rate of passage is decreased and bacterial densities are higher. Improving fermentability of insoluble fibre can increase substrates for the microbiota and there is potential to improve GI health through the stimulatory effects of SCFAs (Bach Knudsen et al., 2012). This may explain why xylanase improved diversity and composition of the microbiota in the large intestine of pigs fed maize fibre (Zhang et al., 2017; Zhang et al., 2018). However, studies evaluating both microbiota composition and phenotypic responses by the host, when given insoluble fibre with xylanase, are unfortunately rare but clearly needed.

Earth's most abundant renewable resources are materials composed of cellulose, hemicellulose and lignin, and they are the main constituents of many industrial products. Thus, carbohydrases have applications well beyond animal nutrition. The role of microbial enzymes in improving fermentation has been around since Ancient Greece, where exogenous enzymes were used in baking, brewing, alcohol production and cheese making. In the 20th century, technology and research in the field of enzymology advanced rapidly and with the development of thermostable enzymes, industrial applications of carbohydrases increased many fold (Dhiman *et al.*, 2008). Today, carbohydrases are utilized by numerous food and non-food sectors: pulp and paper production, bioethanol production, dough production, fruit juice production, production of xylitol sweetener, biostoning in the textile industry, the detergent industry, pharmaceuticals and others (Sunna and Antranikian, 1997; Polizeli *et al.*, 2005; Kuhad *et al.*, 2011).

Cellulase is the third most used enzyme, and the most utilized NSP enzyme in industrial applications (Bajaj and Mahajan, 2019). Xylanase has been categorized as the most industrially important enzyme to research due to the abundance of undegraded xylan found in industrial by-products (Haki and Rakshit, 2003). Many industrial applications require the synergistic action of both cellulase and xylanase, and research of microbial species that can produce these enzymes in tandem at high concentrations, with similar optimum conditions, is in demand by the food, fibre and bioenergy industries (Dhiman *et al.*, 2008; Bajaj and Mahajan, 2019). Conversely, the paper industry has been at the forefront of developing cellulase-free xylanase sources as a means to improve the safety of bleaching pulp for paper production; in 2008, about 30% of the patents related to xylanase awarded in the USA were associated with biobleaching (Loera Corral and Villaseñor-Ortega, 2006). While applications of xylanase and cellulase in industrial processes, and the conditions they are utilized in, are not directly applicable to carbohydrase use in swine

nutrition, their research and technological advancements could help advance their use in the feed industry.

3.8 Future Trends

Carbohydrases emerged in the feed additive market with the intent to improve the utilization of fibre. Today, their role in animal nutrition goes well beyond these original targets, but their efficacy, at least in pigs, is variable and still poorly understood. As such, the future advancement of carbohydrases in the swine industry will require extensive understanding of their *in vivo* mode of action. If the mode of action is correctly elucidated, nutritionists will be able to make more informed decisions about the proper utilization of the right enzyme, from the right source, with the right substrate, in the right situation, and will likely be more successful in achieving an improvement in phenotypic outcomes.

Elucidating the mode of action of carbohydrases will require creative research that reaches beyond the scope of typical digestibility and performance trials. Future studies should consider experimental design conditions that show the greatest promise in efficacy and reproducibility. For example, length of supplementation has emerged as a design variable that appears to have considerable impact on enzyme efficacy. Although the minimum amount of time required is unclear, previous studies might have missed their window of opportunity due to short adaptation periods. Furthermore, there is a need for more encompassing studies that approach mode of action research in a collaborative, multidisciplinary manner, evaluating several modes of action under one set of conditions. Multifaceted research will exponentially improve our understanding of enzymes. Likewise, future studies should provide more comprehensive information on research conditions, such as inclusion of negative controls, analysed composition of all diets, analysed enzyme activities, the health and genetic background of the pigs, description of animal housing and the use of appropriate fibre assays for the fibre types included in the diet (Patience and Petry, 2019).

From recent carbohydrase and pentose metabolism research, one must ask if improved nutrient and energy utilization are the right formulation targets, or is there greater benefit in their ability to improve health and increase survivability of pigs? Carbohydrases' true return on investment may need to include reduction in mortality, ability to beneficially modulate the microbiome and immune system, improve GI barrier integrity, and improve antioxidant capacity and other health measures; these benefits would accrue in addition to improved fibre utilization and growth performance. In fact, some have proposed that carbohydrases could have a role to play in antibiotic-free or antibiotic-reduced programmes (Melo-Duràn et al., 2019); focusing research in this arena could be advantageous to both the enzyme and pork industries.

Carbohydrases have emerged as a positive microbiota modulator through various previously mentioned mechanisms. Recently, advances in the 'prebiotic and stimbiotic' mechanism are promising and may explain multiple phenotypic health responses observed in both pigs and poultry (Bedford, 2019). Continual research on this mechanism of action is warranted, particularly characterizing in situ oligosaccharide production in the pig as relevant analyses become more common and less expensive (Alyassin and Campbell, 2019). As we continue to investigate the GI microbiota, fibre, in situ oligosaccharides and enzymes, it is important that studies delve into the metabolic functions of bacteria, rather than just their taxonomic position or abundance. Furthermore, there is a dearth of understanding of how enzymes modulate the microbiota beyond bacterial origin (e.g. archaea, fungi, protozoa). While these organisms play a much smaller role in microbiota–host homeostasis, they can still have significant implications in microbiome metabolism.

There is still much debate on the correct formulation strategies to adopt when enzymes are being used. At least some of

the variability in enzyme outcomes can be attributed to incorrect formulation of experimental diets (Adeola and Cowieson, 2011). Concurrently, carbohydrase research should focus on both single carbohydrase addition and enzyme blends. Enzyme blends have shown greater efficacy in improving pig performance, but research on single enzyme supplementation is more abundant, largely because of the current enzyme market. The answer to this debate lies within the objective of carbohydrase utilization. If the greater objective is to improve fibre degradation and subsequent utilization, then blends may be more appropriate; but if the objective is to reap the benefits of in situ oligosaccharide production, then single carbohydrase utilization may be more suitable. Enzyme blends, particularly blends that target the degradation of one fibre type, may impair in situ oligosaccharide production (Bedford, 2019). Further basic research, in both enzyme blends and single carbohydrases, will help to pinpoint the right formulation strategy for these products.

3.9   Conclusions

Global food production is facing major challenges in the coming decades due to substantial growth in the human population. At the same time, traditional feed sources utilized by monogastric species are being increasingly used for industrial purposes, the most significant of which at the present time is biofuel production. Consequently, pig and poultry producers are increasing their use of alternative feedstuffs, including co-products of grain processing. The higher fibre content of such ingredients represents a great opportunity for increased use of enzymes in commercial diets. In this regard, the future of the enzyme sector looks very bright.

However, it is clear from the above discussion in this chapter that the traditional view of enzyme use – to enhance fibre utilization and improve diet digestibility – may be too narrow. The prospect of improving animal health through the use of enzymes is becoming a realistic secondary goal. This focus is not only encouraging in its own right, but it fits well with the global trend of reducing the use of subtherapeutic levels of antibiotics in pork production. The tremendous impact of enzymes in the area of environmental protection is already very well established through the use of phytase.

Moving forward, the need to best define the circumstances in which enzymes will be most useful remains foremost in the minds of many nutritionists. This will include everything from the pathogen load on the pigs to many, many aspects of the composition of the diet. Therefore, there remains a need for further research not only to define the optimum conditions for successful use of enzymes, but also for the mode of action of individual enzymes and enzyme blends.

References

Abelilla, J.J. and Stein, H.H. (2019a) Fate of pentoses in the small intestine and hindgut of growing pigs. *Journal of Animal Science* 97, 95. doi: 10.1093/jas/skz122.171

Abelilla, J.J. and Stein, H.H. (2019b) Degradation of dietary fibre in the stomach, small intestine, and large intestine of growing pigs fed corn- or wheat-based diets without or with microbial xylanase. *Journal of Animal Science* 97, 338–352. doi: 10.1093/jas/sky403

Adeola, O. and Cowieson, A.J. (2011) Board-invited review: Opportunities and challenges in using exogenous enzymes to improve nonruminant animal production. *Journal of Animal Science* 89, 3189–3218. doi: 10.2527/jas.2010-3715

Agyekum, A.E., Sands, J.S., Regassa, A., Kiarie, E., Weihrauch, D., *et al.* (2015) Effect of supplementing a fibrous diet with a xylanase and β-glucanase blend on growth performance, intestinal glucose uptake, and transport-associated gene expression in growing pigs. *Journal of Animal Science* 93, 3483–3493. doi: 10.2527/jas.2015-9027

Alyassin, M. and Campbell, G.M. (2019) Challenges and constraints in analysis of oligosaccharides and other fibre components. In: González-Ortiz, G., Bedford, M.R., Bach Knudsen, K.E., Courtin, C.M. and Classen, H.L. (eds) *The Value of Fibre: Engaging the Second Brain for Animal Nutrition*. Wageningen Academic Publishers, Wageningen, the Netherlands, pp. 257–277. doi: 10.3920/978-90-8686-893-3_15

Anguita, M., Canibe, N., Pérez, J.F. and Jensen, B.B. (2006) Influence of the amount of dietary fibre on the available energy from hindgut fermentation in growing pigs: use of cannulated pigs and *in vitro* fermentation. *Journal of Animal Science* 84, 2766–2778. doi: 10.2527/jas.2005-212

Bach Knudsen, K.E. (1997) Carbohydrate and lignin contents of plant materials used in animal feeding. *Animal Feed Science and Technology* 67, 319–338. doi: 10.1016/S0377-8401(97)00009-6

Bach Knudsen, K.E. (2014) Fibre and nonstarch polysaccharide content and variation in common crops used in broiler diets. *Poultry Science* 93, 2380–2393. doi: 10.3382/ps.2014-03902

Bach Knudsen, K.E., Hedemann, M.S. and Lærke, H.N. (2012) The role of carbohydrates in intestinal health of pigs. *Animal Feed Science and Technology* 173, 41–53. doi: 10.1016/j.anifeedsci.2011.12.020

Bajaj, P. and Mahajan, R. (2019) Cellulase and xylanase synergism in industrial biotechnology. *Applied Microbiology and Biotechnology* 103, 8711–8724. doi: 10.1007/s00253-019-10146-0

Beaulieu, A.D., Williams, N.H. and Patience, J.F. (2009) Response to dietary digestible energy concentration in growing pigs fed cereal-grain based diets. *Journal of Animal Science* 87, 965–976.

Bedford, M.R. (2019) Future prospects for non-starch polysaccharide degrading enzymes development in monogastric nutrition. In: González-Ortiz, G., Bedford, M.R., Bach Knudsen, K.E., Courtin, C.M. and Classen, H.L. (eds) *The Value of Fibre: Engaging the Second Brain for Animal Nutrition*. Wageningen Academic Publishers, Wageningen, the Netherlands, pp. 373–383. doi: 10.3920/978-90-8686-893-3_21

Bedford, M.R. and Cowieson, A.J. (2012) Exogenous enzymes and their effects on intestinal microbiology. *Animal Feed Science and Technology* 173, 60–85. doi: 10.1016/j.anifeedsci.2011.12.018

Bhardwaj, N., Kumar, B. and Verma, P. (2019) A detailed overview of xylanases: an emerging biomolecule for current and future perspectives. *Bioresources and Bioprocessing* 6, 40. doi: 10.1186/s40643-019-0276-2

Bourassa, M.W., Alim, I., Bultman, S.J. and Ratan, R.R. (2016) Butyrate, neuroepigenetics and the gut microbiome: can a high fiber diet improve brain health? *Neuroscience Letters* 625, 56–63. doi: 10.1016/j.neulet.2016.02.009

Boyd, R.D., Zier-Rush, C.E., Moeser, A.J., Culbertson, M., Stewart, K.R., *et al.* (2019) Invited review: Innovation through research in the North American pork industry. *Animal* 13, 2951–2966. doi: 10.1017/S1751731119001915

Chen, H.H., Chen, Y.K., Chang, H.C. and Lin, S.Y. (2012) Immunomodulatory effects of xylooligosaccharides. *Food Science and Technology Research* 18, 195–199. doi: 10.3136/fstr.18.195.

Choct, M., Selby, E.A.D., Cadogan, D.J. and Campbell, R.G. (2004) Effect of liquid to feed ratio, steeping time, and enzyme supplementation on the performance of weaner pigs. *Australian Journal of Agricultural Research* 55, 247–252.

Ciolacu, D., Ciolacu, F. and Popa, V.I. (2011) Amorphous cellulose – structure and characterization. *Cellulose Chemistry and Technology* 45, 11–13.

Collins, T., Gerday, C. and Feller, G. (2005) Xylanases, xylanase families and extremophilic xylanases. *FEMS Microbiology Reviews* 29, 3–23. doi: 10.1016/j.femsre.2004.06.005

Courtin, C.M., Swennen, K., Broekaert, W.F., Swennen, Q., Buyse, J., *et al.* (2008) Effects of dietary inclusion of xylooligosaccharides, arabinoxylooligosaccharides and soluble arabinoxylan on the microbial composition of caecal contents of chickens. *Journal of the Science of Food and Agriculture* 88, 2517–2522. doi: 10.1002/jsfa.3373

Cummings, J.H. and Stephen, A.M. (2007) Carbohydrate terminology and classification. *European Journal of Clinical Nutrition* 61, S5–S18. doi: 10.1038/sj.ejcn.1602936

Dale, T., Brameld, J.M., Parr, T. and Bedford, M.R. (2019) Differential effects of fibrolytic enzymes on the *in vitro* release of xylobiose from different cereal types. *Proceedings of the British Society of Animal Science* 10, 222. doi: 10.1017/S2040470019000013

De Lange, C.F.M. and Zhu, C.H. (2012) Liquid feeding corn-based diets to growing pigs: practical considerations and use of co-products. In: Patience, J.F. (ed.) *Feed Efficiency in Swine*. Wageningen Academic Publishers, Wageningen, the Netherlands, pp. 101–129.

De Lange, C.F.M., Pluske, J., Gong, J. and Nyachoti, C.M. (2010) Strategic use of feed ingredients and feed additives to stimulate gut health and development in young pigs. *Livestock Science* 134, 124–132. doi: 10.1016/j.livsci.2010.06.117

De Vries, S., Pustjens, A.M., Schols, H.A., Hendriks, W.H. and Gerrits, W.J.J. (2012) Improving digestive utilization of fiber-rich feedstuffs in pigs and poultry by processing and enzyme technologies: a review. *Animal Feed Science and Technology* 178, 123–138. doi: 10.1016/j.anifeedsci.2012.10.004

Dhiman, S.S., Sharma, J. and Battan, B. (2008) Industrial applications and future prospects of microbial xylanases: a review. *BioResources* 3, 1377–1402.

Dikeman, C.L. and Fahey, G.C. Jr (2006) Viscosity as related to dietary fiber: a review. *Critical Reviews in Food Science and Nutrition* 46, 649–663. doi: 10.1080/10408390500511862

Dodd, D. and Cann, I.K.O. (2009) Enzymatic deconstruction of xylan for biofuel production. *Bioenergy* 1, 2–17. doi: 10.1111/j.1757-1707.2009.01004.x

Duarte, M.E., Zhou, F.X., Dutra, W.M. Jr and Kim, S.W. (2019) Dietary supplementation of xylanase and protease on growth performance, digesta viscosity, nutrient digestibility, immune and oxidative stress status, and gut health of newly weaned pigs. *Animal Nutrition* 5, 351–358. doi: 10.1016/j.aninu.2019.04.005

Durmic, Z., Pethick, D., Mullan, B. and Cranwell, P. (1997) The effects of extrusion and arabinoxylanase in wheat based diets on fermentation in the large intestine and expression of swine dysentery. In: Cranwell, P.D. (ed.) *Manipulating Pig Production VI: Proceedings of the 6th Biennial Conference of the Australasian Pig Science Association, Canberra, Australia*. Australian Pig Science Association, Werribee, Australia, p. 180.

Fisher, C.H. (1989) Anselm Payen: pioneer in natural polymers and industrial chemistry. In: Seymour, R.B., Mark, H.F., Pauling, L., Fisher, C.H. and Stahl, G.A. (eds) *Pioneers in Polymer Science*. Springer, Dordrecht, the Netherlands, pp. 47–61. doi: 10.1007/978-94-009-2407-9

Fouhse, J.M., Zijlstra, R.T. and Willing, B.P. (2016) The role of gut microbiota in the health and disease of pigs. *Animal Frontiers* 6, 30–36. doi: 10.2527/af.2016-0031

Gamauf, C., Metz, B. and Seiboth, B. (2007) Degradation of plant cell wall polymers by fungi. In: Kubicek, C.P. and Druzhinina, I.S. (eds) *The Mycota: Environmental and Microbial Relationships*. Springer, Berlin, pp. 325–340.

González-Ortiz, G., Pérez, J.F., Hermes, R.G., Molist, F., Jiménez-Díaz, R. and Martín-Orúe, S.M. (2014) Screening the ability of natural feed ingredients to interfere with the adherence of enterotoxigenic *Escherichia coli* (ETEC) K88 to the porcine intestinal mucus. *British Journal of Nutrition* 111, 633–642. doi: 10.1017/S0007114513003024

Haki, G.D. and Rakshit, S.K. (2003) Developments in industrially important thermostable enzymes: a review. *Bioresource Technology* 89, 17–34. doi: 10.1016/S0960-8524(03)00033-6

Henrissat, B. (1991) A classification of glycosyl hydrolases based on amino acid sequence similarities. *Biochemical Journal* 280, 309–316. doi: 10.1042/bj2800309

Henry, R.J. (1987) Pentosan and (1 → 3),(1 → 4)-β-glucan concentrations in endosperm and wholegrain of wheat, barley, oats and rye. *Journal of Cereal Science* 6, 253–258. doi: 10.1016/S0733-5210(87)80062-0

Henry, R.J. (1988) The carbohydrates of barley grains – a review. *Journal of the Institute of Brewing* 94, 71–78. doi: 10.1002/j.2050-0416.1988.tb04560.x

Huntley, N.F. and Patience, J.F. (2018) Xylose metabolism in the pig. *PLoS ONE* 13, 10–15. doi: 10.1371/journal.pone.0205913

IUB Enzyme Nomenclature (1992) *Recommendations of the Nomenclature Committee of the International Union of Biochemistry and Molecular Biology on the Nomenclature and Classification of Enzymes.* Academic Press, Orlando, Florida.

Isaacson, R. and Kim, H.B. (2012) The intestinal microbiome of the pig. *Animal Health Research Reviews* 13, 100–109. doi: 10.1017/S1466252312000084

Jaworski, N.W., Lærke, H.N., Bach Knudsen, K.E. and Stein, H.H. (2015) Carbohydrate composition and *in vitro* digestibility of dry matter and nonstarch polysaccharides in corn, sorghum, and wheat and coproducts from these grains. *Journal of Animal Science* 93, 1103–1113. doi: 10.2527/jas2014-8147

Jha, R., Woyengo, T.A., Li, J., Bedford, M.R., Vasanthan, T. and Zijlstra, R.T. (2015) Enzymes enhance degradation of the fibre–starch–protein matrix of distillers dried grains with solubles as revealed by a porcine *in vitro* fermentation model and microscopy. *Journal of Animal Science* 93, 1039–1051. doi: 10.2527/jas.2014-7910

Jones, C.K., Bergstrom, J.R., Tokach, M.D., DeRouchey, J.M., Goodband, R.D., *et al.* (2010) Efficacy of commercial enzymes in diets containing various concentrations and sources of dried distillers grains with solubles for nursery pigs. *Journal of Animal Science* 88, 2084–2091.

Jones, C.K., Frantz, E.L., Bingham, A.C., Bergstrom, J.R., DeRouchey, J.M. and Patience, J.F. (2015) Effects of drought-affected corn and nonstarch polysaccharide enzyme inclusion on nursery growth performance. *Journal of Animal Science* 93, 1703–1709.

Kiarie, E.G., Slominski, B.A., Krause, D.O. and Nyachoti, C.M. (2008) Nonstarch polysaccharide hydrolysis products of soybean and canola meal protect against enterotoxigenic *Escherichia coli* in piglets. *The Journal of Nutrition* 138, 502–508. doi: 10.1093/jn/138.3.502

Kiarie, E., Slominski, B., Krause, D. and Nyachoti, C. (2009a) Acute phase response of piglets fed diets containing non-starch polysaccharide hydrolysis products and egg yolk antibodies following an oral challenge with *Escherichia coli* (K88). *Canadian Journal of Animal Science* 89, 353–360. doi: 10.4141/CJAS09008

Kiarie, E., Slominski, B., Krause, D. and Nyachoti, C. (2009b) Gastrointestinal ecology response of piglets' diets containing non-starch polysaccharide hydrolysis products and egg yolk antibodies following an oral challenge with *Escherichia coli* (K88). *Canadian Journal of Animal Science* 89, 341–352. doi: 10.4141/CJAS09007

Kiarie, E.G., Slominski, B.A. and Nyachoti, C.M. (2010) Effect of products derived from hydrolysis of wheat and flaxseed non starch polysaccharides by carbohydrase enzymes on net absorption in enterotoxigenic *Escherichia coli* (K88) challenged piglet jejunal segments. *Animal Science Journal* 81, 63–71. doi: 10.1111/j.1740-0929.2009.00716.x

Kiarie, E., Romero, L.F. and Nyachoti, C.M. (2013) The role of added feed enzymes in promoting gut health in swine and poultry. *Nutrition Research Reviews* 26, 71–88. doi: 10.1017/S0954422413000048

Kim, B.R., Shin, J., Guevarra, R.B., Lee, J.H., Kim, D.W., *et al.* (2017) Deciphering diversity indices for a better understanding of microbial communities. *Journal of Microbiology and Biotechnology* 27, 2089–2093. doi: 10.4014/jmb.1709.09027

Klemm, D., Heublein, B., Fink, H.-P. and Bohn, A. (2005) Cellulose: fascinating biopolymer and sustainable raw material. *Angewandte Chemie* 44, 3358–3393. doi: 10.1002/anie.200460587

Kuhad, R.C., Gupta, R. and Singh, A. (2011) Microbial cellulases and their industrial applications. *Enzyme Research* 2011, 280696. doi: 10.4061/2011/280696

Lærke, H.N., Arent, S., Dalsgaard, S. and Bach Knudsen, K.E. (2015) Effect of xylanases on ileal viscosity, intestinal fiber modification, and apparent ileal fiber and nutrient digestibility of rye and wheat in growing pigs. *Journal of Animal Science* 93, 4323–4335. doi: 10.2527/jas.2015-9096

Lan, R., Li, T. and Kim, I. (2017) Effects of xylanase supplementation on growth performance, nutrient digestibility, blood parameters, fecal microbiota, fecal score and fecal noxious gas emission of weanling pigs fed corn–soybean meal-based diets. *Animal Science Journal* 88, 1398–1405.

Li, Q.Y. (2018) Impact of dietary fiber and exogenous carbohydrases in weaned pigs. PhD dissertation, Iowa State University, Ames, Iowa.

Li, Q., Gabler, N.K., Loving, C.L., Gould, S.A. and Patience, J.F. (2018a) A dietary carbohydrase blend improved intestinal barrier function and growth rate in weaned pigs fed higher fiber diets. *Journal of Animal Science* 96, 5233–5243. doi: 10.1093/jas/sky383

Li, Q., Schmitz-Esser, S., Loving, C.L., Gabler, N.K., Gould, S.A. and Patience, J.F. (2018b). Exogenous carbohydrases added to a starter diet reduced markers of systemic immune activation and decreased *Lactobacillus* in weaned pigs. *Journal of Animal Science* 97, 1242–1253. doi: 10.1093/jas/sky481

Li, Q., Burrough, E.R., Gabler, N.K., Loving, C.L., Sahin, O., *et al.* (2019) A soluble and highly fermentable dietary fiber with carbohydrases improved gut barrier integrity markers and growth performance in F18 ETEC challenged pigs. *Journal of Animal Science* 97, 2139–2153. doi: 10.1093/jas/skz093

Loera Corral, O. and Villaseñor-Ortega, F. (2006) Xylanases. In: Guevara-González, R.G. and Torres-Pacheco, I. (eds) *Advances in Agricultural and Food Biotechnology*. Research Signpost, Trivandrum, India, pp. 305–322.

Melo-Duràn, D., Solà-Oriol, D., Villagomez-Estrada, S. and Pérez, J.F. (2019) Enzymes as an alternative to antibiotics: an overview. In: González-Ortiz, G., Bedford, M.R., Bach Knudsen, K.E., Courtin, C.M. and Classen, H.L. (eds) *The Value of Fibre: Engaging the Second Brain for Animal Nutrition*. Wageningen Academic Publishers, Wageningen, the Netherlands, pp. 351–371. doi: 10.3920/978-90-8686-893-3_20

Mendis, M., Leclerc, E. and Simsek, S. (2016) Arabinoxylans, gut microbiota and immunity. *Carbohydrate Polymers* 139, 159–166. doi: 10.1016/j.carbpol.2015.11.068

Milo, L.A., Reardon, K.A. and Tappenden, K.A. (2002) Effects of short-chain fatty acid-supplemented total parenteral nutrition on intestinal pro-inflammatory cytokine abundance. *Digestive Diseases and Sciences* 47, 2049–2055. doi: 10.1023/a:1019676929875

Mohanty, S.K. and Swain, M.R. (2019) Bioethanol production from corn and wheat: food, fuel and future. In: Ray, R.C. and Ramachandran, S. (eds) *Bioethanol Production from Food Crops: Sustainable Sources, Interventions, and Challenges*. Academic Press, Cambridge, Massachusetts, pp. 45–59. doi: 10.1016/C2017-0-00234-3

Moran, K., De Lange, C.F.M., Ferket, P., Wilcock, P. and van Heugten, E. (2016) Enzyme supplementation to improve the nutritional value of fibrous feed ingredients in swine diets in dry or liquid form. *Journal of Animal Science* 94, 1031–1040.

Narsing Rao, M.P. and Li, W.J. (2017) Microbial cellulase and xylanase: their sources and applications. In: Shrestha, R. (ed.) *Advances in Biochemistry and Applications in Medicine*. Open Access eBooks, Las Vegas, Nevada, pp. 1–20.

Oakenfull, D. (2000) Physical chemistry of dietary fiber. In: Spiller, G.A. (ed.) *Dietary Fiber in Human Nutrition*, 3rd edn. CRC Press, Boca Raton, Florida, pp. 33–47. doi: 10.1201/9781420038514.ch2.7

Omogbenigun, F.O., Nyachoti, C.M. and Slominski, B.A. (2004) Dietary supplementation with multienzyme preparations improves nutrient utilization and growth performance in weaned pigs. *Journal of Animal Science* 82, 1053–1061.

Oresanya, T.F., Beaulieu, A.D. and Patience, J.F. (2008) Investigations of energy metabolism in weanling barrows: the interaction of dietary energy concentration and daily feed (energy) intake. *Journal of Animal Science* 86, 348–363.

Owusu-Asiedu, A., Simmins, P.H., Brufau, J., Lizardo, R. and Peron, A. (2010) Effect of xylanase and β-glucanase on growth performance and nutrient digestibility in piglets fed wheat–barley-based diets. *Livestock Science* 134, 76–78.

Paloheimo, M., Piironen, J. and Vehmaanperä, J. (2010) Xylanases and cellulases as feed additives. In: Bedford, M.R. and Partridge, G.G. (eds) *Enzymes in Farm Animal Nutrition*. CAB International, Wallingford, Oxfordshire, UK, pp. 12–53.

Patience, J.F. and Petry, A.L. (2019) Susceptibility of fibre to exogenous carbohydrases and impact on performance in swine. In: González-Ortiz, G., Bedford, M.R., Bach Knudsen, K.E., Courtin, C.M. and Classen, H.L. (eds) *The Value of Fibre: Engaging the Second Brain for Animal Nutrition*. Wageningen Academic Publishers, Wageningen, the Netherlands, pp. 99–115. doi: 10.3920/978-90-8686-893-3_5

Pedersen, M.B., Yu, S., Arent, S., Dalsgaard, S., Bach Knudsen, K.E. and Lærke, H.N. (2015) Xylanase increased the ileal digestibility of nonstarch polysaccharides and concentration of low molecular weight nondigestible carbohydrates in pigs fed high levels of wheat distillers dried grains with solubles. *Journal of Animal Science* 93, 2885–2893. doi: 10.2527/jas.2014-8829

Peng, L., Li, Z.-R., Green, R.S., Holzman, I.R., and Lin, J. (2009) Butyrate enhances the intestinal barrier by facilitating tight junction assembly via activation of AMP-activated protein kinase in Caco-2 cell monolayers. *The Journal of Nutrition* 139, 1619–1625. doi: 10.3945/jn.109.104638

Petry, A.L., Huntley, N.F., Bedford, M.R. and Patience, J.F. (2019a) Xylanase improved the nutrient and energy digestibility of diets high in insoluble corn fiber fed to swine following a 36-d dietary adaptation period. *Journal of Animal Science* 96(Suppl. 2), 73–74. doi: 10.1093/jas/skz122.381

Petry, A.L., Masey O'Neill, H.V. and Patience, J.F. (2019b) Xylanase, and the role of digestibility and hindgut fermentation in pigs on energetic differences among high and low energy corn samples. *Journal of Animal Science* 97, 4293–4297. doi: 10.1093/jas/skz261

Polizeli, M.L., Rizzatti, A.C., Monti, R., Terenzi, H.F., Jorge, J.A. and Amorim, D.S. (2005) Xylanases from fungi: properties and industrial applications. *Applied Microbiology and Biotechnology* 67, 577–591. doi: 10.1007/s00253-005-1904-7

Ravn, J.L., Martens, H.J., Pettersson, D. and Pedersen, N.R. (2016) A commercial GH 11 xylanase mediates xylan solubilization and degradation in wheat, rye and barley as demonstrated by microscopy techniques and wet chemistry methods. *Animal Feed Science and Technology* 219, 216–225. doi: 10.1016/j.anifeedsci.2016.06.020

Rios-Covian, D., Gueimonde, M., Duncan, S.H., Flint, H.J. and de los Reyes-Gavilan, C.G. (2015) Enhanced butyrate formation by cross-feeding between *Faecalibacterium prausnitzii* and *Bifidobacterium adolescentis*. *FEMS Microbiology Letters* 362, fnv176. doi: 10.1093/femsle/fnv176

Sadhu, S. and Maiti, T.K. (2013) Cellulase production by bacteria: a review. *Microbiology Research Journal International* 3, 235–258. doi: 10.9734/BMRJ/2013/2367

Samuelsen, A.B., Rieder, A., Grimmer, S., Michaelsen, T.E. and Knutsen, S.H. (2011) Immunomodulatory activity of dietary fiber: arabinoxylan and mixed-linked beta-glucan isolated from barley show modest activities *in vitro*. *International Journal of Molecular Sciences* 12, 570–587. doi: 10.3390/ijms12010570

Stein, H.H. (2019) Multi vs single application of enzymes to degrade fibre in diets for pigs. In: González-Ortiz, G., Bedford, M.R., Bach Knudsen, K.E., Courtin, C.M. and Classen, H.L. (eds) *The Value of Fibre: Engaging the Second Brain for Animal Nutrition*. Wageningen Academic Publishers, Wageningen, the Netherlands, pp. 117–124. doi: 10.3920/978-90-8686-893-3_6

Sunna, A. and Antranikian, G. (1997) Xylanolytic enzymes from fungi and bacteria. *Critical Reviews in Biotechnology* 17, 39–67. doi: 10.3109/07388559709146606

Tervilä-Wilo, A., Parkkonen, T., Morgan, A., Hopeakoski-Nurminen, M., Poutanen, K., *et al.* (1996) *In vitro* digestion of wheat microstructure with xylanase and cellulase from *Trichoderma reesei*. *Journal of Cereal Science* 24, 215–225. doi: 10.1006/jcrs.1996.0054

Thongsomboon, W., Serra, D.O., Possling, A., Hadjineophytou, C., Hengge, R. and Cegelski, L. (2018) Phosphoethanolamine cellulose: a naturally produced chemically modified cellulose. *Science* 359, 334–338. doi: 10.1126/science.aao4096

Tiwari, U.P., Chen, H., Kim, S.W. and Jha, R. (2018) Supplemental effect of xylanase and mannanase on nutrient digestibility and gut health of nursery pigs studied using both *in vivo* and *in vitro* models. *Animal Feed Science and Technology* 245, 77–90. doi: 10.1016/j.anifeedsci.2018.07.002

Torres-Pitarch, A., Manzanillaac, E.G., Gardiner, G.E., O'Doherty, J.V. and Lawlor, P.G. (2019) Systematic review and meta-analysis of the effect of feed enzymes on growth and nutrient digestibility in grow-finisher pigs: effect of enzyme type and cereal source. *Animal Feed Science and Technology* 251, 153–165. doi: 10.1016/j.anifeedsci.2018.12.007

Tsai, T., Dove, C.C., Cline, P.M., Owusu-Asiedu, A., Walsh, M.C. and Azain, M. (2017) The effect of adding xylanase or β-glucanase to diets with corn distillers dried grains with solubles (CDDGS) on growth performance and nutrient digestibility in nursery pigs. *Livestock Science* 197, 46–52.

United Nations (2019) World Population Prospects 2019. United Nations, Department of Economic and Social Affairs, Population Division, New York. Available at: http://population.un.org/wpp/ (accessed 4 May 2020).

USDA (2020) *Grain: World Markets and Trade*. US Department of Agriculture, Foreign Agricultural Service, Washington, DC.

Usui, N., Ray, C., Drongowski, R., Coran, A. and Harmon, C. (1999) The effect of phospholipids and mucin on bacterial internalization in an enterocyte-cell culture model. *Pediatric Surgery International* 15, 150–154. doi: 10.1007/s003830050543

Vila, M.F., Trudeau, M.P., Hung, Y.-T., Zeng, Z., Urriola, P.E., *et al.* (2018) Dietary fiber sources and non-starch polysaccharide-degrading enzymes modify mucin expression and the immune profile of the swine ileum. *PLoS ONE* 13, e0207196. doi: 10.1371/journal.pone.0207196

Wang, W., Archbold, T., Kimber, M.S., Li, J., Lam, J.S. and Fan, M.Z. (2012) The porcine gut microbial metagenomic library for mining novel cellulases established from growing pigs fed cellulose-supplemented high-fat diets. *Journal of Animal Science* 90, 400–402. doi: 10.2527/jas.53942

Yin, Y.L., Baidoo, S.K., Schulze, H. and Simmins, P.H. (2001) Effects of supplementing diets containing hulless barley varieties having different levels of non-starch polysaccharides with β-glucanase and xylanase on the physiological status of the gastrointestinal tract and nutrient digestibility of weaned pigs. *Livestock Production Science* 71, 97–107.

Zeng, Z.K., Trudeau, M., Li, Q.Y., Wang, D.J., Jang, C., *et al.* (2018) Effects of exogenous proteinases and carbohydrases on growth performance in pigs fed diets with corn distillers dried grains with solubles: a meta-analysis. *Journal of Animal Science* 97(Suppl. 3), 307–308.

Zhang, X. and Zhang, Y.P. (2013) Cellulases: characteristics, sources, production, and applications. In: Yang, S., El-Enshasy, H.A. and Thongchul, N. (eds) *Bioprocessing Technologies in Biorefinery for Sustainable Production of Fuels, Chemicals, and Polymers*. Wiley, Hoboken, New Jersey, pp. 131–146. doi: 10.1002/9781118642047.ch8

Zhang, Y.J., Liu, Q., Zhang, W.M., Zhang, Z.J., Wang, W.L. and Zhuang, S. (2017) Gastrointestinal microbial diversity and short-chain fatty acid production in pigs fed different fibrous diets with or without cell wall-degrading enzyme supplementation. *Livestock Science* 207, 105–116. doi: 10.1016/j.livsci.2017.11.017

Zhang, Z., Tun, H.M., Li, R., Gonzalez, B.J., Keenes, H.C., *et al.* (2018) Impact of xylanases on gut microbiota of growing pigs fed corn- or wheat-based diets. *Animal Nutrition* 4, 339–350. doi: 10.1016/j.aninu.2018.06.007

Zijlstra, R.T., Li, S., Owusu-Asiedu, A., Simmins, P.H. and Patience, J.F. (2004) Effect of carbohydrase supplementation of wheat- and canola-meal-based diets on growth performance and nutrient digestibility in group-housed weaned pigs. *Canadian Journal of Animal Science* 84, 689–695.

4 Xylanases, β-Glucanases and Cellulases: Their Relevance in Poultry Nutrition

Michael R. Bedford*

AB Vista, Marlborough, UK

4.1 Introduction: A Brief History of Enzyme Use in Monogastric Feeds

Until recently, fibre, in the form of non-starch polysaccharides (NSPs) and oligosaccharides, has been viewed by monogastric nutritionists as a diluent at best and by many as an antinutrient, the content of which should be limited. High-fibre ingredients are subject to maximum inclusion rates as a consequence. However, the work that started investigating the effect of fibre-degrading enzymes on the performance of poultry initially, and erroneously, targeted starch. In the 1950s, a considerable amount of work was devoted to determining why barley had such a low energy content when its proximate analysis suggested that maize, barley and dehulled barley should be of similar feeding value (Fry *et al.*, 1958). The nitrogen-free extract of both barley and maize were determined to be relatively similar and as a result the differences noted in their nutritional value were assumed to be due to differences in digestibility of the carbohydrate portion. Fine grinding compared with coarse made no difference, suggesting differential access to endosperm contents was not an explanation for this observation, and neither did adding

oat hulls to the maize diet to equilibrate the crude fibre content with the barley diet (Fry *et al.*, 1958). However, addition of tallow to the barley diet did equilibrate performance with the maize diet, suggesting energy availability, and specifically that from the carbohydrate fraction, was indeed the problem (Fry *et al.*, 1958). It should be noted at this point that all diets contained an antibiotic, the relevance of which will be made clear in the next section. Work continued and water-soaking pearled barley prior to feeding was shown to markedly improve bird performance compared with unsoaked material to the point that it was equivalent to maize (Fry *et al.*, 1957). The supposition was that soaking either activated amylolytic enzymes in barley which then pre-digested those carbohydrates that were not well digested by the chick, or it removed an inhibitor. The focus on amylase spurred on investigations employing amylase-rich enzyme sources in barley-based rations and resulted in a marked improvement in performance, suggesting that soaking was indeed activating endogenous starch-degrading enzymes (Jensen, 1957). Later, investigations demonstrated that the focus on amylases was ill-founded since the use of pure, exogenous amylases gave no benefits whereas crude

*Email: mike.bedford@abvista.com

©CAB International 2022. *Enzymes in Farm Animal Nutrition, 3rd Edition* (M. Bedford *et al.* eds)
DOI: 10.1079/9781789241563.0004

preparations did (Willingham *et al.*, 1959). Contaminant activities in the crude amylases were implicated but it was not until 1966 that a comprehensive investigation conclusively proved the target was a soluble, viscous, high-molecular-weight β-glucan and the enzyme of interest was an endo-β-1,3(4)-glucanase (Burnett, 1966). This historical account is of great relevance even today because errors are consistently and currently made in assigning a measured response to a suggested activity with little proof that the response could not equally well be attributed to 'ancillary' and undetermined activities in *any* enzyme product. As a consequence, the pace of development in non-starch polysaccharidases (NSPases) in the 50 years following the seminal work of Burnett (1966) has been hampered by poor experimental design and data interpretation as a result of the incomplete description of most of the NSPase products used in the experiments reported since 1966.

Cellulases, or more precisely β-1,3(4)-glucanases, derived from the brewing industry were first employed commercially in poultry and pig rations in Finland in 1984 to improve the digestibility of barley-based rations (A. Haarisilta, Suomen Rehu, 2000, personal communication). In addition to significantly improved animal performance as was noted in the work in the 1950s, the most obvious commercial benefit was a significant reduction in wet litter (Moran and McGinnis, 1966) and subsequent carcass downgrades and disease. Wet and sticky litter was a hallmark of high inclusion rates in poultry diets of barley, rye and many varieties of wheat (Bedford and Schulze, 1998) as a result of their high extract viscosity, which will be discussed later. The expansion of the commercial feed enzyme business based on β-glucanases targeting barley-based rations was slow due to the relatively small scale of the market. The most obvious commercial target was wheat due to its much greater scale of use and because at the time, in the late 1980s and 1990s, the majority of North European, Canadian and Australian feed wheats were relatively viscous. Thus, with the advent of commercial xylanases in the late 1980s the industry began to expand not just through Northern Europe but throughout the world where wheat could be used in poultry diets in relatively large quantities. Again, the evident reduction in sticky droppings and wet litter accelerated the acceptance of these enzymes in wheat-based diets as it provided an immediate and visual proof of value.

The expansion of NSPases into maize-based diets was a much slower process as there were no visual cues of enzyme efficacy (i.e. with maize the viscosity was much lower, and the litter was already dry in comparison) and the relative improvements in performance were limited and thus deemed less economical. However, with the abolition of antibiotic growth promoters the relative benefit of such enzymes increased (Rosen, 2001) and with the move to more complex (e.g. distillers' dried grains with solubles, wheat middlings, bran, etc.) all-vegetable diets in the traditional maize–soy markets such as the USA, the acceptance of such NSPases also increased. As a result, the uptake of NSPase in maize-based diets increased to the point where, in 2020, most poultry rations contain at least one NSPase.

4.2 Non-Starch Polysaccharide-Degrading Enzymes (NSPases): Factors Affecting the Interpretation of the Literature

4.2.1 Nomenclature and identity

For the purposes of this chapter the focus is on endo-β-1,4-xylanases, β-1,3(4)-glucanases and cellulases, as the remaining main classes (such as mannanases, pectinases, etc.) are dealt with in other chapters. Regardless of the subject, scientific research only has value if it can be repeated, and this relies on precise description of the materials and methods employed. Unfortunately, much of the literature on NSPases fails in this regard even on the most basic of issues, namely the identification and assay of the enzyme used. Nomenclature was first identified as a significant problem in 2002, when it was noted in a comprehensive survey of the literature addressing the topic of 'feed enzymes' that there were 252 generic descriptors of the enzymes used (Rosen, 2002). Within these descriptors were 135 methods of naming single enzyme sources, the remaining 117 being enzymes with between two and 11 components, with most of these activities simply stated but not measured. Very few of these descriptions bore any relationship with the accepted recommendations on enzyme nomenclature at the time. As a result, this makes interpretation of the literature difficult. An example of the problem is given by the many ways of describing the same activity. Xylanase (Barrier-Guillot *et al.*, 1995), pentosanase (Bedford *et al.*, 1991), glycanase (Ravindran *et al.*, 1999), arabinoxylanase (Grootwassink *et al.*, 1989) and hemicellulase (Tahir *et al.*, 2005) have all been used to describe the same enzyme class, which can lead to confusion. The ideal would be a description which leaves no doubt as to the identity of the enzyme since there are enzymological differences between xylanases from different sources that could have a bearing on their utility *in vivo*. For example, identifying an enzyme as being the pI 9 xylanase from *Trichoderma reesei* is precise and far more valuable for interpretation and comparison of trials involving this enzyme than simply stating it is a pentosanase. With the more modern products having undergone genetic modification to improve their suitability for their role (e.g. increased thermostability), it is important to be precise and ideally identify the enzyme on the basis of its new amino acid sequence or declaring where the changes have been made in the wild-type sequence. Virtually all of the literature fails to provide product identity to this degree of precision, and often the description of the product refers to the production organism as much as it does to the source of the enzyme, which is almost irrelevant in describing the enzyme from a functionality viewpoint. As becomes evident from the above, description of a product as a xylanase or glucanase is not the same as describing a product as a vitamin or amino acid. For the latter, the descriptor allows precise identification and comparison with all other work on the same nutrient. For enzymes, the descriptions given merely identify the product as having some activity on an often undefined substrate under conditions irrelevant to the

application in practice. Thus, any conclusions from a review of the NSPase literature have to take account of the uncertainty surrounding the identity of the products used.

4.2.2 Assay

Even if description of the enzyme was complete in all papers, the data are only of value when the amount used is described. This is obvious when considering nutrients such as amino acids or mineral levels which are easily determined, and the amount determined can be directly linked to the function in the animal. The issue with NSPases is that there is no standardized method of analysis even though such an assay was proposed back in the 1990s (Bailey *et al.*, 1992). Methods used vary in temperature, pH, substrate used and the metric of the assay (e.g. colour release from a dyed substrate, viscosity reduction and reducing sugar release). As a result, it is difficult to gauge the amount of enzyme used when comparing two studies where different assays are employed. Even today there are studies describing an assay which cannot be repeated without proprietary standards or substrates being made available, making the units presented meaningless (Cozannet *et al.*, 2017; Chen *et al.*, 2020). A further problem is that the conditions of all *in vitro* assays do not mimic the conditions under which they function. This problem is not unique to NSPases and is in fact a universal problem for all feed enzymes. As a result, the units derived from the assay may have little relationship with the effects in the animal due to differences in pH and ionic strength between these two environments (Bedford and Schulze, 1998), for example, coupled with the lack of information derived from the assay with regard to the proteolytic resilience of the xylanase against endogenous and exogenous proteases (Saleh *et al.*, 2004).

4.2.3 Purity

Modern enzyme production platforms have advanced considerably in the past 20 years and as a result the products available are more specific towards the task at hand, more durable and produced at lower costs. Enzymes that are most fit for purpose are cloned from donor organisms, often improved through evolution techniques and then expressed in a host organism that makes production of the enzyme economic (for details see Vehmaanperä, Chapter 2, this volume, 2022). If produced in a host that has been modified such that it produces only the target activity in quantity, then it is often marketed as a 'monocomponent' enzyme. Nevertheless, even monocomponent enzymes sometimes have contaminating activities that are derived from the production host, with this degree of contamination varying from host to host. At the other end of the scale, some products are produced in hosts that produce a considerable array of their own NSPase enzymes (which may or may not be augmented by a heterologous gene product). They are deliberately marketed in a way to claim the benefits of the side activities of interest and are called 'multi-enzymes' (Sharifi et al., 2014; Cozannet et al., 2018). The challenge with such products is that the activities present can vary from production batch to batch such that the ratios between xylanase and glucanase, for example, can change. The more activities produced, the greater the range in product activity variance. Consistency in response to such products is therefore questionable. Some products are the result of a deliberate blend of two or more monocomponent enzymes to achieve a desired minimum content of the targeted activities in the finished product. Such multicomponent enzymes should be more consistent than their multi-enzyme counterparts from batch to batch. Regardless, such a situation means that even when a product is correctly identified and assayed:

1. There are likely activities other than those declared/assayed which may play a role in the response.
2. The animal response to many of these products should be expected to vary as a result of a shift in key activities between batches of product.

Thus, in summary of this section, it should be recognized that much of the literature is compromised and interpretation made difficult due to poor description of the exact identity of the enzyme used, poor assay description and hence quantification, and lack of information on 'contaminating' activities which may have been responsible for some if not all of the response (positive or negative). As a result, the assignment of a response to a given amount of a given enzyme from almost any paper is open to challenge. An analogy would be feeding fishmeal of unknown origin or composition in an amino-acid-deficient diet and assigning all the benefits to the lysine content of the ingredient. Without full analysis of the diet and the ingredient coupled with knowledge of the requirements of the animal, such a conclusion simply cannot be drawn.

4.3   Mode of Action of NSPases

For many years there have been three modes of action put forward to describe how/why these enzymes work *in vivo*. These relate to the fact that the animal does not produce NSPases but the substrates that the enzymes attack can increase intestinal viscosity, shield endosperm contents from digestion and provide nutrients for stimulation of beneficial bacteria (Bedford and Morgan, 1996; Bedford, 2000a). Two of the mechanisms involve degrading an 'antinutrient' and the third involves provision of a nutrient or prebiotic. There has been little advancement in the understanding of the relevance or dominance of each of these mechanisms since the 1990s, which in many respects reflects the heterogeneity of the products employed and contributes in part to the variance in the responses noted in the literature (Rosen, 2002). Given the caveats noted above, it is worth revisiting these mechanisms with a more challenging approach to determine if there is significant proof that any are dominant or even relevant.

4.3.1   Nutrient encapsulation

Even in finely milled and pelleted feed, a large proportion of the cereal endosperm contents is fully encapsulated in an intact cell wall comprised of NSPs. Typical commercial feed may have a mean particle size of 600–900 µm, which is seen as the optimum for maize- and sorghum-based diets (Amerah *et al.*, 2007), and given the average endosperm cell is only 50–70 µm in diameter, it follows that a large proportion of the cereal endosperm is hidden in the core of each particle, totally intact. Various microscopic explorations have repeatedly shown this to be the case. These cell walls are not digested by the birds' endogenous enzymes, and the gizzard is not capable of breaking open 100% of intact cells as is evidenced by the presence of intact cells within the small intestine (Bedford and Autio, 1996; Parkkonen *et al.*, 1997). It was therefore suggested that more complete penetration of endosperm cells could be effected by supplementation of the diet with NSPases, which should facilitate the destruction of the cell wall matrix thus enabling more efficient ingress of digestive enzymes and hence improving digestibility of the diet. Microscopic evaluation of intestinal contents confirmed that the use of NSPases reduced the number of intact cell walls noted in the jejunum and ileum (Bedford and Autio, 1996). Subsequent *in vitro* work has shown reduction in cell wall integrity when sections of wheat were incubated with a xylanase, for example (Le *et al.*, 2013; Ravn *et al.*, 2017), and the release of starch and protein from ground cereal samples undergoing simulated gastrointestinal digestion processes is increased in the presence of the exogenous NSPase. Thus, the removal of nutrient encapsulation effects of the cell walls seems to be a very plausible and defensible hypothesis.

If this mechanism is indeed dominant, then it has profound implications for the selection of suitable enzymes. The cell walls of cereals are complex and involve many polymeric structures that are linked together by sugar, ester and phenolic bridges to form the composite cell wall (Bach Knudsen, 2014, 2016, 2018). Perforation of such a complex entity clearly would employ many activities, each targeting the main constituents responsible for structural integrity. Multiple enzymes would be required to ensure significant dissolution of the xylan

structures, and similarly multiple enzymes would be needed to degrade the β-glucan, cellulose and other components of the cell wall. A somewhat laminated structure, whereby the xylan 'coats' the β-glucan component in barley endosperm cell walls, indicates that complete dissolution needs both enzyme classes to be present in sufficient quantity so as to effect this destruction in a timely manner (Langenaeken *et al.*, 2020). Delivery of such a complex mixture of enzymes is not without challenges given that each of the activities has its own idiosyncrasy with regard to optimum pH, temperature, stability to feed manufacture and endogenous proteases and pH shifts, and ability to function in the varying ionic strengths of the gastrointestinal tract. However, if cell wall destruction is the key mechanism by which NSPases function, then complex mixtures providing activities that approximate the cell wall composition of the total diet should outperform all other products. Given this was the case, then all new product development should and would have focused on the evolution and production of all the key activities needed so the enzymes survive all the challenges of feed manufacture and passage through the intestinal tract. However, this has not happened, and deeper scrutiny of the data and interpretation of the results from papers supporting the nutrient encapsulation hypothesis suggest there may be significant flaws in this proposal. The problems relate to both the *in vivo* and *in vitro* data and are listed below.

4.3.1.1 In vivo *data*

Microscopic analysis of the small intestinal contents where it is clear that NSPase supplementation of the diet has increased the extent of cell wall disruption is by far the most convincing data in support of this theory. However, two points are worth noting:

1. Some of the most convincing work reported the effects of a very pure xylanase on wheat cell wall destruction *in vivo* in broilers as early as the crop and gizzard in particular (Bedford and Autio, 1996). However, the time and pH constraints of the digestive tract are such that the added enzyme had no chance to disrupt the cell walls to the extent noted *in vivo* given the dosage fed to the birds. As will be noted below, the scale of *in vivo* cell wall destruction reported cannot be replicated even in an optimized *in vitro* environment with the enzyme levels and activities used in the field.

2. The enzyme used was a fairly pure pI 9 xylanase from *T. reesei* with no appreciable side activities (Bedford and Autio, 1996), which challenges the concept that cell wall destruction requires a combination of enzyme activities.

4.3.1.2   In vitro *data*

1. Most of the *in vitro* protocols use incubation processes that do not replicate the gastrointestinal tract from a viewpoint of residence time, pH or protease presence (Li *et al.*, 2004). *In vitro* simulations where pepsin and pancreatin were employed noted almost all endosperm protein had disappeared by the time the material had finished the pepsin step, and all starch was gone at the end of the small intestinal step (Parkkonen *et al.*, 1997). Further doubt was cast on the suggested 'barrier effect' of the endosperm cell wall to digestive enzymes since it was noted there was no additional release of their contents *in vitro* (Tervila-Wilo *et al.*, 1996) when cell-wall-degrading enzymes were added. These results suggest that the cereal grain cell walls do not prevent access to their contents by endogenous digestive enzymes that is proposed in this mechanism, at least as far as the endosperm is concerned.

2. *In vitro* incubations of the target cereal with NSPases rarely if ever show the same degree of cell wall puncture that is noted *in vivo* (Tervila-Wilo *et al.*, 1996; Le *et al.*, 2013; Ravn *et al.*, 2017) when a commercially relevant dose of enzyme is used. Cell wall degradation is shown to take place, but the effects noted are very limited (Morgan *et al.*, 1995), and in some cases even when tenfold the commercial dose was employed, only marginal degradation of the cell walls was noted after 3 h of incubation (Ravn *et al.*, 2017). A telling observation was that after simulated crop, gizzard and 60 min simulated

small intestinal digestion, the addition of the equivalent to four times the commercial dose of xylanase resulted in no effect on wheat microstructure (Parkkonen *et al.*, 1997). This was the same enzyme used *in vivo* where significant cell wall destruction was noted as early as the gizzard (Bedford and Autio, 1996). One recent paper used 200 to 20,000 times the commercial dose of an enzyme and noted some marginal additional benefit in dissolution of cell wall material when extra xylanase and arabinofuranosidase activity was present, but these effects were markedly reduced when the assay was undertaken during simulated gastric and intestinal digestion (Vangsøe *et al.*, 2020).

3. Related to point 1 above, for this mechanism to be relevant, cell wall dissolution needs to take place very early on in the digestive tract so that assimilation of the contents can be realized by the bird. Hence any simulation that cannot show significant effects by the stage of the gizzard or very early on in the small intestinal simulation is not particularly supportive of this mechanism.

4.3.1.3   *Resolution of* in vitro *with* in vivo *data*

The degree of hydrolysis of cell walls can also be approximated by measurement of the digestibility of constituent NSPs. Presumably the greater the 'digestibility' of the water-unextracted arabinoxylan (WU-AX), then the greater the degree of hydrolysis of the cell walls. Even in the absence of an exogenous NSPase, the digestibility of WU-AX increases with age as a result of what is presumed to be an increasingly competent microbiome (Bautil *et al.*, 2019). At 35 days of age as much as 25% of the WU-AX had been 'digested' (Bautil *et al.*, 2019). The application of xylanases has been shown to increase digestibility of the WU-AX in wheat-based diets in a dose-dependent manner (Bautil, 2020). However, the effect of the enzyme decreased substantially with age to the extent that at 36 days of age the digestibility of WU-AX in birds fed the commercial dose of the enzyme was no different to the control (Bautil, 2020). The interaction of efficacy with age is interesting as it suggests the 'cell wall' effects decline with age and indeed is not a relevant mechanism in older animals.

Regardless, it is clear that addition of NSPases increases the proportion of disrupted cells noted in small intestinal and even gizzard digesta (Bedford and Autio, 1996). In both pigs and poultry, the vast majority of intact cells from wheat were from the aleurone layer followed by the embryo root, embryo leaf and scutellum. Intact endosperm cells represented less than 2% of total intact wheat cells (Torrallardona et al., 2000). In the case of the work with pigs, when either of two xylanases were added to these diets, the number of intact cells fell to approximately 60% that of the control, suggesting the enzymes were clearly aiding in the destruction of some, but by no means all, of the intact cells, and indeed it appeared the preferential targets were of aleurone origin. The likelihood that exogenous NSPases focus most of their attention on the aleurone layer in particular is also suggested by the particularly low arabinose to xylose (A:X) ratio of this tissue in wheat (Vangsøe et al., 2019). Most endoxylanases, particularly family 11 endoxylanases, attack unsubstituted stretches of xylan in the arabinoxylan molecule, which would suggest that tissues with particularly low A:X ratios such as the aleurone layer would be most susceptible. This is tempered by the fact that these cell walls are also mostly insoluble and are more heavily esterified than starchy endosperm arabinoxylan (Bach Knudsen, 2014; Vangsøe et al., 2019). Nevertheless, several pieces of research have shown that xylanase treatment of wheat, for example, can result in significant release of soluble arabinoxylans, and indeed arabinoxylo-oligosaccharides (AXOS), and that by far the majority of this is derived from the aleurone layer (Vangsøe et al., 2019) not the endosperm which tends to have a higher A:X ratio. Thus, the cell wall mechanism is likely not relevant for the starchy endosperm.

4.3.1.4   Comparison of effects in maize versus wheat

Much of the work purporting to support the nutrient encapsulation mode of action has been conducted on wheat-based diets which are known to be far more susceptible to xylanase action than maize. The extension of wheat-derived data to maize-based diets, whether flawed in design or not, is not justified however due to the much greater intransigence of maize NSPs to hydrolysis compared with wheat (Dale et al., 2020). Indeed, in vivo microscopy of intestinal contents in the presence and absence of xylanase showed no additional cell wall disruption as a result of enzyme addition although it was noted that glucose transporter gene expression was increased after 3 weeks of feeding of the enzyme (Lee et al., 2017), suggesting that enzyme addition had augmented starch digestion by some other mechanism.

4.3.1.5   Consequences for enzyme development

In conclusion for this section, it appears that the evidence supporting the cell wall mechanism is far from conclusive and in fact is open to considerable doubt by the challenges laid out above. If these challenges are justified and the cell wall mechanism is not relevant, then this has significant implications for the development of 'next-generation' NSPases. Adherence to this particular mechanism would evolve significantly more complex enzyme candidates to enable optimization of this process and probably yield products which are significantly less effective in dealing with the two remaining mechanisms to be considered. Indeed, some authors suggest feed enzymes should also consider the protein meal components of the diet (De Keyser et al., 2018), which adds even further levels of complexity and divergence from products that can address the remaining mechanisms. Ironically, much of the work that supports complex enzymes for the cell wall mechanism rarely if ever compares the complex enzyme with the individual components (Masey O'Neill et al., 2014; Menezes-Blackburn and Greiner, 2015; De Keyser et al., 2018), reinforcing the point that the case is yet to be made for this mechanism.

4.3.2 Viscosity

Viscosity was probably the first mechanism to gain much traction as a result of Burnett's (1966) work with barley, but it was several years later before studies identified that this was also the case in other cereal grains, particularly rye (Grootwassink et al., 1989). A proportion of the fibre making up the cell walls of the endosperm is soluble; some of this soluble material is of high molecular weight and has the capacity to create viscous solutions if concentrations are high enough. Correlated with intestinal viscosity is the presence of sticky droppings and wet litter, a phenomenon which was often the case with the wheat varieties used in Northern Europe in the early 1990s. The proportion and type of fibre that is both soluble and of high molecular weight and therefore viscous varies between and within cereals. Generally, rye is the most viscous, followed by barley, triticale, oats and wheat, with the least viscous being maize then sorghum (Bedford, 1996). The majority of the viscous fibre is arabinoxylan in rye, triticale, wheat, maize and sorghum, with the mixed-linked β-glucans being responsible in barley and oats (Bedford, 1996), and most of the viscous fibre is derived from the endosperm cell walls (Ward and Marquardt, 1987). As noted above, however, there is a great deal of variation even within a cereal species and in some cases, there may be some samples of wheat or barley that are more viscous than some samples of rye. Regardless of the source of the viscous fibre, the impact it has on the rate of digestion is proportional to the viscosity created in the digestive tract. The tenet of the mechanism is that the more viscous a solution, the poorer the efficiency of mixing and the slower the rate of diffusion of solutes. Hence digestion is compromised as it depends upon vigorous mixing of the contents and rapid, random movement of enzymes and their soluble products. Many studies have shown correlations between measured intestinal viscosity and digestibility of nutrients and performance of the broiler and layer (Smulikowska, 1998; Danicke et al., 2000b; Langhout et al., 2000; Alzueta et al., 2003). This is especially true for saturated

fats, which are particularly dependent upon the vigorous mixing of emulsifiers, fat droplets, bile acids and lipase for efficient micelle formation and subsequent digestion. This process is disproportionately compromised when the aqueous phase of the digesta is viscous (Pasquier et al., 1996). Consequently, diets containing high concentrations of longer chain length, saturated fats are far more susceptible to viscosity than those containing low levels of fat or unsaturated fats (Ward and Marquardt, 1983). Moreover, significant energy is then expended on activities such as pancreatic enzyme synthesis (Silva et al., 1997) and release, intestinal growth (Wu et al., 2004) and turnover of cells (Silva and Smithard, 1996)/proteins (Danicke et al., 2000a) in an attempt to maximize nutrient extraction under such circumstances that the conversion of digestible to net energy is compromised, although such responses are not universally noted (Wu and Ravindran, 2004). Since the viscosity of the digesta is exponentially related to the concentration of the higher-molecular-weight solutes, only a few, strategically central 'cuts' in the polymer by the relevant endo-acting enzyme are required to radically reduce molecular weight and thus viscosity. This mechanism has been shown to be relevant in in vitro digestion models as well (Bedford and Classen, 1993; Murphy et al., 2010) and thus was seen as being the primary mechanism of action of NSPases when used in diets containing the more viscous cereals.

The viscosity mechanism has stood the test of time and has even been suggested to be relevant in low-viscosity maize-based diets when supplemental fat levels are moderate to high (Coelho and Troescher, 2018; Troesher and Coelho, 2018). However, several papers have failed to establish clear-cut relationships between enzyme use, viscosity and performance (Geraert et al., 2001; McCracken et al., 2001; Amerah et al., 2008; Lamp et al., 2015). Some enzymes have been shown to have no effect (Bautil, 2020) or even increase intestinal viscosity but at the same time improve performance of the bird, which clearly challenges the universality of this hypothesis. Several interacting factors have been identified that may explain such anomalies and include:

1. Health status. Viscosity has been shown to be much lower in cocci-infected broilers (Waldenstedt *et al.*, 2000) and hence this may mute any enzyme-derived reduction in viscosity and limit the scope for a response in growth rate or efficiency driven by viscosity reduction per se. However, it is generally accepted that stressed birds or poor-performing birds tend to respond more to the addition of an enzyme; perhaps if this is so in the case of cocci-infected chicks, then it is not through the viscosity mechanism.

2. Linked to the above, the relevance of viscosity is far less evident in germ-free compared with conventional chickens (Langhout *et al.*, 2000). Many potential explanations for this phenomenon have been discussed elsewhere but they all relate to the fact that the microbiome's ability to extract dietary nutrients is proportional to the viscosity of the digesta (as this delays the host's digestion, providing more for the resident microbiome) (Bedford, 2000b; Bedford and Fothergill, 2002; Bedford and Cowieson, 2012). Indeed, the effects of viscous diets when fed to germ-free birds are negligible compared with the effects in their conventional counterparts (Smits and Annison, 1996; Langhout *et al.*, 2000), which suggests the delay in nutrient digestion per se can be overcome if there is no resident microbiome to take advantage of the slow digestion rate. Conversely, a viscous diet exposes the bird to disease outbreaks by providing a more conducive environment for pathogens to invade (Jia *et al.*, 2009). Overlaid on this is the observation that some species of bacteria are able to produce bile-salt-degrading enzymes (Feighner and Dashkevicz, 1988), especially under viscous conditions, thus markedly reducing the digestibility of fat compared with other nutrients (Maisonnier *et al.*, 2003) and disproportionately exacerbating the negative effect of viscosity if such species are present. As a consequence, the impact of viscosity on performance is greater under more challenging conditions.

3. The gastric environment can have a profound influence on the subsequent viscosity in the small intestine. *In vitro* work has shown that a lower pH in the gastric phase of a two-phase digestion process results in a disproportionately higher viscosity of the aqueous phase in the small intestinal stage of digestion (Murphy *et al.*, 2010). Many dietary factors can influence both the pH and residence time in the gizzard and thus subsequent intestinal viscosity. Such factors include structural (Sacranie *et al.*, 2012, 2017) and fermentable fibre (Singh *et al.*, 2012), fat (Mateos and Sell, 1980; Mateos *et al.*, 1982; Smulikowska, 1998) and dietary calcium, or more importantly limestone levels (Walk *et al.*, 2012).

4. Age. Several papers suggest that viscosity increases with age to a maximum at approximately 3 weeks of age, followed by a decline thereafter (Petersen *et al.*, 1999; Fischer, 2003; Bautil *et al.*, 2019). This is assumed to be due to the ileal microbiome producing xylanases in sufficient quantity to release soluble, viscous arabinoxylans from the insoluble arabinoxylan matrix of the cell walls (Bautil *et al.*, 2019). This capacity increases with age of the broiler and development of the microbiome, and at a critical point, achieved at approximately 3 weeks of age, the enzymatic array produced is of sufficient capacity to break down the viscous arabinoxylans faster than they are released and hence viscosity drops. Thus, the impact of a viscosity-reducing enzyme on the digestion of nutrients, particularly fat, increases and then reduces with age (Smulikowska, 1998). There also seems to be an effect of fat type on viscosity, with the more saturated fats apparently delaying transit and holding digesta in the gastric environment longer. This enables dissolution of more insoluble fibres into viscous, soluble fibres (Smulikowska, 1998), as discussed in point 3 above, thus further increasing viscosity.

There are many other factors involved in moderating the viscosity of the intestinal tract or mitigating its effects such that there will never be a universal and consistent relationship between an absolute viscosity value and the performance depression noted. For example, thermal processing of a diet (pelleting or extrusion) is known to elevate intestinal viscosity proportionally with the temperature of the process (Silversides and Bedford, 1999; Svihus *et al.*, 2000; Creswell and Bedford, 2005; Coelho and Troescher,

2018) in wheat-, rye- and maize-based diets due to destruction of endogenous NSPase activity and disruption of the insoluble matrix which facilitates dissolution of greater quantities of viscous fibres. The effects of thermal processing of barley on subsequent intestinal viscosity seem to be significantly muted, however, indicating a differential response to pelleting dependent upon the cereal employed (Svihus *et al.*, 2000; Lamp *et al.*, 2015). Regardless, it does appear that for conventionally reared chickens, development of a viscous digesta is clearly associated with depressed performance and its reduction by use of the relevant NSPase most often is coincident with improved performance. As a result, the viscosity mechanism is still relevant today. If this were the only relevant mechanism, then the evolution of enzymes to better address this issue could be quite different from that of the nutrient encapsulation mechanism.

4.3.2.1   Consequences for enzyme development

For optimal viscosity reduction, the enzyme should clearly be able to reduce the molecular weight of the offending fractions as quickly as possible. Thus, enzymes which are endo-acting on the backbone of the polymer and able to tolerate a reasonable degree of steric interference from any substitutions along the backbone are clearly favoured. An argument is made that most xylanases will stall at some point on substituted regions of the backbone and hence removal of the side chains will facilitate more rapid depolymerization. As a result, the utility of accessory enzyme activities such as arabinofuranosidase and feruloyl esterase in the depolymerization of arabinoxylans is often discussed. While *in vitro* and *in vivo* evidence has been presented (Lei *et al.*, 2016; Cozannet *et al.*, 2017) in support of such a hypothesis, both fail to specifically address the synergy question due to lack of in-feed analysis of all relevant components, or lack of a true factorial nature of the treatments, or both, as discussed in detail earlier (Masey O'Neill *et al.*, 2014; Menezes-Blackburn and Greiner, 2015). In brief, no paper to date has categorically

shown that the 'accessory' enzymes are pure and do not contribute other activities – such as endoxylanase – as well; and critically, the dose chosen for the endoxylanase alone is not proven to be optimal in the absence of the accessory enzymes. As a result, the response to the accessory enzymes may be due in part to contaminating activities. In-feed analysis of all enzyme components in all diets is critically missing in all cases and thus leaves the question regarding the identity of the next-generation enzyme(s) for viscosity reduction *in vivo* unanswered to date.

4.3.3   Prebiotic effects

The third mechanism ascribed to NSPases and the least discussed is the prebiotic mechanism. Prebiotics were first defined by Gibson and Roberfroid (1995) thus: 'A prebiotic is a nondigestible food ingredient that beneficially affects the host by selectively stimulating the growth and/or activity of one or a limited number of bacteria in the colon, and thus improves host health'. The concept was, and still is, that the prebiotics generated are quantitatively fermented to volatile fatty acids (VFAs) which exert their benefits directly. Such VFAs can be produced directly from fermentation of the oligosaccharide or via further metabolism (cross-feeding) of the initial products of oligosaccharide metabolism (Moreno *et al.*, 2017).

The early barley, rye and then wheat work was very much focused on the viscosity and to a lesser extent the nutrient encapsulation mechanism, and since these seemed to explain the experimental observations made in the trials to the satisfaction of the authors, the prebiotic mechanism was not raised or considered as a serious contender. Indeed, the first reference to this mechanism came quite late in feed enzyme research (Morgan *et al.*, 1995) and even then, it was not presented as a serious contender. This is despite the fact that there was significant prebiotic research focusing on human health in the 1990s (Steer *et al.*, 2000) which largely focused on the beneficial effects of the fructo-oligosaccharides (FOS) derived from inulin (Simmering and Blaut, 2001). In poultry the focus also started with FOS as they were shown to be able to stimulate the growth of bacterial species that competed with *Salmonella* (Oyarzabal and Conner, 1995) without providing sustenance to the *Salmonella* themselves (Oyarzabal *et al.*, 1995). The oligosaccharides derived from NSPase hydrolysis of xylans, glucans and mannans have not been widely considered as prebiotics until more recently.

4.3.3.1 Manno-oligosaccharides (MOS)

Manno-oligosaccharides (MOS) derived from plant mannan hydrolysis have been shown to be utilized by beneficial species such as *Bifidobacteria* and *Lactobacilli* and as such their production could be considered a pre-biotic mechanism for this enzyme (Shastak *et al.*, 2015). A search for literature relating to MOS versus xylo-oligosaccharides (XOS) versus gluco-oligosaccharides (GOS) in poultry diets yields more hits on MOS than on XOS and GOS combined, suggesting this is a well-researched topic. However, the major-ity of the literature on MOS is not relevant for describing the effects of endo-β-1,4-mannanases in poultry diets. This is be-cause the vast majority of such work has in-vestigated the effects of yeast cell-wall-derived mannan fractions and not those from hydro-lysed plant materials. Yeast cell wall man-nans have a completely different backbone structure (α rather than β linkages) and are also polysaccharides rather than oligosac-charides (Torrecillas *et al.*, 2014; Chacher *et al.*, 2017), despite their almost universal description as oligosaccharides in the litera-ture. They are consistently termed as MOS when they are mostly polysaccharides and thus far less capable of being fermented than their β-1,4-oligosaccharide counterparts. This results in the prebiotic literature concerning MOS making confusing and irrelevant com-parisons between the effects of dietary en-domannanases and yeast-derived mannan polysaccharides. There is little doubt that hydrolysed mannans from plant cell wall material will be fermented readily but their contribution to the overall response to added mannanases is relatively poorly researched

and understood. Furthermore, the proposal that mannans derived from some ingredients, such as soybean meal, can act as immune stimulants, thus creating inflammatory re-sponses, further clouds the understanding of the value of the oligosaccharides derived from their hydrolysis to MOS because this will be coincident with the removal of the immunological effect (Shastak *et al.*, 2015). Consequently, the true value of MOS derived from plant fibre is largely unknown.

4.3.3.2 Gluco-oligosaccharides (GOS)

Studies on GOS are limited. Hydrolysis of β-glucans present in hull-less barley-rich diets resulted in the production of GOS and higher-molecular-weight, soluble β-glucans in the ileal digesta of broilers. This did not influ-ence short-chain fatty acid (SCFA) production in the ileum but did elevate them in the caeca, suggesting that fermentation was in the large intestine only (Karunaratne *et al.*, 2021). More-over, the effect of increasing concentrations of β-glucanase was to depress performance in younger birds, suggesting that some degree of maturation of the microbiome is required be-fore advantage can be taken of these prebiotic compounds. In older animals the majority of the soluble β-glucans are fermented before they reach the large intestine, suggesting their utility as a caecal prebiotic may be age-related.

4.3.3.3 Arabinoxylo-oligosaccharides (AXOS) and xylo-oligosaccharides (XOS)

As noted above, the XOS and AXOS gener-ated by endoxylanase activity were not con-sidered as good prebiotic candidates until the late 1990s (Campbell *et al.*, 1997; Vazquez *et al.*, 2000). Nevertheless, in the last 15 years there has been increasing interest in the use of XOS and AXOS either produced and fed as additives or derived from endox-ylanase hydrolysis of dietary xylans and arabinoxylans, respectively (Courtin *et al.*, 2008; Eeckhaut *et al.*, 2008; Bautil *et al.*, 2019, 2020; Dale *et al.*, 2019, 2020). How-ever, recent observations suggest the AXOS and XOS and other oligosaccharides generated by NSPases or added directly to the diet are likely not acting as classic prebiotics but as what are termed 'stimbiotics'. This term is used to describe the effects of a non-digested, fermentable oligosaccharide which is fed at levels that could never quantitatively alter the SCFA levels in the intestine but is present in sufficient quantities to provide a stimulus to resident fibre-degrading species to increase their capacity to digest dietary fibre that otherwise would have been voided. The most striking evidence to support such a concept came from a study in which feeding a 0.5% AXOS product to broilers was shown not only to accelerate ileal but also caecal hydrolysis of the total arabinoxylan present in the diet (Bautil *et al.*, 2020). In other words, the added oligosaccharide was not simply a source of fermentable fuel but was accelerating fermentation of dietary insoluble and soluble arabinoxylans. Previous work had intimated such an effect when the caecal microbiome from xylanase-fed birds was shown to have a radically enhanced ability to digest xylose, XOS and polymeric arabinoxylan in an *ex vivo* test compared with the microbiome harvested from control birds (Bedford and Apajalahti, 2018). In both cases, the increment in fibre digestion achieved vastly exceeds the quantity of oligosaccharide added or generated. Further evidence of such a microbiome developmental effect is provided by the observation that *in ovo* injection of DP4 XOS (but interestingly not DP3 XOS or DP3 and DP4 MOS) resulted in changes in the subsequent adult bird caecal VFA contents (Singh *et al.*, 2019). The fact that only 3 mg of the oligosaccharide was administered and that this was prior to hatch clearly indicates there are some long-term effects these products can have on the microbiome which are not related to their quantitative fermentation into energy-yielding and/or hormonal-stimulating VFAs, and that the structure of the oligosaccharide is critical in explaining its efficacy.

4.3.3.4 Consequences of a prebiotic versus a stimbiotic

Prebiotics alter the structure and metabolism of the microbiome largely by presenting it with all the fuel needed to effect this change, and this change should be noticeable almost immediately upon feeding. Stimbiotics, by their very nature, cannot quantitatively influence the VFA environment directly, but by selecting for and stimulating the activity of bacterial species which can degrade the most difficult substrates (that otherwise would have been voided), they facilitate the capture of a greater proportion of the gross energy from the fibre fraction of the diet. This obviously has performance benefits but coupled with this effect is the suggestion that with the additional VFAs generated, particularly butyrate, there is endocrine feedback via peptide YY and other entero-hormones (Masey O'Neill *et al.*, 2012; Singh *et al.*, 2012) which delays gastric emptying, enabling more extensive peptic digestion and thus facilitating a more complete digestion of the whole diet. This is reflected in the observation that the digestibility of all amino acids is improved by NSPase addition in a manner directly proportional to their presence in the undigested fraction, regardless of whether the diet is maize-, wheat- or rye-based (Cowieson and Bedford, 2009).

4.3.3.5 Benefits of a more complete fibre digestion

In addition to the points made above, the health of the lower intestine is very much dependent upon the balance between fermentable carbohydrate and protein. Carbohydrate is fermented in preference to protein by many species, but if they are not adapted to the particular carbohydrate substrates available then they will switch to protein putrefaction which results in the production of damaging amines, indoles and ammonia (Rinttila and Apajalahti, 2013). As the most rapidly fermentable carbohydrate sources are stripped out of the digesta with passage through the intestinal tract, the caeca and colon are left with the most intransigent and slow-to-ferment substrates (Gibson and Roberfroid, 1995; Bach Knudsen, 2014). These substrates are the arabinoxylans and cellulose, the latter being too intransigent for significant fermentation to take place. Even arabinoxylans vary in their fermentability, with insoluble, lignified and highly substituted xylan backbones being much slower to ferment (Bach Knudsen,

2014, 2016; Bautil *et al.*, 2020) and as a result constituting the bulk of the faeces (Bach Knudsen, 2016). The challenge is therefore to develop and maintain a population of hindgut species that can adequately ferment the available substrates as they evolve with time and thus minimize the likelihood of protein putrefaction.

Since the arabinoxylans also constitute the vast majority of the intransigent but potentially fermentable fibre in typical poultry rations (Bach Knudsen, 2014), this highlights why AXOS and XOS above all other stimbiotics should be most effective in improving overall energy extraction from the fibre fraction of the diet. The exact structure and chain length of these 'signalling' molecules required to optimize this response is still not clear and the focus of significant research streams at present.

4.3.3.6 Consequences for enzyme development

If the above mechanism were to dominate in the majority of poultry diets, then the characteristics of the enzyme required are quite distinct from those required for the nutrient encapsulation method. The goal is the provision of oligosaccharides of a particular chain length and degree of substitution, all of which has yet to be precisely identified, but nevertheless the selected enzyme should produce these end products and avoid overprocessing them to constituent sugars. Consequently, exoacting enzymes should be avoided at all costs, particularly if they reduce the chain length of the oligosaccharide, and even debranching enzymes, such as arabinofuranosidase, may be undesirable if the end goal is the production of AXOS rather than XOS.

4.4 The Future

Increasing global restrictions on antibiotic use in farm animals have prompted a significant upsurge in interest in the role of fibre in controlling intestinal health. Central to this is the recognition that there are beneficial and detrimental types of fibre with regard to how they interact with the nutrition of both the host animal and the microbiome and thus subsequent intestinal health. Of all the feed additives in use today, the NSPases have the most dramatic effect on this aspect of intestinal health, whether it be through reduction of viscosity, reduced nutrient encapsulation or provision of fermentable oligosaccharides. The further development of this enzyme sector requires resolution of which mechanism(s) dominate(s) so that the next generation of enzymes has improved characteristics with regard to both substrate and product specificity.

References

Alzueta, C., Centeno, C., Cutuli, M.T., Ortiz, L.T., Rebole, A., *et al.* (2003) Effect of whole and demucilaged linseed in broiler chicken diets on digesta viscosity, nutrient utilisation and intestinal microflora. *British Poultry Science* 44, 67–74.

Amerah, A.M., Ravindran, V., Lentle, R.G. and Thomas, D.G. (2007) Feed particle size: implications on the digestions and performance of poultry. *World's Poultry Science Journal* 63, 439–453.

Amerah, A.M., Ravindran, V., Lentle, R.G. and Thomas, D.G. (2008) Influence of particle size and xylanase supplementation on the performance, energy utilisation, digestive parameters and digesta viscosity of broiler starters. *British Poultry Science* 49, 455–462.

Bach Knudsen, K.E. (2014) Fiber and nonstarch polysaccharide content and variation in common crops used in broiler diets. *Poultry Science* 93, 2380–2393.

Bach Knudsen, K.E. (2016) Carbohydrates in pig nutrition – recent advances. *Journal of Animal Science* 94, 1–11.

Bach Knudsen, K.E. (2018) Dietary fibre analyses in a nutritional and physiological context – past and present. *Proceedings of the Society of Nutrition and Physiology* 27, 189–192.

Bailey, M.J., Biely, P. and Poutanen, K. (1992) Interlaboratory testing of methods for assay of xylanase activity. *Journal of Biotechnology* 23, 257–270.

Barrier-Guillot, B., Bedford, M.R., Metayer, J.P. and Gatel, F. (1995) Effect of xylanase on the feeding value of wheat-based diets from different wheat varieties for broilers. In: *Proceedings of the WPSA 10th European*

Symposium on Poultry Nutrition, Antalya, Turkey, 15–19 October 1995. World's Poultry Science Association, Beekbergen, the Netherlands, pp. 324–325.

Bautil, A. (2020) Arabinoxylan digestion and endoxylanase functionality in ageing broilers fed wheat-based diets. PhD thesis, KU Leuven, Leuven, Belgium.

Bautil, A., Verspreet, J., Courtin, C.M., Buyse, J., Goos, P. and Bedford, M.R. (2019) Age-related arabinoxylan hydrolysis and fermentation in the gastrointestinal tract of broilers fed wheat-based diets. *Poultry Science* 98, 4606–4621.

Bautil, A., Verspreet, J., Buyse, J., Goos, P., Bedford, M.R. and Courtin, C.M. (2020) Arabinoxylan-oligosaccharides kick-start arabinoxylan digestion in the aging broiler. *Poultry Science* 99, 2555–2565.

Bedford, M.R. (1996) The effect of enzymes on digestion. *Journal of Applied Poultry Research* 5, 370–378.

Bedford, M.R. (2000a) Exogenous enzymes in monogastric nutrition – their current value and future benefits. *Animal Feed Science and Technology* 86, 1–13.

Bedford, M.R. (2000b) Removal of antibiotic growth promoters from poultry diets: implications and strategies to minimise subsequent problems. *World's Poultry Science Journal* 56, 347–365.

Bedford, M.R. and Apajalahti, J. (2018) Exposure of a broiler to a xylanase for 35d increases the capacity of cecal microbiome to ferment soluble xylan. *Poultry Science* 97, 98–99.

Bedford, M.R. and Autio, K. (1996) Microscopic examination of feed and digesta from wheat-fed broiler chickens and its relation to bird performance. *Poultry Science* 75, 1.

Bedford, M.R. and Classen, H.L. (1993) An *in vitro* assay for prediction of broiler intestinal viscosity and growth when fed rye-based diets in the presence of exogenous enzymes. *Poultry Science* 72, 137–143.

Bedford, M.R. and Cowieson, A.J. (2012) Exogenous enzymes and their effects on intestinal microbiology. *Animal Feed Science and Technology* 173, 76–85.

Bedford, M.R. and Fothergill, A. (2002) Alternatives to antibiotics – nutritional strategies to manage microfloral populations. In: *Proceedings of the 38th Eastern Nutrition Conference, Guelph, Ontario, Canada, 9–10 May 2002.* Animal Nutrition Society of Canada, Ottawa, pp. 65–79.

Bedford, M.R. and Morgan, A.J. (1996) The use of enzymes in poultry diets. *World's Poultry Science Journal* 52, 61–68.

Bedford, M.R. and Schulze, H. (1998) Exogenous enzymes for pigs and poultry. *Nutrition Research Reviews* 11, 91–114.

Bedford, M.R., Classen, H.L. and Campbell, G.L. (1991) The effect of pelleting, salt, and pentosanase on the viscosity of intestinal contents and the performance of broilers fed rye. *Poultry Science* 70, 1571–1577.

Burnett, G.S. (1966) Studies of viscosity as the probable factor involved in the improvement of certain barleys for chickens by enzyme supplementation. *British Poultry Science* 7, 55–75.

Campbell, J.M., Fahey, G. Jr and Wolf, B.W. (1997) Selected indigestible oligosaccharides affect large bowel mass, cecal and fecal short-chain fatty acids, pH and microflora in rats. *The Journal of Nutrition* 127, 130–136.

Chacher, M.F.A., Kamran, Z., Ahsan, U., Ahmad, S., Koutoulis, K.C., *et al.* (2017) Use of mannan oligosaccharide in broiler diets: an overview of underlying mechanisms. *World's Poultry Science Journal* 73, 831–844.

Chen, H., Zhang, S. and Kim, S.W. (2020) Effects of supplemental xylanase on health of the small intestine in nursery pigs fed diets with corn distillers' dried grains with solubles. *Journal of Animal Science* 98, skaa185.

Coelho, M. and Troescher, A. (2018) Effect of a NSPase enzyme, Natugrain TS, on feed passage rate, jejunum viscosity, energy release and performance on broilers fed corn/soy diets processed at variable conditions. *Poultry Science* 97, 85.

Courtin, C.M., Broekaert, W.F., Swennen, K., Lescroart, O., Onagbesan, O., *et al.* (2008) Dietary inclusion of wheat bran arabinoxylooligosaccharides induces beneficial nutritional effects in chickens. *Cereal Chemistry* 85, 607–613.

Cowieson, A.J. and Bedford, M.R. (2009) The effect of phytase and carbohydrase on ileal amino acid digestibility in monogastric diets: complimentary mode of action? *World's Poultry Science Journal* 65, 609–624.

Cozannet, P., Kidd, M.T., Neto, R.M. and Geraert, P.A. (2017) Next-generation non-starch polysaccharide-degrading, multi-carbohydrase complex rich in xylanase and arabinofuranosidase to enhance broiler feed digestibility. *Poultry Science* 96, 2743–2750.

Cozannet, P., Kidd, M.T., Yacoubi, N., Geraert, P.-A. and Preynat, A. (2018) Dietary energy and amino acid enhancement from a multi-enzyme preparation. *Journal of Applied Poultry Research* 28, 136–144.

Creswell, D. and Bedford, M.R. (2005) High pelleting temperatures reduce broiler performance. In: *Proceedings of the 18th Australian Poultry Science Symposium, Sydney, Australia, 20–22 February 2006.* Poultry Research Foundation, Sydney, Australia, pp. 1–6.

Dale, T., Brameld, J.M., Parr, T. and Bedford, M.R. (2019) Differential effects of fibrolytic enzymes on the *in vitro* release of xylobiose from different cereal types. *Proceedings of the British Society of Animal Science* 10, 222.

Dale, T., Hannay, I., Bedford, M.R., Tucker, G.A., Brameld, J.M. and Parr, T. (2020) The effects of exogenous xylanase supplementation on the *in vivo* generation of xylooligosaccharides and monosaccharides in broilers fed a wheat-based feed. *British Poultry Science* 61, 471–481.

Danicke, S., Bottcher, W., Jeroch, H., Thielebein, J. and Simon, O. (2000a) Replacement of soybean oil with tallow in rye-based diets without xylanase increases protein synthesis in small intestine of broilers. *The Journal of Nutrition* 130, 827–834.

Danicke, S., Jeroch, H., Bottcher, W. and Simon, O. (2000b) Interactions between dietary fat type and enzyme supplementation in broiler diets with high pentosan contents: effects on precaecal and total tract digestibility of fatty acids, metabolizability of gross energy, digesta viscosity and weights of small intestine. *Animal Feed Science and Technology* 84, 279–294.

De Keyser, K., Dierick, N., Kuterna, L., Maigret, O., Kaczmarek, S., *et al.* (2018) Non-starch polysaccharide degrading enzymes in corn and wheat-based broiler diets: dual activity for major substrates. *Journal of Agricultural Science and Technology* 8, 76–88.

Eeckhaut, V., Van Immerseel, F., Dewulf, J., Pasmans, F., Haesebrouck, F., *et al.* (2008) Arabinoxylooligosaccharides from wheat bran inhibit *Salmonella* colonization in broiler chickens. *Poultry Science* 87, 2329–2334.

Feighner, S.D. and Dashkevicz, M.P. (1988) Effect of dietary carbohydrates on bacterial cholyltaurine hydrolase in poultry intestinal homogenates. *Applied and Environmental Microbiology* 54, 337–342.

Fischer, E.N. (2003) Interrelationship of diet fibre and endoxylanase with bacteria in the chicken gut. PhD thesis, University of Saskatchewan, Saskatoon, Canada.

Fry, R.E., Allred, J.B., Jensen, L.S. and McGinnis, J. (1957) Influence of water-treatment on nutritional value of barley. *Proceedings of the Society of Experimental Biology and Medicine* 95, 249–251.

Fry, R.E., Allred, J.B., Jensen, L.S. and McGinnis, J. (1958) Effect of pearling barley and of different supplements to diets containing barley on chick growth and feed efficiency. *Poultry Science* 37, 281–288.

Geraert, P.P., Rouffineau, F. and Barrier-Guillot, B. (2001) Non-starch polysaccharide enzymes and viscosity: the relationship revisited. *Australian Poultry Science Symposium Proceedings* 13, 208–211.

Gibson, G.R. and Roberfroid, M.B. (1995) Dietary modulation of the human colonic microbiota: introducing the concept of prebiotics. *The Journal of Nutrition* 125, 1401–1412.

Grootwassink, J.W.D., Campbell, G.L. and Classen, H.L. (1989) Fractionation of crude pentosanase (arabinoxylanase) for improvement of the nutritional value of rye diets for broiler chickens. *Journal of the Science of Food and Agriculture* 46, 289–300.

Jensen, L.S. (1957) Improvement in the nutritional value of barley for chicks by enzyme supplementation. *Poultry Science* 36, 919–921.

Jia, W., Slominski, B.A., Bruce, H.L., Blank, G., Crow, G. and Jones, O. (2009) Effects of diet type and enzyme addition on growth performance and gut health of broiler chickens during subclinical *Clostridium perfringens* challenge. *Poultry Science* 88, 132–140.

Karunaratne, N.D., Newkirk, R.W., Ames, N.P., Van Kessel, A.G., Bedford, M.R. and Classen, H.L. (2021) Hulless barley and β-glucanase affect ileal digesta soluble beta-glucan molecular weight and digestive tract characteristics of coccidiosis-vaccinated broilers. *Animal Nutrition* 7, 595–608.

Lamp, A.E., Evans, A.M. and Moritz, J.S. (2015) The effects of pelleting and glucanase supplementation in hulled barley based diets on feed manufacture, broiler performance and digesta viscosity. *Journal of Applied Poultry Research* 24, 295–303.

Langenaeken, N.A., Ieven, P., Hedlund, E.G., Kyomugasho, C., Van De Walle, D., *et al.* (2020) Arabinoxylan, β-glucan and pectin in barley and malt endosperm cell walls: a microstructure study using CLSM and cryo-SEM. *The Plant Journal* 103, 1477–1489.

Langhout, D.J., Schutte, J.B., De Jong, J., Sloetjes, H., Verstegen, M.W.A. and Tamminga, S. (2000) Effect of viscosity on digestion of nutrients in conventional and germ-free chicks. *British Journal of Nutrition* 83, 533–540.

Le, D.M., Fojan, P., Azem, E., Pettersson, D. and Pedersen, N.R. (2013) Visualization of the anticaging effect of Ronozyme WX xylanase on wheat substrates. *Cereal Chemistry* 90, 439–444.

Lee, S.A., Wiseman, J., Masey O'Neill, H.V., Scholey, D.V., Burton, E.J. and Hill, S.E. (2017) Understanding the direct and indirect mechanisms of xylanase action on starch digestion in broilers. *Journal of World's Poultry Research* 7, 35–47.

Lei, Z., Shao, Y., Yin, X., Yin, D., Guo, Y. and Yuan, J. (2016) Combination of xylanase and debranching enzyme specific to wheat arabinoxylan improve the growth performance and gut health of broilers. *Journal of Agricultural and Food Chemistry* 64, 4932–4942.

Li, W.F., Sun, J.Y. and Xu, Z.R. (2004) Effects of NSP degrading enzyme on *in vitro* digestion of barley. *Asian-Australasian Journal of Animal Sciences* 17, 122–126.

Maisonnier, S., Gomez, J., Bree, A., Berri, C., Baeza, E. and Carre, B. (2003) Effects of microflora status, dietary bile salts and guar gum on lipid digestibility, intestinal bile salts, and histomorphology in broiler chickens. *Poultry Science* 82, 805–814.

Masey O'Neill, H.V., Haldar, S. and Bedford, M.R. (2012) The role of peptide YY in the mode of action of dietary xylanase. *Poultry Science* 91, T122.

Masey O'Neill, H.V., Smith, J.A. and Bedford, M.R. (2014) Multicarbohydrase enzymes for non-ruminants. *Asian-Australasian Journal of Animal Sciences* 27, 290–301.

Mateos, G.G. and Sell, J.L. (1980) Influence of graded levels of fat on utilization of pure carbohydrate by the laying hen. *The Journal of Nutrition* 110, 1894–1903.

Mateos, G.G., Sell, J.L. and Eastwood, J.A. (1982) Rate of food passage (transit time) is influenced by level of supplemental fat. *Poultry Science* 61, 94–100.

McCracken, K.J., Bedford, M.R. and Stewart, R.A. (2001) Effects of variety, the 1B/1R translocation and xylanase supplementation on nutritive value of wheat for broilers. *British Poultry Science* 42, 638–642.

Menezes-Blackburn, D. and Greiner, R. (2015) Enzymes used in animal feed: leading technologies and forthcoming developments. In: Cirillo, G., Spizzirri, U.G. and Iemma, F. (eds) *Functional Polymers in Food Science: From Technology to Biology*, vol. 2: *Food Processing*. Wiley, Hoboken, New Jersey, pp. 47–73.

Moran, J.E.T. and McGinnis, J. (1966) A comparison of corn and barley for the developing turkey and the effect of antibiotic and enzyme supplementation. *Poultry Science* 45, 636–639.

Moreno, F.J., Corzo, N., Montilla, A., Villamiel, M. and Olano, A. (2017) Current state and latest advances in the concept, production and functionality of prebiotic oligosaccharides. *Current Opinion in Food Science* 13, 50–55.

Morgan, A.J., Bedford, M.R., Tervila-Wilo, A., Autio, K., Hopeakoski-Nurminen, M., *et al.* (1995) How enzymes improve the nutritional value of wheat. *Zootecnica International* (April), 44–48.

Murphy, T.C., McCracken, K.J., McCann, M.E.E., George, J. and Bedford, M.R. (2010) Broiler performance and *in vivo* viscosity as influenced by a range of xylanases, varying in ability to effect wheat *in vitro* viscosity. *British Poultry Science* 50, 716–724.

Oyarzabal, O.A. and Conner, D.E. (1995) *In vitro* fructooligosaccharide utilisation and inhibition of *Salmonella* spp. by selected bacteria. *Poultry Science* 74, 1418–1425.

Oyarzabal, O.A., Conner, D.E. and Blevins, W.T. (1995) Fructooligosaccharide utilisation by salmonellae and potential direct-fed microbial bacteria for poultry. *Journal of Food Protection* 58, 1192–1196.

Parkkonen, T., Tervila-Wilo, A., Hopeakoski-Nurminen, M., Morgan, A.J., Poutanen, K. and Autio, K. (1997) Changes in wheat microstructure following *in vitro* digestion. *Acta Agriculturae Scandinavica, Section B – Soil & Plant Science* 47, 43–47.

Pasquier, B., Armand, M., Guillon, F., Castelain, C., Borel, P., *et al.* (1996) Viscous soluble dietary fibers alter emulsification and lipolysis of triacylglycerols in duodenal medium *in vitro*. *The Journal of Nutritional Biochemistry* 7, 293–302.

Petersen, S.T., Wiseman, J. and Bedford, M.R. (1999) Effects of age and diet on the viscosity of intestinal contents in broiler chicks. *British Poultry Science* 40, 364–370.

Ravindran, V., Selle, P.H. and Bryden, W.L. (1999) Effects of phytase supplementation, individually and in combination with glycanase on the nutritive value of wheat and barley. *Poultry Science* 78, 1588–1595.

Ravn, J.L., Thogersen, J.C., Eklof, J., Pettersson, D., Ducatelle, R., *et al.* (2017) GH11 xylanase increases prebiotic oligosaccharides from wheat bran favouring butyrate-producing bacteria *in vitro*. *Animal Feed Science and Technology* 226, 113–123.

Rinttila, T. and Apajalahti, J. (2013) Intestinal microbiota and metabolites – implications for broiler chicken health and performance. *Journal of Applied Poultry Research* 22, 647–658.

Rosen, G.D. (2001) Multi-factorial efficacy evaluation of alternatives to antimicrobials in pronutrition. *British Poultry Science* 42, S104–S105.

Rosen, G.D. (2002) Exogenous enzymes as pro-nutrients in broiler diets. In: Garnsworthy, P.C. and Wiseman, J. (eds) *Recent Advances in Animal Nutrition 2002*, 1st edn. Nottingham University Press, Nottingham, UK, pp. 89–103.

Sacranie, A., Svihus, B., Denstadli, V., Iji, P.A. and Choct, M. (2012) The effect of insoluble fibre and intermittent feeding on gizzard development, gut motility and performance in broiler chickens. *Australian Poultry Science Symposium* 23, 24–27.

Sacranie, A., Adiya, X., Mydland, L.T. and Svihus, B. (2017) Effect of intermittent feeding and oat hulls to improve phytase efficacy and digestive function in broiler chickens. *British Poultry Science* 58, 442–451.

Saleh, F., Ohtsuka, A., Tanaka, T. and Hayashi, K. (2004) Carbohydrases are digested by proteases present in enzyme preparations during *in vitro* digestion. *Journal of Poultry Science* 41, 229–235.

Sharifi, S.D., Golestani, G., Yaghobfar, A., Khadem, A. and Pashazanussi, H. (2014) Effects of supplementing a multienzyme to broiler diets containing a high level of wheat or canola meal on intestinal morphology and performance of chicks. *Journal of Applied Poultry Research* 22, 671–679.

Shastak, Y., Ader, P., Feuerstein, D., Ruehle, R. and Matuschek, M. (2015) β-Mannan and mannanase in poultry nutrition. *World's Poultry Science Journal* 71, 161–174.

Silva, S.S.P. and Smithard, R.R. (1996) Exogenous enzymes in broiler diets: crypt cell proliferation, digesta viscosity, short chain fatty acids and xylanase in the jejunum. *British Poultry Science* 37(Suppl.), S77–S79.

Silva, S.S.P., Gilbert, H.J. and Smithard, R.R. (1997) Exogenous polysaccharides do not improve digestion of fat and protein by increasing trypsin or lipase activities in the small intestine. *British Poultry Science* 38(Suppl.), S39–S40.

Silversides, F.G. and Bedford, M.R. (1999) Effect of pelleting temperature on the recovery and efficacy of a xylanase enzyme in wheat-based diets. *Poultry Science* 78, 1184–1190.

Simmering, R. and Blaut, M. (2001) Pro- and prebiotics – the tasty guardian angels? *Applied Microbiology and Biotechnology* 55, 19–28.

Singh, A., Masey O'Neill, H.V., Ghosh, T.K., Bedford, M.R. and Haldar, S. (2012) Effects of xylanase supplementation on performance, total volatile fatty acids and selected bacterial populations in caeca, metabolic indices and peptide YY concentrations in serum of broiler chickens fed energy restricted maize–soybean based diets. *Animal Feed Science and Technology* 177, 194–203.

Singh, A., Tiwari, U.P., Mishra, B. and Jha, R. (2019) Comparative effects of *in ovo* injection of oligosaccharides (xylotriose, xylotetraose, mannotriose, and mannotetraose) on growth performance and gut health parameters of broilers. *Poultry Science* 98(E-Suppl. 1), 181.

Smits, C.H.M. and Annison, G. (1996) Non-starch plant polysaccharides in broiler nutrition – towards a physiologically valid approach to their determination. *World's Poultry Science Journal* 52, 203–221.

Smulikowska, S. (1998) Relationship between the stage of digestive tract development in chicks and the effect of viscosity reducing enzymes on fat digestion. *Journal of Animal and Feed Sciences* 7, 125–134.

Steer, T., Carpenter, H., Tuohy, K. and Gibson, G.R. (2000) Perspectives on the role of the human gut microbiota and its modulation by pro- and prebiotics. *Nutrition Research Reviews* 13, 229–254.

Svihus, B., Edvardsen, D.H., Bedford, M.R. and Gullord, M. (2000) Effects of methods of analysis and heat treatment on viscosity of wheat, barley and oats. *Animal Feed Science and Technology* 88, 1–12.

Tahir, M., Saleh, F., Ohtsuka, A. and Hayashi, K. (2005) Synergistic effect of cellulase and hemicellulase on nutrient utilisation and performance in broilers fed a corn–soybean meal diet. *Animal Science Journal* 76, 559–565.

Tervila-Wilo, A., Parkkonen, T., Morgan, A.J., Hopeakoski-Nurminen, M., Poutanen, K., *et al.* (1996) *In vitro* digestion of wheat microstructure with xylanase and cellulase from *Trichoderma reesei*. *Journal of Cereal Science* 24, 215–225.

Torrallardona, D., Nielsen, J.E. and Braufau, J. (2000) Apparent ileal digestibility of protein and amino acids in wheat supplemented with enzymes for growing pigs. In: Lindberg, J.E. and Ogle, B. (eds) *Digestive Physiology of Pigs. Proceedings of the 8th Symposium, Swedish University of Agricultural Sciences, Uppsala, Sweden, 20–22 June 2000.* CAB International, Wallingford, UK, pp. 184–186.

Torrecillas, S., Montero, D. and Izquierdo, M. (2014) Improved health and growth of fish fed mannan oligosaccharides: potential mode of action. *Fish & Shellfish Immunology* 36, 525–544.

Troesher, A. and Coelho, M. (2018) Assessment of a NSPase enzyme, Natugrain TS, dose titration on jejunum viscosity, IDE and necrotic enteritis lesion scores on birds challenged with coccidiosis vaccine and *Clostridium perfringens* and 28-day bird performance on corn/soy diets. *Poultry Science* 97, 155–156.

Vangsøe, C.T., Sørensen, J.F. and Bach Knudsen, K.E. (2019) Aleurone cells are the primary contributor to arabinoxylan oligosaccharide production from wheat bran after treatment with cell wall-degrading enzymes. *International Journal of Food Science & Technology* 54, 2847–2853.

Vangsøe, C.T., Nørskov, N.P., Devaux, M.-F., Bonnin, E. and Bach Knudsen, K.E. (2020) A carbohydrase complex rich in xylanases and arabinofuranosidases affects the autofluorescence signal and liberates phenolic acids from the cell wall matrix in wheat, maize, and rice bran: an *in vitro* digestion study. *Journal of Agricultural and Food Chemistry* 68, 9878–9887.

Vazquez, M.J., Alonso, J.L., Dominguez, H. and Parajo, J.C. (2000) Xylooligosaccharides: manufacture and applications. *Trends in Food Science & Technology* 11, 387–393.

Vehmaanperä, J. (2022) Feed enzymes: enzymology, biochemistry, and production on an industrial scale. In: Bedford, M.R., Partridge, G.G., Hruby, M. and Walk, C.L. (eds) *Enzymes in Farm Animal Nutrition*, 3rd edn. CAB International, Wallingford, UK, pp. 10–32.

Waldenstedt, L., Elwinger, K., Lunden, A., Thebo, P. and Bedford, M.R. (2000) Intestinal digesta viscosity decreases during coccidial infection in broilers. *British Poultry Science* 41, 459–464.

Walk, C.L., Bedford, M.R. and McElroy, A.P. (2012) Influence of limestone and phytase on broiler performance, gastrointestinal pH and apparent ileal nutrient digestibility. *Poultry Science* 91, 1371–1378.

Ward, A.T. and Marquardt, R.R. (1983) The effect of saturation, chain length of pure triglycerides, and age of bird on the utilization of rye diets. *Poultry Science* 62, 1054–1062.

Ward, A.T. and Marquardt, R.R. (1987) Antinutritional activity of a water-soluble pentosan-rich fraction from rye grain. *Poultry Science* 66, 1665–1674.

Willingham, H.E., Jensen, L.S. and McGinnis, J. (1959) Studies on the role of enzyme supplements and water treatment for improving the nutritional value of barley. *Poultry Science* 38, 539–544.

Wu, Y.B. and Ravindran, V. (2004) Influence of whole wheat inclusion and xylanase supplementation on the performance, digestive tract measurements and carcass characteristics of broiler chickens. *Animal Feed Science and Technology* 116, 129–139.

Wu, Y.B., Ravindran, V., Thomas, D.G., Birtles, M.J. and Hendriks, W.H. (2004) Influence of phytase and xylanase, individually or in combination, on performance, apparent metabolisable energy, digestive tract measurements and gut morphology in broilers fed wheat-based diets containing adequate level of phosphorus. *British Poultry Science* 45, 76–84.

5 Mannanase, α-Galactosidase and Pectinase: Minor Players or Yet to be Exploited?

Jason T. Lee[1]* and Kyle D. Brown[2]

[1]*CJ Bio America, Downers Grove, Illinois, USA;* [2]*Texas A&M University, College Station, Texas, USA*

5.1 Introduction: β-Mannan

Structural plant material consists of cellulose, hemicellulose and lignin with an approximate representation of 2:1:1. Cellulose is present as insoluble bundles of tightly packed polysaccharide chains providing strength and rigidity to cell walls, whereas lignin acts as an amorphous aromatic-rich barrier to microbial degradation. Hemicelluloses are intertwined with cellulose and lignin completing the matrix and providing cell wall resistance to microbial degradation yet enough flexibility to allow movement and growth (Van Zyl *et al.*, 2010). Hemicelluloses are linear and branched polysaccharides composed of D-xylose, D-galactose, D-mannose, D-glucose and L-arabinose. Hemicelluloses are classified according to the major monosaccharide present in the polymer backbone, such as xylans, galactans and mannans (Gray *et al.*, 2006). Mannan as a hemicellulosic polysaccharide is second to xylan in abundance (McCleary, 1988). The family of mannans comprises four subfamilies: glucomannan, galactomannan, galactoglucomannan and pure mannans (Petkowicz *et al.*, 2001). Mannan and heteromannans are a part of the hemicellulose fraction of the cell wall in all leguminous plants (Reid, 1985) including soybean meal (SBM), sesame meal, palm kernel meal, copra meal and guar meal (Dhawan and Kaur, 2007). SBM's β-mannans are linear polysaccharides formed from repeating β-1,4-mannose and α-1,6-galactose molecules bound to the β-mannan backbone (Jackson *et al.*, 2004). β-Mannan content of some typically used grains is presented in Table 5.1.

Dietary non-starch polysaccharides (NSPs) are indigestible by poultry but represent a potential energy source that can be utilized with the addition of enzymes (Meng *et al.*, 2005). Aside from representing a potential energy source, the presence of dietary NSPs, which are indigestible by monogastric animals, can result in increased intestinal viscosity, reduced nutrient digestibility, increased feed conversion ratio (FCR) and ultimately decreased bird performance (Bedford and Classen, 1992; Bedford and Morgan, 1996; Lázaro *et al.*, 2003). SBM is a primary source of vegetable protein and contains 3% soluble NSPs and 16% insoluble NSPs (Irish and Balnave, 1993), consisting mainly of mannans and galactomannans (Slominski, 2011). β-Mannan, or galactomannan, is a polysaccharide and has repeating units of mannose containing galactose and/

*Email: jason.lee2@cj.net

©CAB International 2022. *Enzymes in Farm Animal Nutrition, 3rd Edition* (M. Bedford *et al.* eds)
DOI: 10.1079/9781789241563.0005

Table 5.1. Approximate content of β-mannan in some feedstuffs. (From Dierick, 1989; Shastak et al., 2015.)

Feedstuff	β-Mannan content (g/kg)	Reference
Palm kernel meal	367	Sundu et al. (2006a)
Guar meal		
Germ fraction	56	Lee et al. (2004)
Hull fraction	98	Lee et al. (2004)
Combined	87	Lee et al. (2004)
Copra meal	250	Sundu et al. (2006b)
SBM (44% CP)	16	Hsiao et al. (2006)
SBM (48% CP)	13	Hsiao et al. (2006)
Rye	6.1	Dierick (1989)
Barley	4.3	Dierick (1989)
Rapeseed meal	4.5	Dierick (1989)
Wheat	0.9	Dierick (1989)
Maize	0.8	Dierick (1989)
Bakery meal	1.0	Dierick (1989)
Maize DDGS	2.7	Dierick (1989)

SBM, soybean meal; CP, crude protein; DDGS, distillers dried grains with solubles.

or glucose (Carpita and McCann, 2000; Hsiao et al., 2006). Galactomannan content in dehulled SBM has been reported at levels from 1.02 to 1.51% (Hsiao et al., 2006). Although galactomannan content of SBM is in low concentrations, it is a concern for nutritionists because it has antinutritive properties. Mannans are surface components of multiple pathogens, and the innate immune system reacts to antigens on these pathogens. Mannans in the diet can stimulate the innate immune system and lead to a purposeless energy-draining immune response (Hsiao et al., 2006).

The main component of mannan is D-mannose, a six-carbon sugar. Due to the heterogeneity and complex chemical nature of plant mannans, its breakdown into simple sugars, to be readily used as an energy source, is not possible by monogastric animals as it requires the synergistic action of endo-1,4-β-mannanases and exo-acting β-mannosidases (Dhawan and Kaur, 2007) and β-glucosidases (Moreira and Filho, 2008). Endo-β-mannanases are ubiquitous in nature and are endohydrolases that cleave the internal glycosidic bonds of the mannan backbone, producing β-1,4-manno-oligosaccharides (Chauhan et al., 2012). The degree of hydrolysis is influenced by numerous factors including the substitution extent and distribution of galactose in the

D-mannan backbone (Stalbrand et al., 1993), the acetylation degree (McCleary, 1991), the β-mannanase source, e.g. bacterial, fungal, etc. (McCleary, 1979), and the quantity of enzyme. The most important mannan- and galactomannan-cleaving enzymes for animal nutrition are endo-β-mannanase and α-galactosidases since feedstuffs used in avian nutrition contain galactomannan and/or linear mannans (Shastak et al., 2015).

There are currently many applications for mannanases in industrial processes. Mannanases are used mainly for improving the quality of food, in feeds and aiding in enzymatic bleaching of soft wood pulps in the paper and pulp industries (Dhawan and Kaur, 2007). Specific applications include extraction of lignin from wood fibres in the paper industry, reducing the viscosity of coffee extracts, stain-removing boosters in the detergent industry, enhancing the flow of oil and gas, oil extraction of coconut meat, degradation of thickening agents, as well as improvement in the nutritional value of animal feed. There are numerous published investigations into the effect of β-mannanase on poultry performance and feed digestibility (Jackson et al., 1999, 2002a, 2004; Odetallah et al., 2002; Lee et al., 2003a; Daskiran et al., 2004; Wu et al., 2005; Li et al., 2010); however, more recently investigators have focused on dual enzyme application (Williams *et al.*, 2014), minimizing the potential of a feed-induced immune response (Arsenault *et al.*, 2017) and determining a minimum substrate level (galactomannan) present to elicit a negative impact on the animal (Latham *et al.*, 2018).

5.2   Modes of Action

To determine the long-term viability and potential usefulness of a β-mannanase in monogastric production systems, nutritionists must consider the modes of actions and the potential benefits to their production systems. There have been multiple modes of action proposed and defined for β-mannanase; these include reduction of viscosity in the gastrointestinal (GI) tract of the animal, the suppression of harmful microorganism proliferation in the GI tract and the reduction of a feed-induced immune response due to the presence of galactomannan in the plant-based ingredients. As a result of these modes of action, β-mannanases improve nutrient digestibility and utilization and increase animal growth performance and efficiency.

The negative impact of elevated digesta viscosity in the GI tract of animals on nutrient absorption and performance has been well documented (Smits *et al.*, 1997; Lee *et al.*, 2003a,b; Latham *et al.*, 2018). Increasing viscosity compromises the ability of the GI tract to physically mix digesta (Edwards *et al.*, 1988), impairing the diffusion and convective transport of digestive enzymes within the GI tract (Almirall *et al.*, 1995) and reducing the contact intensity of nutrients and their respective digestive secretions (Choct and Annison, 1992), leading to reductions in nutrient digestion and absorption (Kratzer *et al.*, 1967; Maisonnier *et al.*, 2001). Galactomannans of leguminous plants such as guar can absorb high amounts of water, similar to soluble arabinoxylans and β-glucans, forming high-viscosity digesta. Elevated levels of soluble galactomannan increased the *in vitro* viscosity of feed (Lee *et al.*, 2009), reduced glucose absorption in the porcine jejunum from 74.2 to 41.4% (Rainbird *et al.*, 1984) and increased FCR

from 1.757 to 1.868 in broiler chickens (Latham *et al.*, 2018). Highly viscous mannans may slow gastric emptying, affect the mixing of substrate with digestive enzymes and reduce the contact of nutrients with enterocytes (Read, 1986). However, not all linear galactomannans are soluble in water. Water-insoluble linear mannans with a very low degree of galactose substitution, such as those in palm kernel meal (Dusterhoft *et al.*, 1992), would not form any viscous solution in the digestive tract. Thus, the structure of the mannan itself determines the potential negative impact that it may present as a result of increasing intestinal viscosity.

β-Mannanase effectively hydrolyses galactomannan and reduces intestinal viscosity in animals fed diets containing soluble galactomannan. In a review, Shastak *et al.* (2015) indicated that β-mannanase added to diets containing greater than 8 g galactomannan from guar/kg will reduce intestinal viscosity. More recently, Latham *et al.* (2018) demonstrated that as little as 1.5 g guar galactomannan/kg was sufficient to increase intestinal viscosity and the supplementation of β-mannanase eliminated this increase in viscosity. In addition to the negative influences of viscosity recently described, continuous feeding of a highly viscous ingredient will increase intestinal mass (Smits *et al.*, 1997; Lee *et al.*, 2003a) as the animal attempts to adapt to the decreased absorption rate. While the GI tract uses 20% of all dietary energy to maintain digestion and absorption (Weurding *et al.*, 2003), an increase in tissue mass would increase the basal metabolism requirement and negatively impact feed efficiency (Lee *et al.*, 2003a). Therefore, the benefit of feeding β-mannanase in diets containing soluble galactomannan is not only reducing intestinal viscosity, thereby increasing nutrient utilization through enhancing nutrient contact with the intestinal wall, but also reducing basal metabolism as an effect of intestinal mass reduction and improving performance (Shastak *et al.*, 2015). However, galactomannans present in SBM, which is the most widely used vegetable protein source for poultry, have not been linked to increases in intestinal viscosity, possibly as the result of differences in structure, solubility and/or concentration as compared with guar and copra (Gullon *et al.*, 2009).

The hydroxylation of mannans with β-mannanase results in the production of short β-1,4-manno-oligosaccharides and D-mannose. These products can potentially be used as an energy source for the host as short-chain fatty acids following fermentation, bind to mannose-specific binding sites on pathogenic bacteria preventing their attachment to and colonization of the GI tract (Ofek *et al.*, 1977), or function as a prebiotic (Kiarie *et al.*, 2013) for the proliferation of bifidobacteria and lactobacilli (Asano *et al.*, 2001). For example, β-mannanase inclusion in a maize–SBM–guar meal-based moult-inducing diet reduced *Salmonella enteritidis* colonization in late-phase laying hens following a controlled challenged compared with an enzyme-free diet (Gutierrez *et al.*, 2008). These documented impacts of β-mannanase explain the effects observed by Jackson *et al.* (2003) during a control challenge of *Eimeria* and *Clostridium perfringens* in broilers fed a maize–SBM-based diet. In multiple experiments, β-mannanase supplementation reduced the severity of challenge as verified by improvements in growth performance and reduced intestinal lesion development compared with broilers fed enzyme-free diets, and the β-mannanase-supplemented broilers were similar to broilers fed the antibiotic bacitractin methylene disalicilate.

Dale *et al.* (2008) demonstrated that the presence of β-mannan in SBM can stimulate an innate immune response, termed a feed-induced immune response, which can negatively impact the performance of the animal. This plant-derived β-mannan is viewed as a pathogen-associated molecular pattern analogue for poultry, resulting in an innate immune response leading to the energy-costly activation and proliferation of monocytes and macrophages and subsequent cytokine production. β-Mannanase supplementation to SBM-based diets improved energy utilization in broilers and laying hens (Wu *et al.*, 2005) which was attributed to a reduction in immune activation, and this was confirmed by lower relative immune organ weights (Li *et al.*, 2010). More recently, Arsenault *et al.*

(2017) used kinome analysis to determine the influence of β-mannan and β-mannanase on immune and metabolic gut responses in broilers and observed that increasing β-mannan concentration by 3 g/kg altered a number of immune processes, confirming that a feed-induced immune response is initiated by β-mannan. Negative impacts of feeding SBM to swine have also been reported. Cromwell (1999) noted that feeding a soy-based ration to early weaned pigs led to reduced feed intake and slower rates of growth from the initiation of an inflammatory response in the intestine. The inclusion of β-mannanase reduced the activation of these pathways while also activating additional pathways associated with carbohydrate metabolism (insulin signalling), growth (ErbB pathway), adipose responses (adipocytokine signalling) and protein metabolism (mTOR pathway), suggesting improvement in digestion and gut barrier function with β-mannanase. These changes in immune and metabolic activity correlated with the observed improved efficiency and growth of broilers (Latham *et al.*, 2018).

The final mode of action of β-mannanase is the typical NSP-degrading function resulting in improved digestibility, similar to xylanase supplementation. NSPs decrease nutrient digestibility through the 'cage effect' – the encapsulation of nutrients such as starch and protein inside the endosperm (Bedford, 1993; Slominski, 2011). However, the cage effect of β-mannans may not have a large impact in legumes as only a minor portion of some high-mannose type *N*-glycans are linked to the storage of glycoproteins (Kimura *et al.*, 1997). Even though this mechanism may not bear significant responsibility in the feeding of β-mannanase, multiple researchers have documented increases in amino acid digestibility (Ferreira *et al.*, 2016) and energy digestibility (Daskiran *et al.*, 2004; Ferreira *et al.*, 2016; Latham *et al.*, 2018) with the inclusion of β-mannanase in diets containing elevated amounts of β-mannan. However, Latham *et al.* (2016) did not observe a benefit of β-mannanase inclusion on ileal digestible energy in broilers but did observe body weight (BW) and feed conversion improvements presumably associated with the other modes of action previously discussed.

5.3 Application

The documented modes of action described above must lend themselves to measurable improvements in animal performance for continued market expansion and use of β-mannanases in monogastric feeds. Jackson *et al.* (2004) demonstrated a significant 4.4% increase in BW and a 3.7% improvement in FCR in 42-day-old broilers fed a maize–soy-based diet when β-mannanase was added into the control diet. Similarly, Daskiran *et al.* (2004) observed a significant 2.9% improvement in FCR with the addition of β-mannanase to a maize–soy-based diet which included an animal protein blend at 5% in 14-day-old broilers. Improvements in flock uniformity have also been reported with a decreased in-flock coefficient of variation by 19% (Jackson *et al.*, 2005) and 26% (Piao *et al.*, 2003). More recently, Latham *et al.* (2016) reported a significant 2.2% increase in BW and a 1.5% improvement in FCR at 42 days of age with the supplementation of β-mannanase into a broiler diet based on maize–soy–meat and bone meal (MBM)–distillers' dried grains with solubles. These results suggest that β-mannanase improves broiler performance in maize–soy-based diets; however, its efficacy is dependent on available substrate. While none of the above publications analysed for galactomannan present in the diets, the reported performance enhancement correlated with the level of SBM in the diet. Diets containing higher levels of β-mannan allow for a higher benefit on performance (Daskiran *et al.*, 2004; Latham *et al.*, 2018); however, diets which lack sufficient levels of β-mannan-containing ingredients do not show a benefit of β-mannanase inclusion (Latham *et al.*, 2018). In general, diets containing in excess of 25% SBM tend to show beneficial effects of β-mannanase inclusion while those with less than 20% typically show minimal responses.

In addition to performance benefits, benefits on intestinal maturation and disease resistance have been reported (Jackson *et al.*, 2003; Saki *et al.*, 2005) in broilers. β-Mannanase inclusion has been shown to increase duodenal villus height as well as decrease epithelial thickness and goblet cell

numbers (Adibmoradi and Mehri, 2007). This reduced goblet cell number would be expected to lower mucin production and endogenous nitrogen losses while improving nutrient absorption with decreased epithelial thickness. The GI tract influences combined with the antimicrobial properties of hydrolysis (prebiotic and mannose binding) may be responsible for the reduction in lesion scores attributed to *Eimeria* and *C. perfringens* challenge in broilers fed β-mannanase (Jackson *et al.*, 2003). Reductions in observed mortality have also been reported in broilers (Klein *et al.*, 2015) and swine (O'Quinn *et al.*, 2002).

Opportunities also exist to capitalize on the advantages of feeding β-mannanase to turkeys and laying hens. Interestingly, the amount of SBM in turkey and laying hen diets and thus the potential β-mannan content varies considerably; however, benefits have been reported in both. Jackson *et al.* (2002b, 2008) reported BW increases of 4.9% in 18-week-old toms and 5.8% in 20-week-old toms with a conversion improvement of 20 points. This is a similar response to that reported by Odetallah *et al.* (2002) with main effect improvement in BW of 2% and 9-point improvement in FCR.

Benefits of β-mannanase inclusion in laying hen diets have also been described in multiple reports. In maize–SBM diets, significant increases in egg laying rate and early egg weight in diets of varying energy level have been reported by Jackson *et al.* (1999). Egg laying rate was increased by 0.70, 1.07 and 1.50% compared with the control diet for the second, third and fourth 6-week cycles evaluated. The advantage of enzyme inclusion over the control increased as the age of the birds increased as well from 30 weeks of age to 66 weeks of age. All of the diets had in excess of 20% SBM and the authors attributed the separation of egg production level with increasing age to the enzyme's ability to delay the post-peak decline in productivity through the stimulation of insulin secretion. Wu *et al.* (2005) reported observed improvements in egg production and egg mass with a 4.4% improvement in egg feed conversion.

In addition, multiple experiments have been conducted with β-mannanase supplementation into the diets of pigs of various ages and sizes. In these studies, β-mannanase supplementation resulted in a 4.0% improvement, a 4.8% improvement and a 4.2% improvement in FCR of 6.25, 13.6 and 109 kg BW pigs, respectively (Pettey *et al.*, 2002). Other researchers have reported similar observations with a 3% improvement in feed conversion (Hahn *et al.*, 1995) and a 4.6–5.5% improvement in FCR (Kim *et al.*, 2003). FCR improvements have been correlated to increased energy and dry matter (DM) digestibility (Upadhaya *et al.*, 2016a; Kim *et al.*, 2017). However, the animals' response to β-mannanase supplementation may be more variable in swine than in poultry, with multiple reports showing no advantage in performance or digestibility (Kwon and Kim, 2015; Upadhaya *et al.*, 2016b; Huntley *et al.*, 2018).

As noted above, and with any enzyme, the presence of substrate in the diet is the determining factor in effectiveness and benefit. Additionally, a complete feed contains many NSPs that require multiple enzymes for complete hydrolysis. Therefore, some recent investigations aimed to evaluate the inclusion of β-mannanase in combination with a commercial non-starch polysaccharide-degrading enzyme (NSPase) targeting maize arabinoxylan in a continuous feeding regime or intermittently with β-mannanase in the early diets when SBM is in higher concentration and an

NSPase targeting arabinoxylan in the later feeds of broilers. Klein *et al.* (2015) demonstrated continuous feeding of β-mannanase and an NSPase in maize- and soy-based diets was necessary to reach statistical similarity in final FCR to the control diet following an energy reduction of 131 kcal/kg. These results indicate there is a sub-additive effect of dual administration of β-mannanase and NSPases in low-energy broiler diets (Table 5.2).

While Klein *et al.* (2015) demonstrated a sub-additive relationship between β-mannanase and NSPase, continuous feeding of both enzymes may prove to not be economically feasible compared with feeding only one of the enzymes individually. Typically, β-mannanase targets substrates in US broiler diets associated with SBM while xylanases or NSPases target substrates in the same diet associated with the maize fraction. As broilers age and diets are changed from starter to grower to finisher, the amount of SBM in the diet decreases and the amount of maize increases. Therefore, the diet that contains the highest level of substrate for β-mannanase would be the starter diet and the highest level of substrate for a xylanase would be in the final diets of grow out. Williams *et al.* (2014) evaluated the intermittent feeding of β-mannanase and NSPase in an effort to target the substrate present in the diet according to age

Table 5.2. Mortality-corrected feed conversion ratio (FCR) and cumulative FCR of broilers fed diets reduced in energy and supplemented with a cocktail of NSPase[a] and β-mannanase[b] separately and in combination (Experiment 2). (From Klein *et al.*, 2015.)

Treatment	FCR Starter (days 1–14)	FCR Grower (days 15–27)	FCR Finisher (days 28–41)	FCR Cumulative (days 1–41)	Mortality (%)
Positive control	1.251[B]	1.465[B]	1.995[B]	1.678[C]	5.0[A]
Negative control	1.296[A]	1.510[A]	2.056[A]	1.737[A]	3.1[A,B]
β-Mannanase	1.282[A]	1.499[A]	2.018[B]	1.716[A,B]	1.8[B]
NSPase	1.285[A]	1.4990[A]	2.010[B]	1.706[B]	2.8[A,B]
β-Mannanase/NSPase[c]	1.272[A,B]	1.502[A]	1.994[B]	1.699[B,C]	4.7[A,B]
P value	0.047	0.049	0.019	<0.001	0.037
Pooled SEM	0.004	0.005	0.008	0.005	0.4

SEM, standard error of the mean.
[a]Enspira®, Enzyvia LLC, Sheridan, Indiana (113.5 g/ton).
[b]Hemicell® L, Elanco Animal Health, Greenfield, Indiana (100 ml/ton).
[c]Both enzymes were fed continuously.
[A–C]Mean values within a column with unlike upper-case superscript letters are significantly different at $P < 0.05$.

with a more economical strategy combined to dual administration as conducted by Klein *et al.* (2015). A five-phase feeding programme was fed with the first two diets containing the inclusion of β-mannanase and the last three diets containing an NSPase. Additional treatments included a positive and negative control with energy separation and birds fed the β-mannanase or NSPase separately for the entirety of the grow out. In this experiment, the potential impact of switching the dietary exogenous enzymes was unknown and the possibilities ranged from beneficial, to no impact and even potential negative impacts associated with the enzyme switching, the concomitant effect on oligosaccharides produced in the GI tract and the downstream effect on changing the microbiota. Results of the experiment are presented in Table 5.3. Williams *et al.* (2014) observed no negative impact of enzyme switching on the performance or yield of the broilers. Interestingly, the broilers that were switched from β-mannanase to NSPase on day 21 of age were the heaviest broilers at the conclusion of the experiment and had an elevated BW gain from 22 to 47 days of age compared with the positive control (high energy) diet. These broilers also expressed a 2-point reduction in FCR compared with the high-energy diet and each of the enzymes when fed separately.

β-Mannanase application has been extensively studied and has shown consistent beneficial results in performance of monogastric animals; however, the magnitude of the benefit is tied to the amount of dietary β-mannan. Some reports do not show improvements in digestibility while others do and this lack of consistency with a clearly defined mode of action may draw scepticism from some researchers and nutritionists. Nevertheless, most recent evaluations focusing on further understanding and describing the mechanism of action, in particular around the feed-induced immune response of β-mannans, are continuing to define the energy sparing mode of action that is likely responsible for the lack of digestibility improvements in many reports. These same reports do show an improvement in performance however and this may

be due to the benefits of β-mannanase to reduce or alleviate the β-mannan-induced immune response. Other recent investigations have focused on strategies of dual and intermittent application aimed at generating data for practising nutritionists to determine if and how β-mannanase can work in their production systems.

5.4 α-Galactosidase

SBM, which is used as the predominant dietary protein source for monogastric animals in most poultry- and swine-producing countries, contains 63 g soluble NSPs/kg DM and 154 g insoluble NSPs/kg DM (Kocher *et al.*, 2002) with significant concentrations of galactose-containing carbohydrates. These carbohydrates have relatively poor digestibility when fed to monogastric animals, with digestibility coefficients of approximately 52 and 72% for chickens and swine, respectively. The poor digestibility can be attributed to the composition of the carbohydrate fraction, which is comprised of nearly equal amounts of various polysaccharides and oligosaccharides (Table 5.4). The polysaccharide and oligosaccharide content comprises approximately 15 to 18% of SBM. Other than sucrose, the relative digestibility of each polysaccharide and oligosaccharide by monogastric animals is poor. These indigestible polysaccharides and oligosaccharides represent a potential energy source for a growing monogastric animal if digestible. Due to the more extensive GI tract and potential for microbial fermentation in swine, the digestibility is elevated compared with poultry. Soybeans contain three main types of oligosaccharides – verbascose, stachyose and raffinose – comprising a combined 6% of SBM which, as previously mentioned, are poorly digestible in monogastric animals due to the absence of endogenous α-galactosidase activity (Gitzelmann and Auricchio, 1965). The accumulation of these oligosaccharides results in fluid retention and increased flow rate of digesta, which will have a negative impact on nutrient digestibility and absorption (Wiggins, 1984). These oligosaccharides limit

Table 5.3. Average body weight (BW), weight gain (WG) and feed conversion ratio (FCR) of male broilers fed low-energy diets with the inclusion of β-mannanase[a], NSPase[b] and intermittent application of β-mannanase/NSPase. (From Williams *et al.*, 2014.)

Treatment (days 1–21)	Treatment (days 22–47)	BW (g) (day 10)	BW (g) (day 21)	BW (kg) (day 32)	BW (kg) (day 40)	BW (kg) (day 47)	WG (kg) (days 1–21)	WG (kg) (days 22–47)	FCR (days 1–47)
Positive control	Positive control	234.3[A]	890.1[A]	1.788[A]	2.474[A]	2.938[A]	0.848[A]	2.048[B]	1.814[B]
Negative control	Negative control	163.6[B]	591.3[B]	1.297[B]	1.946[B]	2.409[B]	0.549[B]	1.818[C]	1.878[A]
β-Mannanase	β-Mannanase	226.0[A]	863.8[A]	1.758[A]	2.446[A]	2.923[A]	0.820[A]	2.064[A,B]	1.824[B]
NSPase	β-Mannanase	–	–	1.796[A]	2.528[A]	3.054[A]	–	2.190[A]	1.798[B]
NSPase	NSPase	220.3[A]	848.2[A]	1.776[A]	2.508[A]	2.959[A]	0.806[A]	2.110[A,B]	1.816[B]
SEM		0.004	0.018	0.033	0.036	0.041	0.018	0.028	0.010
P value		<0.001	<0.001	<0.001	<0.001	<0.001	<0.001	<0.001	<0.001

SEM, standard error of the mean.

[a]Hemicell® HT, Elanco Animal Health, Greenfield, Indiana (363.2 g/ton).

[b]Enspira®, Enzyvia LLC, Sheridan, Indiana (113.5 g/ton).

[A–C]Mean values within a column with unlike upper-case superscript letters are significantly different at $P \leq 0.05$.

Table 5.4. Carbohydrate content of dehulled soybean meal. (From Honig and Rackis, 1979.)

Carbohydrate	Percentage (by weight)
Polysaccharide content (total)	15–18
Acidic polysaccharides	8–10
Arabinogalactans	5
Cellulosic material	1–2
Starch	0.5
Oligosaccharide content (total)	15
Sucrose	6–8
Stachyose	4–5
Raffinose	1–2

the energy value of SBM to monogastric animals. Coon *et al.* (1990) reported a 21% increase in the true metabolizable energy (TME) value of oligosaccharide-free SBM combined with a 50% reduction in passage time. Parsons *et al.* (2000) reported a 9.8% higher TME value in SBM with lower levels of total raffinose, stachyose and galactinol.

The lack of endogenously produced α-galactosidase in monogastric animals and the high concentration of polysaccharides and oligosaccharides provide an exogenous enzymatic opportunity to increase digestibility and performance. However, reports have been published with varying results on digestibility. For example, incubation of SBM with α-galactosidase decreased the α-galactoside concentration from 6.5 to 1.43% but did not significantly increase the TME value of the meal when fed to adult roosters (Irish *et al.*, 1995). However, a similar study with α-galactosidase treatment of SBM degraded raffinose and stachyose by 55 and 70%, respectively, and reported that this degradation increased the TME value by 12% but was not sufficient to elicit a chick performance response (Graham *et al.*, 2002). Meanwhile, other studies have reported benefits of α-galactosidase on energy digestibility and performance level (Knap *et al.*, 1996; Ghazi *et al.*, 2003). Wang *et al.* (2005) reported increases in dietary TME value and increases in digestibility of methionine and cysteine along with calcium and phosphorus in diets containing α-galactosidase. Similar digestibility results have been reported in swine, with improvements in oligosaccharide

degradation (Smiricky *et al.*, 2002) as well as additional benefits of energy and amino acid digestibility when additional stachyose was added to the diet (Pan *et al.*, 2002).

The adoption of a nutritional strategy will depend on the confidence of the nutritionist or company regarding that strategy and the consistency of a response. Multiple research teams have conducted series of experiments to evaluate the potential of α-galactosidase to improve digestibility and enhance performance in monogastric animals. Kidd *et al.* (2001a,b) conducted a total of four experiments to determine the effect of a liquid blend with primary activity of α-galactosidase (additional activities included α-amylase, β-glucanase, protease, xylanase and cellulose) on broiler performance and observed significant improvements in FCR in two of the four experiments with no influence on BW gain. In one of the experiments, a significant improvement of 6% in FCR combined with a significant reduction in mortality (6%) was reported when added in a maize–soy diet. In the second experiment, a significant 1.5% reduction in FCR was reported when added to a maize–soy diet in 42-day-old chickens. In a series of experiments to evaluate the influence of α-galactosidase on broiler performance containing different energy levels (Waldroup *et al.*, 2005) and enzyme inclusion levels (Waldroup *et al.*, 2006), the research team reported no effect of α-galactosidase inclusion on broiler performance. However, more recently Zhang *et al.* (2010) evaluated the inclusion of α-galactosidase in broiler diets containing dehulled SBM and varying in energy level. The researchers reported a significant increase in metabolizable energy (ME) with the inclusion of α-galactosidase at 2.1%, a significant increase in BW (2%) and a significant improvement in FCR (3%) at 42 days of age with no interaction present between the enzyme and dietary energy level. Similarly, Shang *et al.* (2018) reported that α-galactosidase inclusion significantly improved energy and protein digestibility, as well as increased several essential amino acids, which led to increased average daily BW gain in a 28-day swine experiment beginning with 7 kg piglets.

The supplementation of α-galactosidase in monogastric diets containing SBM merits consideration as the presence of the substrate and opportunity for oligosaccharide degradation and improved nutrient digestibility is a viable mode of action. It stands to reason the opportunity may be greater in poultry than in swine due to the large difference in ME value between the two species. The low ME value of SBM in poultry should provide an opportunity for markedly increased energy digestibility which would potentially increase the ME value of soy, remove the potentially negative impact of indigestible oligosaccharides and improve performance of the animal. However, review of the literature indicates inconsistent results in both poultry and swine, although the vast majority of research is dated. The continued investigation, development and selection of α-galactosidases may reduce or eliminate this variability in response. Currently, the most viable approach for the use of α-galactosidase may be as a component in a multi-enzyme complex. Jasek *et al.* (2018) investigated the effect of an enzyme complex containing α-galactosidase and xylanase when supplemented to maize–soy–MBM– bakery diets varying in nutrient concentration (energy and amino acids) and reported the enzyme complex significantly increased energy digestibility by 2.8% and crude protein (CP) digestibility by 3.8% with increased digestibility of all essential amino acids in 21-day-old broilers (Table 5.5). This complementary approach may currently be the most viable approach for an α-galactosidase in monogastric nutrition; however, with continued development, an independent enzyme application may be viable under the right circumstances.

5.5 Pectinase

Chemically, pectin substances are complex colloidal acid polysaccharides, with a backbone of galacturonic acid residues linked by α-1,4 linkages. The side chains of the pectin molecule consist of L-rhamnose, arabinose, galactose and xylose. The carboxyl groups of galacturonic acid are partially esterified by methyl groups and partially or completely neutralized by sodium, potassium or ammonium ions (Kashyap *et al.*, 2001). Pectin is structurally and functionally the most complex polysaccharide in the plant cell wall (Mohnen, 2008). The concentration of pectin varies considerably throughout feedstuffs. Malathi and Devegowda (2001) reported the pectin and total NSP contents of a variety of potential feedstuffs for monogastric animals (Table 5.6). Pectinolytic enzymes are a group of enzymes which hydrolyse pectin and can be divided into hydrolases and lyases (Sakai *et al.*, 1993).

The *in vitro* assays contacted by Malathi and Devegowda (2001) used a two-stage *in vitro* digestion to better simulate the digestive tract of a bird. In their research, multiple enzyme combinations were evaluated and with regard to SBM, the addition of pectinase into the combination led to a further reduction in *in vitro* viscosity and higher total sugar release than combinations without pectinase; however, similar reductions in viscosity were not observed when adding the enzymes into broiler feed samples. As expected, enzyme addition through an *in vitro* system increased the total sugars released during the digestion period, with the highest again being the combination that contained pectinase. Similar results were reported by Kocher *et al.* (2002), who observed increased sugar release with a multi-enzyme containing pectinase supplementation of SBM.

Tahir *et al.* (2008) developed a model using the amount of free galacturonic acid as an index or marker for pectin hydrolysis and determined the impact of single and multi-enzymes on galacturonic acid concentration. The model correlated galacturonic acid concentration to CP and DM digestibility with R^2 values for each model of 0.75 and 0.97, respectively. These researchers evaluated the impact of purified cellulase, hemicellulase, pectinase and their combinations when added to a maize–SBM-based diet in an *in vitro* assay. Individual inclusions of each enzyme did not benefit CP or DM digestibility; however, hemicellulase did increase galacturonic acid compared with the control diet.

Table 5.5. Apparent ileal amino acid (AA) and energy digestibility (%) of male broilers fed a positive control (PC) or a negative control (NC) diet with or without supplementation of α-galactosidase enzyme. The NC diet contained a 2.5% reduction in apparent metabolizable energy and digestible AAs. (From Jasek et al., 2018.)

Diet	Enzyme	Thr	Cys	Val	Met	Ile	Leu	Lys	Arg	Trp	Total AA	IDE (kcal/kg)
PC	Control	68.8	62.1	72.7	86.3	75.4	70.5	80.5	86.2	80.9	76.5	3174.3
NC	Control	67.0	60.6	72.0	85.7	74.6	70.6	80.1	86.4	78.1	76.0	3109.9
PC	Enzyme[a]	73.0	68.4	77.6	89.4	79.7	75.1	83.5	88.5	84.8	80.6	3304.4
NC	Enzyme[a]	69.1	65.7	73.7	88.5	75.6	71.1	81.3	87.0	80.7	77.8	3167.5
Diet												
PC		70.8[A]	65.2[A]	75.1[A]	87.8[A]	77.5[A]	72.7[A]	82.0[A]	87.3[A]	82.8[A]	78.5[A]	0.752[A]
NC		68.0[B]	63.1[A]	72.8[B]	87.0[A]	75.1[B]	70.8[A]	80.7[A]	86.7[A]	79.3[B]	76.9[A]	0.734[A]
Enzyme												
Control		67.9[B]	61.4[B]	72.3[B]	86.0[B]	75.0[B]	70.5[B]	80.3[B]	86.3[A]	79.5[B]	76.3[B]	0.729[B]
Enzyme[a]		71.0[A]	67.1[A]	75.6[A]	88.9[A]	77.7[A]	73.1[A]	82.4[A]	87.8[A]	82.7[A]	79.2[A]	0.755[A]
P value												
Diet		0.050	0.211	0.056	0.276	0.030	0.155	0.175	0.367	<0.001	0.118	0.091
Enzyme		0.031	0.001	0.009	<0.001	0.021	0.049	0.035	0.063	0.001	0.008	0.030
Diet × Enzyme		0.454	0.739	0.192	0.847	0.140	0.144	0.362	0.245	0.482	0.275	0.235
Pooled SEM		0.8	0.9	0.7	0.4	0.6	0.7	0.5	0.4	0.5	0.6	0.006

IDE, ileal digestible energy; SEM, standard error of the mean.

[a]AlphaGal™, Kerry Inc., Beloit, Wisconsin.

[A,B]In the separate Diet and Enzyme comparisons, mean values within a column with unlike upper-case superscript letters are significantly different at $P < 0.05$.

Table 5.6. Total pentosan, cellulose, pectin and total NSP content (%) of different feed ingredients[a]. (From Malathi and Devegowda, 2001.)

Ingredient	Total pentosan	Cellulose	Pectin	Total NSP
Maize	5.35	3.12	1.00	9.32
Sorghum	2.77	4.21	1.66	9.75
De-oiled rice bran	10.65	15.20	7.25	59.97
Soybean meal	4.21	5.75	6.16	29.02
Peanut meal	6.11	6.55	11.60	29.50
Sunflower meal	11.01	22.67	4.92	41.34
Rapeseed meal	8.85	14.21	8.86	39.79

[a]Each value represents the mean of triplicate analysis.

Furthermore, when combining the enzymes, benefits in CP and DM digestibility as well as galacturonic acid were observed with hemicellulase + pectinase, cellulase + hemicellulose, and cellulase + hemicellulase + pectinase compared with the control. The combination of all three single enzymes resulted in increased digestibility and galacturonic acid concentration compared with all combinations containing only two enzymes. These results demonstrate the importance of hemicellulose as no combination without hemicellulase resulted in differences from the control and confirm the benefit of pectinase to maximize digestibility.

In a follow-up *in vivo* study to the *in vitro* assay, Tahir *et al.* (2008) evaluated the use of only a combination multi-enzyme of cellulase, hemicellulase and pectinase as these were more efficacious in the *in vitro* evaluation compared with individual enzyme inclusion. The researchers evaluated a low-protein diet (2% less CP than the control diet) with enzyme addition. Enzymatic inclusion in both the control diet and the low-protein diet resulted in increased BW gain, reduced FCR, increased carcass yield, and increased protein digestibility and DM digestibility. Enzymatic addition to the low-protein diet resulted in similar growth performance and digestibility to the control diet without enzyme, indicating this combination of enzymes was capable of compensating for a reduction in CP.

A similar study from the same research team (Tahir *et al.*, 2006) evaluated multiple combinations of cellulase, hemicellulase and pectinase on broiler performance and digestibility. Addition of three combinations,

including cellulase + pectinase, hemicellulase + pectinase, and hemicellulase + cellulase + pectinase, increased protein digestibility, DM digestibility, apparent metabolizable energy (AME) and carcass yield, while pectinase alone was unable to significantly influence any of these parameters. Similarly, Igbasan *et al.* (1997) reported that increasing the level of pectinase was unable to improve broiler performance when fed a diet containing peas; however, the addition of α-galactosidase to the lowest level of pectinase tended to increase BW gain ($P = 0.06$), confirming the need for additional enzyme activity aside from pectinase for consistent improvement.

These observations of enzyme combinations including pectinase increasing digestibility compared with single or multi-enzymes without pectinase in diets with varying ingredient profiles have also been reported by other researchers. In the evaluation of defatted flaxseed meal, enzyme combinations of cellulase, pectinase, xylanase, glucanase and mannanase were more effective in NSP degradation than when included individually. Compared with the control, the inclusion of the enzyme combination degraded 35% of the NSPs present following *in vitro* application (Slominski *et al.*, 2006). When evaluating the combination of cellulase + pectinase + xylanase + glucanase, increased TME_n of defatted flaxseed meal from 2717 to 3750 kcal/kg in adult roosters, decreased FCR in broiler chicks by 3.5 points and increased AME_n of the diet from 2701 to 2846 kcal/kg were observed. Similar results were found when adding these enzymes to canola seed (Meng *et al.*, 2006). Meng and Slominski (2005) demonstrated the benefits of the inclusion of a multi-enzyme containing xylanase, glucanase, pectinase, cellulase, mannanase and galactanase on performance and/or NSP and nutrient digestibility in maize diets containing SBM, canola meal or peas as the protein source. Improvements in FCR of 4 points were reported with the SBM while reductions of 50 to 55% in digesta NSP content and increases in starch digestibility between 1.5 and 2.5% were reported for diets containing peas, canola and SBM.

In general, published reports investigating the use of enzyme combinations containing pectinase are viable as multiple published reports describe observed advantages in nutrient digestibility, growth performance and carcass yield (Meng and Slominski, 2005; Saleh *et al.*, 2005; Meng *et al.*, 2006; Slominski *et al.*, 2006; Tahir *et al.*, 2006, 2008). The dietary components in these reports vary and included protein sources such as SBM, canola, flaxseed meal and peas. However, other reports indicate a lack of individual activity of pectinase or no impact of a multi-enzyme which contained pectinase (Zyla *et al.*, 1996; Igbasan and Guenter, 1997). Regardless, the numerous published data reporting beneficial impacts all have pectinase in the form of a multi-enzyme complex combined with other carbohydrases. *In vitro* assays demonstrate the potential of pectinase inclusion in multi-enzyme products for further sugar release and NSP degradation. However, the translation of these *in vitro* assays to consistent improvement in growth performance has not materialized. Interestingly, the vast majority of the published literature regarding pectinase inclusion in monogastric animal feeds is more than a decade old. The lack of recent work either indicates an obstacle to expand pectinase use such as cost or efficacy or a lack of innovation, advancement and technology.

5.6　Conclusion

As there are now more than 30 years of published research data on carbohydrase use in monogastric nutrition, we must reflect on where we have been and where we are going. At this juncture, an overwhelming adoption of carbohydrases in poultry diets has taken place globally over the past decade. The vast majority of the enzymes currently used are xylanase based; however, many contain additional activities such as mannanase, galactosidase, glucanase, cellulase, hemicellulase and/or pectinase although the main focus is on xylanase. The main reason for this centres around reliability, consistency and price. Increased competition in this market has resulted in more consistent, efficacious and cost-effective products in which formulating nutritionists trust, although xylanase mainly targets NSPs present in cereal grains (maize and wheat) which do comprise the majority of a monogastric diet. However, a large concentration of NSPs is present in SBM which represents a potential source of additional nutrients for the animal and is mainly responsible for the low ME value of SBM and other protein sources.

We have just discussed the vast amount of research that has focused on β-mannanase, α-galactosidase and pectinase. These enzymes are clearly more efficacious in poultry as compared with swine presently and the authors believe this will hold true for the foreseeable future. The inconsistent results in swine currently represent a barrier to widespread adoption; however, they also represent an opportunity for development of enzymes with more consistent and predictive responses.

Within each enzyme, numerous research reports demonstrate enzymatic efficacy and animal benefit and allude to circumstances in which these enzymes provide a benefit to the animal. At this juncture, β-mannanase is the only one of the three enzymes that has currently demonstrated the ability to provide consistent and predictable digestibility and performance improvement when fed as a single-source enzyme. However, as demonstrated by Latham *et al.* (2018), diets low in β-mannan (β-mannan concentrations are low in SBM) do not respond to inclusions of β-mannanase due to lack of available substrate. Therefore, nutritionists must consider ingredient profile and concentration to determine the potential benefit that β-mannanase will provide them. Williams *et al.* (2014) demonstrated a feeding strategy in which β-mannanase can be fed early during grow out when SBM levels are higher in the diet and switch to a xylanase-based enzyme in the final diets of the commercial broiler as SBM and β-mannan levels drop.

Regarding α-galactosidase and pectinase, the research is fairly definitive in the fact that these two enzymes in the current industry would not be successful if fed as a single enzyme but can have value when included in a multi-enzyme product. Jasek *et al.* (2018) demonstrated the results of feeding a multi-enzyme product that contains α-galactosidase on amino acid and energy digestibility. Similarly, Tahir *et al.* (2006, 2008) and Slominski *et al.* (2006) demonstrated the digestibility and performance benefits of enzyme combinations that contain pectinase over individual enzyme feeding. Currently the role for α-galactosidase and pectinase is in a complementary role and the authors do not expect that to change dramatically over the coming decade. However, as the industry continues to strive to improve efficiency combined with

reducing the environmental impact and production footprint, the authors believe the development and advancement of enzyme technology of complementary enzymes such as α-galactosidase and pectinase will continue. Continued market competition and research and development will lead to improved *in vivo* efficacy and increased enzyme production yield which should lead to reduced production costs, putting these complementary enzymes in a position for inclusion in more multi-enzyme products. Although there are some trends that may apply stress to development, such as the move towards lower-CP diets that reduce the amount of SBM and other protein ingredients in the diet, continued genetic selection and improvement combined with addition of by-product meals and protein alternatives will impact the amounts of substrates that these enzymes target in future diets. Overall, the authors believe the opportunities outweigh the potential risks and that exponential growth potential exists within these classes of enzymes, although growth will likely be as components within multi-enzyme products.

References

Adibmoradi, M. and Mehri, M. (2007) Effects of β-mannanase on broiler performance and gut morphology. In: *Proceedings of the 16th European Symposium on Poultry Nutrition, Strasbourg, France, 26–30 August 2007*. World's Poultry Science Association, Beekbergen, the Netherlands, pp. 471–474.

Almirall, M., Fransesch, M., Perez-Vendrell, A., Brufau, D. and Esteve-Garcia, E. (1995) The differences in intestinal viscosity produced by barley and β-glucanase alter digesta enzyme activities and ileal nutrient digestibilities more in broiler chicks than in cocks. *The Journal of Nutrition* 125, 947–955.

Arsenault, R., Kogut, M., Latham, R., Carter, B. and Lee, J.T. (2017) Broilers fed β-mannanase display reduced gut feed-induced immune response signaling. *Poultry Science* 96, 4307–4316.

Asano, I., Nakamura, Y., Hoshino, H., Aoki, K., Fujii, S., *et al.* (2001) Use of mannooligosaccharides from coffee mannan by intestinal bacteria. *Nippon Nogeikagaku Kaishi* 75, 1077–1083.

Bedford, M.R. (1993) Mode of action of feed enzymes. *Journal of Applied Poultry Research* 2, 85–92.

Bedford, M.R. and Classen, H.L. (1992) Reduction of intestinal viscosity through manipulation of dietary rye and pentosanase concentration is effected through changes in the carbohydrate composition of the intestinal aqueous phase and results in improved growth rate and food conversion efficiency of broiler chicks. *The Journal of Nutrition* 122, 560–569.

Bedford, M.R. and Morgan, A.J. (1996) The use of enzymes in poultry diets. *World's Poultry Science Journal* 52, 61–68.

Carpita, N. and McCann, M. (2000) The cell wall in biochemistry and molecular biology of plants. In: Buchanan, B.B., Gruissem, W. and Jones, R. (eds) *Biochemistry and Molecular Biology of Plants*. American Society of Plant Physiologists, Rockville, Maryland, pp. 52–108.

Chauhan, P., Puri, N., Sharma, P. and Gupta, N. (2012) Mannanases: microbial sources, production, properties and potential biotechnological applications. *Applied Microbiology and Biotechnology* 93, 1817–1830.

Choct, M. and Annison, G. (1992) The inhibition of nutrient digestion by wheat pentosans. *British Poultry Science* 67, 123–132.

Coon, C., Leske, K., Akavanichan, O. and Cheng, T. (1990) Effect of oligosaccharide-free soybean meal on true metabolizable energy and fiber digestion in adult roosters. *Poultry Science* 69, 787–793.

Cromwell, G. (1999) Soybean meal – the 'gold standard'. *The Farmer's Pride, KPPA News* 11(20), 10 November.

Dale, N., Anderson, D. and Hsiao, H. (2008) Identification of an inflammatory compound for chicks in soybean meal. *Poultry Science* 87(Suppl. 1), 153.

Daskiran, M., Teeter, R., Fodge, D. and Hsiao, H. (2004) An evaluation of endo-β-D-mannanase (Hemicell) effects on broiler performance and energy use in diets varying in β-mannan content. *Poultry Science* 83, 662–668.

Dhawan, S. and Kaur, J. (2007) Microbial mannanases: an overview of production and applications. *Critical Reviews in Biotechnology* 27, 197–216.

Dierick, N.A. (1989) Biotechnology aids to improve feed and feed digestion: enzyme and fermentation. *Archives of Animal Nutrition* 39, 241–246.

Dusterhoft, E., Posthumus, M. and Voragen, A. (1992) Non-starch polysaccharides from sunflower meal and palm kernel meal preparation of cell wall material and extraction of polysaccharide fractions. *Journal of the Science of Food and Agriculture* 59, 151–160.

Edwards, C., Johnson, I. and Read, N. (1988) Do viscous polysaccharides slow absorption by inhibiting diffusion or convection? *European Journal of Clinical Nutrition* 42, 306–312.

Ferreira, H. Jr, Hannas, M., Albino, L., Rostagno, H., Neme, R., *et al.* (2016) Effect of the addition of β-mannanase on the performance, metabolizable energy, amino acid digestibility coefficients, and immune functions of broilers fed different nutritional levels. *Poultry Science* 95, 1848–1857.

Ghazi, S., Rooke, J. and Galbraith, H. (2003) Improvement in nutritive value of soybean meal by protease and α-galactosidase treatment in broiler cockerels and broiler chicks. *British Poultry Science* 44, 410–418.

Gitzelmann, R. and Auricchio, S. (1965) The handling of soy α-galactosidase by a normal and galactosemic child. *Pediatrics* 36, 231–232.

Graham, K., Kerley, M., Firman, J. and Allee, G. (2002) The effect of enzyme treatment of soybean meal on oligosaccharide disappearance and chick growth performance. *Poultry Science* 81, 1014–1019.

Gray, K., Zhao, L. and Emptage, M. (2006) Bioethanol. *Current Opinion in Chemical Biology* 10, 141–146.

Gullon, P., Gullon, B., Moure, A., Alonso, J., Dominguez, H. and Parajo, J. (2009) Biological properties of mannans and mannan-derived products. In: Charalampopoulos, D. and Rastall, R. (eds) *Prebiotics and Probiotics Science and Technology*. Springer, New York, pp. 559–566.

Gutierrez, O., Zhang, C., Caldwell, D., Carey, J., Cartwright, A. and Bailey, C. (2008) Guar meal diets as an alternative approach to inducing molt and improving *Salmonella enteritidis* resistance in late-phase laying hens. *Poultry Science* 87, 536–540.

Hahn, J., Gahl, M., Giesemann, M., Holzgraefe, D. and Fodge, D. (1995) Diet type and feed form effects on the performance of finishing swine fed beta-mannanase enzyme product Hemicell. *Journal of Animal Science* 73(Suppl. 1), 175.

Honig, D. and Rackis, J. (1979) Determination of the total pepsin-pancreatin indigestible content (dietary fiber) of soybean products, wheat bran, and corn bran. *Journal of Agricultural and Food Chemistry* 27, 1262–1266.

Hsiao, H., Anderson, D. and Dale, N. (2006) Levels of β-mannan in soybean meal. *Poultry Science* 85, 1430–1432.

Huntley, N., Nyachoti, C. and Patience, J. (2018) Lipopolysaccharide immune stimulation but not β-mannanase supplementation affects maintenance energy requirements in young weaned pigs. *Journal of Animal Science and Biotechnology* 9, 47.

Igbasan, F. and Guenter, W. (1997) The influence of micronization, dehulling, and enzyme supplementation on the nutritional value of peas for laying hens. *Poultry Science* 6, 331–337.

Igbasan, F., Guenter, W. and Slominski, B. (1997) The effect of pectinase and alpha-galactosidase supplementation on the nutritive value of peas for broiler chickens. *Canadian Journal of Animal Science* 77, 537–539.

Irish, G.G. and Balnave, D. (1993) Non-starch polysaccharides and broiler performance on diets containing soybean meal as the sole protein concentrate. *Australian Journal of Agricultural Research* 44, 1483–1499.

Irish, G., Barbour, G., Classen, H., Tyler, R. and Bedford, M. (1995) Removal of α-galactosides of sucrose from soybean meal using either ethanol extraction or exogenous α-galactosidase and broiler performance. *Poultry Science* 74, 1484–1494.

Jackson, M., Fodge, D. and Hsiao, H. (1999) Effects of β-mannanase in corn–soybean meal diets on laying hen performance. *Poultry Science* 78, 1737–1741.

Jackson, M., James, R., Anderson, D. and Hsiao, H. (2002a) Improvement of body weight uniformity in turkey using β-mannanase (Hemicell). *Poultry Science* 81(Suppl. 1), 42.

Jackson, M., James, R., Hsiao, H., Krueger, K. and Mathis, G. (2002b) Effects of β-mannanase (Hemicell) on performance, carcass characteristics, and body weight uniformity in commercial tom turkeys. *Poultry Science* 81(Suppl. 1), 23.

Jackson, M., Anderson, D., Hsiao, H., Mathis, G. and Fodge, D. (2003) Beneficial effect of β-mannanase feed enzyme on performance of chicks challenged with *Eimeria* sp. and *Clostridium perfringens*. *Avian Diseases* 47, 759–763.

Jackson, M., Geronian, K., Knox, A., McNab, J. and McCartney, E. (2004) A dose–response study with the feed enzyme β-mannanase in broilers provided with corn–soybean meal-based diets in the absence of antibiotic growth promoters. *Poultry Science* 83, 1992–1996.

Jackson, M., Anderson, D., Hsiao, H., Jin, F. and Mathis, G. (2005) Effect of β-mannanase (Hemicell) on performance and body weight uniformity in broiler chickens provided with corn–soybean meal diets and economic ramifications. *Poultry Science* 84(Suppl. 1), 82.

Jackson, M., Greenwood, M., Stephens, K. and Mathis, G. (2008) An estimation of the energy value of β-mannanase (Hemicell feed enzyme) in turkey toms under practical conditions using varying energy levels. *Poultry Science* 87(Suppl. 1), 161.

Jasek, A., Latham, R., Manon, A., Llamas-Moya, S., Adhikari, R., et al. (2018) Impact of a multicarbohydrase containing α-galactosidase and xylanase on ileal digestible energy, crude protein digestibility, and ileal amino acid digestibility in broiler chickens. *Poultry Science* 97, 3149–3155.

Kashyap, D., Vohra, P., Chopra, S. and Tewari, R. (2001) Applications of pectinases in the commercial sector: a review. *Bioresource Technology* 77, 215–227.

Kiarie, E., Romero, L. and Nyachoti, C. (2013) The role of added feed enzymes in promoting gut health in swine and poultry. *Nutrition Research Reviews* 26, 71–88.

Kidd, M., Morgan, G., Price, C., Welch, P., Brinkhaus, F. and Fontana, E. (2001a) Enzyme supplementation to corn and soybean meal diets for broilers. *Journal of Applied Poultry Research* 10, 65–70.

Kidd, M., Morgan, G., Zumwalt, C., Price, C., Welch, P., et al. (2001b) α-Galactosidase enzyme supplementation to corn and soybean meal broiler diets. *Journal of Applied Poultry Research* 10, 186–193.

Kim, I., Kim, J., Hong, J., Kwon, O., Min, B. and Lee, W. (2003) Effects of β-mannanase enzyme addition on swine performance fed low and high energy diets without antibiotics. In: *Proceedings of the 9th International Symposium on Digestive Physiology in Pigs, Banff, Alberta, Canada, 14–18 May 2003*. University of Alberta, Alberta, Canada, pp. 302–304.

Kim, J., Ingale, S., Hosseindoust, A., Lee, S., Lee, J. and Chae, B. (2017) Effects of mannan level and β-mannanase supplementation on growth performance, apparent total tract digestibility and blood metabolites of growing pigs. *Animal* 11, 202–208.

Kimura, Y., Ohno, A. and Takagi, S. (1997) Structural analysis of N-glycans of storage glycoproteins in soybean seed. *Bioscience, Biotechnology & Biochemistry* 61, 1866–1871.

Klein, J., Williams, M., Brown, B., Rao, S. and Lee, J.T. (2015) Effects of dietary inclusion of a cocktail NSPase and β-mannanase separately and in combination in low energy diets on broiler performance and processing parameters. *Journal of Applied Poultry Research* 24, 489–501.

Knap, K., Ohmann, H. and Dale, N. (1996) Improved bioavailability of energy and growth performance from adding α-galactosidase (from *Aspergillus* sp.) to soybean meal-based diets. *Proceedings of the Australian Poultry Science Symposium* 8, 153–156.

Kocher, A., Choct, M., Porter, M. and Broz, J. (2002) Effects of feed enzymes on nutritive value of soybean meal by broilers. *British Poultry Science* 43, 54–63.

Kratzer, F., Rajagurer, R. and Vohra, P. (1967) The effect of polysaccharides on energy utilization, nitrogen retention and fat absorption in chickens. *Poultry Science* 46, 1489–1493.

Kwon, W. and Kim, B. (2015) Effects of supplemental β-mannanase on digestible energy and metabolizable energy contents of copra expellers and palm kernel expellers fed to pigs. *Asian-Australian Journal of Animal Science* 28, 1014–1019.

Latham, R., Williams, M., Smith, K., Stringfellow, K., Clemente, S., et al. (2016) Effect of β-mannanase inclusion on growth performance, ileal digestible energy, and intestinal viscosity of male broilers fed a reduced-energy diet. *Journal of Applied Poultry Research* 25, 40–47.

Latham, R., Williams, M., Walters, H., Carter, B. and Lee, J.T. (2018) Efficacy of β-mannanase on broiler growth performance and energy utilization in the presence of increasing dietary galactomannan. *Poultry Science* 97, 549–556.

Lázaro, R., Garcia, M., Aranibar, M.J. and Mateos, G.G. (2003) Effect of enzyme addition to wheat-, barley- and rye-based diets on nutrient digestibility and performance of laying hens. *British Poultry Science* 44, 256–265.

Lee, J.T., Bailey, C. and Cartwright, A. (2003a) β-Mannanase ameliorates viscosity-associated depression of growth in broiler chickens fed guar germ and hull fractions. *Poultry Science* 82, 1925–1931.

Lee, J.T., Bailey, C. and Cartwright, A. (2003b) Guar meal germ and hull fractions differently affect growth performance and intestinal viscosity of broiler chickens. *Poultry Science* 82, 1589–1595.

Lee, J.T., Connor-Appleton, S., Haq, A., Bailey, C. and Cartwright, A. (2004) Quantitative measurement of negligible trypsin inhibitor activity and nutrient analysis of guar meal fraction. *Journal of Agricultural and Food Chemistry* 52, 6492–6495.

Lee, J.T., Bailey, C. and Cartwright, A. (2009) *In vitro* viscosity as a function of guar meal and β-mannanase content of feeds. *International Journal of Poultry Science* 8, 715–719.

Li, Y., Chen, X., Chen, Y., Li, Z. and Cao, Y. (2010) Effects of β-mannanase expressed by *Pichia pastoris* in corn–soybean meal diets on broiler performance, nutrient digestibility, energy utilization and immuno-globulin levels. *Animal Feed Science and Technology* 159, 59–67.

Maisonnier, S., Gomez, J. and Carre, B. (2001) Nutrient digestibility and intestinal viscosities in broiler chickens fed on wheat diets, as compared to corn diets with added guar gum. *British Poultry Science* 42, 102–110.

Malathi, V. and Devegowda, G. (2001) *In vitro* evaluation of nonstarch polysaccharide digestibility of feed ingredients by enzymes. *Poultry Science* 80, 302–305.

McCleary, B. (1979) Modes of action of β-mannanase enzymes of diverse origin on legume seed galactomannans. *Phytochemistry* 18, 757–763.

McCleary, B.V. (1988) β-Mannanase. *Methods in Enzymology* 160, 596–610.

McCleary, B. (1991) Comparison of endolytic hydrolases that depolymerize 1,4-/3-β-mannan, 1,5-α-L-arabinan and 1,4-β-D-galactan. In: Leaham, G.F. and Himmel, M.E. (eds) *Enzymes in Biomass Conversion.* American Chemical Society, Washington, DC, pp. 437–449.

Meng, X. and Slominski, B. (2005) Nutritive values of corn, soybean meal, canola meal, and peas for broiler chickens as affected by a multicarbohydrase preparation of cell wall degrading enzymes. *Poultry Science* 84, 1242–1251.

Meng, X., Slominski, B.A., Nyachoti, C.M., Campbell, L.D. and Guenter, W. (2005) Degradation of cell wall polysaccharides by combinations of carbohydrase enzymes and their effect on nutrient utilization and broiler chicken performance. *Poultry Science* 84, 37–47.

Meng, X., Slominski, B., Campbell, L., Guenter, W. and Jones, O. (2006) The use of enzyme technology for improved energy utilization from full-fat oilseeds. Part I: Canola seed. *Poultry Science* 85, 1025–1030.

Mohnen, D. (2008) Pectin structure and biosynthesis. *Current Opinion in Plant Biology* 11, 266–277.

Moreira, L. and Filho, E. (2008) An overview of mannan structure and mannan-degrading enzyme systems. *Applied Microbiology and Biotechnology* 79, 165–178.

Odetallah, N., Ferket, P., Grimes, J. and McNaughton, J. (2002) Effect of mannan-endo-1,4-β-mannosidase on the growth performance of turkey fed diets containing 44 and 48% crude protein soybean meal. *Poultry Science* 81, 1322–1331.

Ofek, I., Mirelman, D. and Sharon, N. (1977) Adherence of *Escherichia coli* to human mucosal cells mediated by mannose receptors. *Nature* 265, 623–625.

O'Quinn, P., Funderburke, D., Funderburke, C. and James, R. (2002) Influence of dietary supplementation with β-mannanase on performance of finishing pigs in a commercial system. *Journal of Animal Science* 80(Suppl. 2), 65.

Pan, B., Li, D., Piao, X., Zhang, L. and Guo, L. (2002) Effect of dietary supplementation with α-galactosidase preparation and stachyose on growth performance, nutrient digestibility and intestinal bacterial populations of piglets. *Archiv für Tierernahrung* 56, 327–337.

Parsons, C., Zhang, Y. and Araba, M. (2000) Nutritional evaluation of soybean meals varying in oligosaccharide content. *Poultry Science* 79, 1127–1131.

Petkowicz, C., Reicher, F., Chanzy, H., Taravel, F. and Vuong, R. (2001) Linear mannan in the endosperm of *Schizolobium amazonicum*. *Carbohydrate Polymers* 44, 107–112.

Pettey, L., Carter, S., Senne, B. and Shriver, J. (2002) Effects of β-mannanase addition to corn–soybean meal diets on growth performance, carcass traits, and nutrient digestibility of weaning and growing-finishing pigs. *Journal of Animal Science* 80, 1012–1019.

Piao, X., Wang, C., Li, D., Gong, L., Xu, G. and Kang, X. (2003) Effects of β-mannanase (Hemicell) on broiler performance and flock uniformity fed normal and low energy diets with and without antibiotics. *Poultry Science* 82(Suppl. 1), 29.

Rainbird, A., Low, A. and Zebrowska, T. (1984) Effect of guar gum on glucose and water absorption from isolated loops of jejunum in conscious growing pigs. *British Journal of Nutrition* 52, 489–498.

Read, N. (1986) Dietary fiber and bowel transit. In: Vahouny, G. and Kritchevsky, D. (eds) *Dietary Fiber: Basic and Clinical Aspects*. Plenum Press, New York, pp. 91–100.

Reid, J.S.G. (1985) Cell wall storage carbohydrates in seeds: biochemistry of the seed gums and hemicelluloses. *Advances in Botanical Research* 11, 125–155.

Sakai, T., Sakamoto, T., Hallaert, J. and Vandamme, E. (1993) Pectin, pectinase, and protopectinase. Production, properties, and application. *Advances in Applied Microbiology* 39, 213–294.

Saki, A., Mazugi, M. and Kemyab, A. (2005) Effect of mannanase on broiler performance, ileal and *in vitro* protein digestibility, uric acid and litter moisture in broiler feeding. *International Journal of Poultry Science* 4, 21–26.

Saleh, F., Tahir, M., Ohtsuka, A. and Havashi, K. (2005) A mixture of pure cellulase, hemicellulase and pectinase improves broiler performance. *British Poultry Science* 46, 602–606.

Shang, Q., Ma, X., Li, M., Zhang, L., Hu, J. and Piao, X. (2018) Effects of α-galactosidase supplementation on nutrient digestibility, growth performance, intestinal morphology and digestive enzyme activities in weaned pigs. *Animal Feed Science and Technology* 236, 45–56.

Shastak, Y., Ader, P., Feuerstein, D., Ruehle, R. and Matuschek, M. (2015) β-Mannan and mannanase in poultry nutrition. *World's Poultry Science Journal* 71, 161–174.

Slominski, B.A. (2011) Recent advances in research on enzymes for poultry diets. *Poultry Science* 90, 2013–2023.

Slominski, B., Meng, X., Campbell, L., Guenter, W. and Jones, O. (2006) The use of enzyme technology for improved energy utilization from full-fat oilseeds. Part II: Flaxseed. *Poultry Science* 85, 1031–1037.

Smiricky, M., Grieshop, C., Albin, D., Wubben, J. and Fahey, G. (2002) The influence of soy oligosaccharides on apparent and true ileal amino acid digestibilities and fecal consistency in growing pigs. *Journal of Animal Science* 80, 2433–2441.

Smits, C., Veldman, A., Verstegen, M. and Beynen, A. (1997) Dietary carboxymethylcellulose with high instead of low viscosity reduces macronutrient digestion in broiler chickens. *The Journal of Nutrition* 127, 483–487.

Stalbrand, H., Siika-Aho, M., Tenkanen, M. and Viikari, L. (1993) Purification and characterization of two β-mannanases from *Trichoderma reesei*. *Journal of Biotechnology* 29, 229–242.

Sundu, B., Kumar, A. and Dingle, J. (2006a) Palm kernel meal in broiler diets: effect on chicken performance and health. *World's Poultry Science Journal* 62, 316–325.

Sundu, B., Kumar, A. and Dingle, J. (2006b) Response of broiler chicks fed increasing levels of copra meal and enzymes. *International Journal of Poultry Science* 5, 13–18.

Tahir, M., Saleh, F., Ohtsuka, A. and Hayashi, K. (2006) Pectinase plays an important role in stimulating digestibility of a corn–soybean meal diet in broilers. *The Journal of Poultry Science* 43, 323–329.

Tahir, M., Saleh, F., Ohtsuka, A. and Hayashi, K. (2008) An effective combination of carbohydrases that enables reduction of dietary protein in broilers: importance of hemicellulase. *Poultry Science* 87, 713–718.

Upadhaya, S., Park, J., Lee, J. and Kim, I. (2016a) Ileal digestibility of nutrients and amino acids in low quality soybean meal sources treated with β-mannanase for growing pigs. *Animal* 10, 1148–1154.

Upadhaya, S., Park, J., Lee, J. and Kim, I. (2016b) Efficacy of β-mannanase supplementation to corn–soya bean meal-based diets on growth performance, nutrient digestibility, blood urea nitrogen, fecal coliform, and lactic acid bacteria and fecal noxious gas emission in growing pigs. *Archives of Animal Nutrition* 70, 33–43.

Van Zyl, W.H., Rose, S.H., Trollope, K. and Gorgens, J. (2010) Fungal β-mannanases: mannan hydrolysis, heterologous production and biotechnological applications. *Process Biology* 45, 1203–1213.

Waldroup, P., Fritts, C., Keen, C. and Yan, F. (2005) The effect of α-galactosidase enzyme with and without Avizyme 1502 on performance of broilers fed diets based on corn and soybean meal. *International Journal of Poultry Science* 4, 920–937.

Waldroup, P., Keen, C., Yan, F. and Zhang, K. (2006) The effect of levels of α-galactosidase enzyme on performance of broilers fed diets based on corn and soybean meal. *Journal of Applied Poultry Research* 15, 48–57.

Wang, C., Lu, W., Li, D. and Xing, J. (2005) Effects of alpha-galactosidase supplementation to corn–soybean meal diets on nutrient utilization, performance, serum indices and organ weight in broilers. *Asian-Australian Journal of Animal Science* 18, 1761–1768.

Weurding, R., Enting, H. and Verstegen, M. (2003) The relation between starch digestion rate and amino acid level for broiler chickens. *Poultry Science* 82, 279–284.

Wiggins, H. (1984) Nutritional value of sugars and related compounds undigested in the small gut. *Proceedings of the Nutrition Society* 43, 69–85.

Williams, M.P., Brown, B., Rao, S. and Lee, J.T. (2014) Evaluation of beta-mannanase and NSP-degrading enzyme inclusion separately or intermittently in reduced energy diets fed to male broilers on performance parameters and carcass yield. *Journal of Applied Poultry Research* 23, 715–723.

Wu, G., Bryant, M., Voitle, R. and Roland, D. (2005) Effect of β-mannanase in corn–soy diets on commercial leghorns in second-cycle hens. *Poultry Science* 84, 894–897.

Zhang, B., Cao, Y., Chen, Y., Li, Y., Qiao, S. and Ma, Y. (2010) Effects of α-galactosidase supplementation on performance and energy metabolism for broilers fed corn-non-dehulled soybean meal diets. *Asian-Australian Journal of Animal Science* 23, 1340–1347.

Zyla, K., Ledoux, D., Kujawski, M. and Veum, T. (1996) The efficacy of an enzymatic cocktail and a fungal mycelium in dephosphorylating corn–soybean meal-based feeds to growing turkeys. *Poultry Science* 75, 381–387.

6 Starch- and Protein-Degrading Enzymes in Non-Ruminant Animal Production

Aaron J. Cowieson[1]*, Laerke T. Haahr[2] and Lars K. Skov[2]
[1]DSM Nutritional Products, Kaiseraugst, Switzerland;
[2]Novozymes A/S, Lyngby, Denmark

6.1 Introduction

Exogenous feed enzymes have been used commercially to enhance environmental and economic sustainability of non-ruminant production animal systems since the 1980s. A substantial research effort has been made over the past four decades to generate actionable insights into mode of action and complementarity of effect to enable their optimal use at the end user level. Considerable efforts have been made with regard to the non-starch polysaccharide-degrading enzymes and phytase, where their value as monocomponent enzymes has been systematically explored. However, the usefulness of proteases and amylases has received considerably less attention and much of the research has been oriented around their value as part of enzyme admixtures where their value contribution is inferred but not always explicitly determined. In the last decade monocomponent amylases and proteases have been launched, which has enabled research into these activities without the confounding effects of adjacent enzymes. While exogenous amylases and proteases have the potential to significantly improve animal performance and the digestibility of energy and amino acids, the mode of action

is not fully defined. Furthermore, given that commercial nutritionists are faced with an array of at least six or seven major exogenous enzyme classes, the assembly of admixtures of enzymes to achieve optimal return on investment is not trivial. The objective of this chapter is to provide background on exogenous amylases and proteases and to explore main effect drivers for *in vivo* response. Literature evidence is presented and considers mode of action, variability of effect and factors that may be considered when exploring the usefulness of these underexploited enzyme activities.

6.2 Biochemistry and Enzymology of Exogenous Amylases

Starch is the main energy source in cereals that are fed to non-ruminant production animals. Starch is present as starch granules and consists of two α-1,4-biopolymers of glucose, amylose and amylopectin (Fig. 6.1). The starch granules need to be opened up and the glucose polymers need to be converted into small oligosaccharides before they can be absorbed and utilized as an energy source

*Email: aaron.cowieson@dsm.com

©CAB International 2022. *Enzymes in Farm Animal Nutrition, 3rd Edition* (M. Bedford *et al.* eds)
DOI: 10.1079/9781789241563.0006

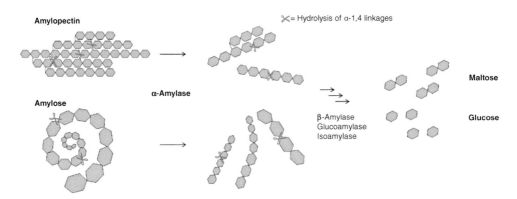

Fig. 6.1. Overview of the enzymes involved in hydrolysis of branched amylopectin (top) and unbranched amylose (bottom) into maltose and glucose. (Created by Novozymes 2021.)

by the animals. In nature (when grains are sprouting or when grains are digested by animals) several enzymes are involved in this process. The enzymes involved in the hydrolysis of the biopolymers (linear amylose and branched amylopectin) are called amylolytic enzymes and include: α-amylase (EC 3.2.1.1), β-amylase (EC 3.2.1.2), cyclodextrin glycosyltransferase (EC 2.4.1.19), glucoamylase (EC 3.2.1.3), α-glucosidase (EC 3.2.1.20) and pullulanase (EC 3.2.1.41) (Wong, 1995; Horváthová *et al.*, 2001). α-Amylases are mid-sized enzymes with about 500 amino acid residues in a single peptide chain. They are known to be Ca^{2+}-dependent and are generally stable molecules. Amylase (originally called diastase) was discovered and isolated in 1833 (Payen and Persoz, 1833) and is today used in many industrial applications to break down starch into smaller sugars. α-Amylases have a cleft-like active site (Fig. 6.2) and can attack the biopolymer (amylose or amylopectin) at many positions. They are so-called endo-acting enzymes. Most α-amylases are found in the glycoside hydrolase family 13 (GH13), but a few are found in the related families 70 and 77 (Horváthová *et al.*, 2001; Lombard *et al.*, 2014).

GH13 is a huge family with more than 86,000 sequences (http://www.cazy.org/GH13.html, accessed 15 September 2021). It is in this family that the endogenous α-amylases from chickens, pigs and humans are found, and where current commercial feed amylases originate. The GH13 family has been further divided into subfamilies that to some extent separate the many enzyme activities found here (Stam *et al.*, 2006). Currently 25 EC numbers are listed in GH13, and α-amylases are found in subfamilies 1, 2, 5–7, 15, 19, 24, 27, 28 and 32. Figure 6.3 illustrates the separation into different subfamilies using three-dimensional structures of α-amylases as found in the Protein Data Bank (https://www.rcsb.org/, accessed 15 September 2021). Nine subfamilies are represented with structures, and they mainly separate according to taxonomic class; for example, subfamily 6 (GH13_6) contains α-amylases from barley and rice, whereas GH13_24 contains mammalian amylases (saliva and pancreatic from humans and pigs). Chicken (*Gallus gallus*) has only the pancreatic homologue and this is also found in GH13_24. Current commercial animal feed amylases are all from bacteria and found in subfamily 5.

6.3 Starch Digestion and the Potential of Exogenous Amylases

The majority of dietary digestible energy in the diets of pigs and poultry is delivered to the animal by ingestion of starch from cereals (Cowieson, 2005). Starch is a heterogeneous polymer of glucose with a complex and variable crystalline macrostructure (Tester *et al.*, 2004). Glucose monomers are connected by α-1,4 or α-1,6 bonds, forming amylose or

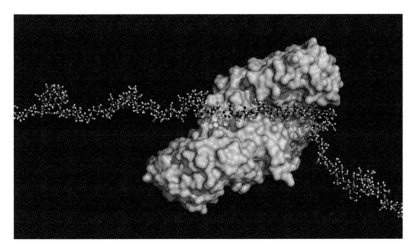

Fig. 6.2. Surface representation (in yellow) of a GH13_5 α-amylase with an amylose fragment (white = hydrogen, black = carbon and red = oxygen) docked into the cleft-like active site. (Created by Novozymes 2021.)

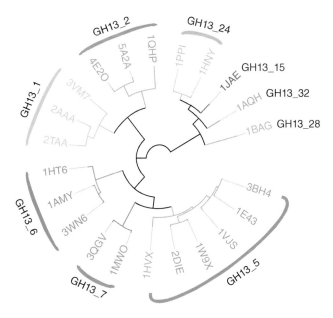

Fig. 6.3. Phylogenetic tree of GH13 α-amylases (EC 3.2.1.1) with publicly known three-dimensional structure (indicated by Protein Data Bank entries (https://www.rcsb.org/, accessed 15 September 2021); sequences that are more than 95% identical are represented as one entry). The sequences separate into different subfamilies and are coloured by taxonomy: Bacilli (light blue) in GH13_2, GH13_5 and GH13_28; *Eurotiomycetes* (light green) in GH13_1; *Lilliopsida* (red) in GH13_6; Thermococci (olive green) in GH13_7; Mammalia (light violet) in GH13_24; Insecta (dark violet) in GH13_15; and Gammaproteobacteria (green) in GH13_32. (Created by Novozymes 2021.)

amylopectin, respectively. Starches with a substantial concentration of amylopectin are referred to as 'waxy', whereas those with a dominant concentration of amylose are described as 'normal' or 'amylo'. Starches with a high ratio of amylopectin to amylose tend to be more amorphous and soluble and so are more readily digestible by livestock

(Moran, 1982). In cereal grains such as maize or wheat, starch does not exist in isolation from other macroscopic structures in the seed. Indeed, starch granules are usually tightly packed in a protein 'envelope' and the extent to which this occurs confers important physicochemical properties to the seed. In cases where the starch is tightly associated with protein the starch is referred to as 'vitreous' and is usually mechanically hard and nutritionally poor. Alternatively, 'floury' starch is friable, loosely associated with protein and typically more readily solubilized and digested (Gibbon *et al.*, 2003; Cowieson, 2005). Thus, while starch may be considered a moderately simple polymer (relative to protein), there is considerable heterogeneity in presentation, association with adjacent macromolecules, solubility and concentration that confers important mechanical, chemical and nutritional characteristics that directly influence feeding value.

In swine, starch digestion is initiated in the mouth via the function of salivary amylase, whereas in poultry starch digestion begins when ingested starch encounters pancreatic amylase in the small intestine (Moran, 1985). Polymeric starch is rapidly degraded to dextrins of variable molecular weight and these oligosaccharides are further hydrolysed to glucose monomers by brush-border maltase and isomaltase prior to absorption by the intestinal enterocytes (Moran, 1985). In non-ruminant livestock species the digestion of starch is relatively high compared with alternative macronutrients such as protein or lipid and may reach 98–100% in some cases. However, evidence for incomplete starch digestion exists (Wiseman *et al.*, 2000) and this may be associated with various factors such as animal age, pancreatic output, feed processing conditions, dietary antinutrient content or intestinal development (Uni *et al.*, 1998; Svihus *et al.*, 2005; Itani and Svihus, 2019).

A significant determinant in the effectiveness of starch digestion may be the extent to which the intestine can process ingested starch over time. Krogdahl and Sell (1989) reported that pancreatic amylase output rose rapidly in the first week post-hatch in chicks, which putatively suggests that older animals may have a greater capacity to degrade dietary starch compared with their neonatal counterparts. However, Croom *et al.* (1999) noted that while intestinal maturity increases with age qualitatively, quantitatively this does not keep pace with the substantial rise in body weight or in feed intake over the life of the animal. Indeed, pancreatic weight relative to body weight reaches a maximum around 14 days post-hatch and declines rapidly thereafter. These factors are important when considering the targeted use of exogenous amylases or other interventions intended to augment endogenous starch digestion in animals and may explain why variable effects of exogenous amylase have been reported in the literature.

Use of monocomponent exogenous amylases in non-ruminant animal production has not received as much attention in the scientific literature compared with alternative carbohydrases such as arabinoxylanase or β-glucanase. However, several studies have been reported and a summary of major results can be found in Table 6.1. Generally, improvements in weight gain and feed conversion from about 2 to 4% have been observed although these effects vary depending on the experimental conditions (age, duration, maize source, etc.). Effects on digestibility of energy of about 80–200 kcal/kg have also been noted and these appear to be greater when measured at the ileal level (as opposed to total tract assessment). Interestingly, exogenous amylase addition to poultry diets has been shown to reduce endogenous amylase secretion and alter intestinal morphology (Mahagna *et al.*, 1995; Gracia *et al.*, 2003; Onderci *et al.*, 2006; Jiang *et al.*, 2008), which is suggestive of nutrient sparing effects that may beneficially influence animal performance. Thus, the effects of exogenous amylase may be mediated both via direct increases in the digestibility of dietary starch and also by augmentation of endogenous enzyme function and intervention in both secretory and absorptive machinery. Future work on exogenous amylase for non-ruminant animal production should focus on exploring variability in effect associated with cereal quality, animal age, gut health and net energy. Further research on variance in

Table 6.1. Overview of the effect of exogenous microbial amylase on poultry performance, nutrient digestibility and intestinal function.

Reference	Species	Diet	Duration	Weight gain effect (%)	FCR effect (%)	Digestibility effect (%)
Stefanello et al. (2015)	Broiler (Cobb 500)	Maize–SBM	Days 14–25	+0.14	–3.0	IDE: +2.7 AME: +2.1
Stefanello et al. (2019)	Broiler (Cobb 500)	Maize–SBM or Maize–SBM + additional maize	Days 14–25	NR	NR	IDE: +5.9 AME: +3.6
De Faria Castro et al. (2020)	Broiler (Cobb 500)	Maize–SBM	Days 21–42	+7.2	–10.7	NR
Yin et al. (2018)	Broiler (Cobb 500)	Maize–SBM– maize gluten meal	Days 5–16	+1.3	–0.7	Ileal starch: +1.7
Stefanello et al. (2017)	Broiler (Cobb 500)	Maize–SBM	Days 1–40	+1.5	–0.1	AME: +3[b]
Vieira et al. (2015)	Broiler (Cobb 500)	Maize–SBM	Days 1–40	+2.0	–0.1	AME: +2.3[b]
Gracia et al. (2003)	Broiler (Cobb 500)	Maize–SBM	Days 1–42	+4.7	–0.1	Ileal starch: +1.6 AME: +2.4
Ritz et al. (1995)	Turkey (Nicholas)	Maize–SBM– fishmeal– MBM	Days 1–35	+2.9	–6.5	NR
Jiang et al. (2008)	Broiler (Arbor Acre)	Maize–SBM	Days 1–21	+4.5	–0.06	NR
Onderci et al. (2006)[a]	Broiler (Cobb 500)	Maize–SBM– fishmeal	Days 1–42	+0.4	–3.0	Total tract dry matter: +2.2

FCR, feed conversion ratio; SBM, soybean meal; MBM, meat and bone meal; NR, not reported; IDE, ileal digestible energy; AME, apparent metabolizable energy.
[a]This study involved feeding a bacterial culture that expressed α-amylase activity.
[b]Determined by regression against an AME titration, not measured.

the capacity to digest starch at the level of the individual animal would also be useful and is largely missing from the scientific literature today.

6.4   Biochemistry and Enzymology of Exogenous Proteases

Proteases are enzymes that are capable of degrading protein. Proteins are large biomolecules built from long linear chains of amino acid residues, called polypeptides. The amino acid residues are joined together by peptide bonds connecting the carboxyl group of one amino acid to the amino group of the next amino acid in the chain. Each of the 20 amino acids has a different side group which varies in size, shape, charge, hydrophobicity and reactivity. The sequence of amino acid residues in a polypeptide chain determines the three-dimensional structure and properties of the protein and is defined by the nucleotide sequence of the gene.

Proteins are an essential nutrient required for the nutrition of all animals. In feed for production animals, protein is a major cost driver. In a typical broiler diet around half the protein will come from protein meals such as soybean meal and rapeseed meal, which contain high concentrations of protein (35–50%), while the other half will come from cereal grains such as maize and wheat which have a lower concentration of protein (8–15%). The protein quality varies between different feed ingredients primarily due to the differences in amino acid composition and protein availability (digestibility), which can also be influenced by processing and various other factors.

As mentioned earlier, proteases are enzymes which are capable of degrading protein by hydrolysing the peptide bonds between amino acid residues, basically cutting the long polypeptide chains into smaller pieces. Proteases constitute a huge enzyme class which differs significantly in both sequence and structure, so that an impressive diversity in terms of functionality (such as specificity, stability, temperature and pH profiles) is found within the protease space. Proteases are categorized into different protease families and subfamilies based on their sequence homology. The six main protease families are called serine, metallo, cysteine, aspartic, glutamic and threonine proteases (Barrett *et al.*, 2012). The names of the protease families refer to the amino acid (or metal ion) in the active site where hydrolysis of peptide bonds takes place and is not descriptive of the substrate specificity of a given protease. Within each main family there are several subfamilies. Furthermore, proteases are grouped into exo- and endopeptidases. Exopeptidases including di- and tripeptidyl peptidases cleave from the end of protein chains, releasing single amino acids, dipeptides or tripeptides. Exopeptidases are categorized as carboxy- or aminopeptidases depending on whether they cleave from the carboxy or amino terminus of the polypeptide. Endopeptidases cleave within the protein chains, releasing and solubilizing larger protein fragments. The site of cleavage for both endo- and exopeptidases further depends on the specificity of the protease. Very specific proteases exclusively cleave next to certain amino acids, limiting the number of cuts in a protein chain, whereas proteases with a broad specificity have substantially more opportunity to catalyse hydrolytic events. Proteases are typically also divided into acid, neutral or alkaline proteases based on their pH optimum, meaning the pH at which they have the highest activity. Acid proteases are most active at low pH and have potential for hydrolysing protein during gastric digestion, while neutral or slightly alkaline proteases will be most active in the small and large intestine. An overview of the major endogenous proteases involved in protein digestion can be found in Table 6.2.

Pepsin is an aspartic endoprotease with broad specificity but is most efficient in cleaving peptide bonds between large hydrophobic amino acids such as phenylalanine and leucine (Tang, 1963; Fruton, 1976). It is an acid protease, suitable to the conditions in the gastric phase of the animal, where pH is low. Trypsin, chymotrypsin and elastase are all endoproteases of the serine protease family and work optimally at pH around 7–9, suitable for the neutral environment in the small intestine (duodenum, jejunum and ileum). Trypsin has a high substrate specificity and primarily hydrolyses peptide bonds next to basic amino acids such as lysine and arginine (Barrett *et al.*, 2012). Chymotrypsin preferably cleaves next to aromatic amino acids such as phenylalanine, tyrosine and tryptophan (Bergmann and Fruton, 1941; Desnuelle, 1960), while elastase hydrolyses at the site of uncharged small amino acids such as alanine, glycine and serine (Bieth, 1978).

Table 6.2. Overview of the major endogenous proteases involved in protein digestion in monogastric animals. (From McDonald *et al.*, 2010.)

Protease	Endo/exo	Protease family	Specificity	Site of action
Pepsin	Endo	Aspartic	Phenylalanine, tyrosine, leucine	Stomach/proventriculus/gizzard
Trypsin	Endo	Serine	Lysine, arginine	Intestines
Chymotrypsin	Endo	Serine	Phenylalanine, tyrosine, tryptophan	Intestines
Elastase	Endo	Serine	Alanine, glycine, serine	Intestines
Carboxypeptidase A	Exo	Metallo	Aromatic or non-polar side chains	Intestines
Carboxypeptidase B	Exo	Metallo	Arginine, lysine	Intestines

The endoprotease activity from pepsin and the three major pancreatic proteases trypsin, chymotrypsin and elastase releases smaller oligopeptides, which are further degraded by exopeptidases, such as carboxypeptidase A and carboxypeptidase B, both coming from the metalloprotease family. The action of these enzymes is aligned so that the endopeptidases produce peptides with C-terminal amino acids, which then become substrates for the exopeptidases. As an example, trypsin produces peptides with basic C-terminal amino acids that are particularly suited for the action of carboxypeptidase B (Folk *et al.*, 1960; Tan and Eaton, 1995).

To regulate protease activity in the gastrointestinal tract, most endogenous proteases are expressed as inactive pro-enzymes which need to be activated, typically by a combination of protease activity and certain conditions (e.g. low pH). The spectrum of endogenous proteases generally offers a diverse and quite effective protein digestion in animals. However, as the animal farming industry evolves, focus on reduced feed costs and sustainability increases, and with that the need for a uniform and consistently high protein digestion grows. The use of exogenous proteases offers the potential to aid endogenous proteases with activities or properties that either synergize with endogenous proteases or supplement what the animals cannot offer themselves. As an example, the major feed source, soybean meal, depending on processing conditions, often contains critical amounts of trypsin inhibitor. Trypsin inhibitors are proteins that, as the name implies, effectively inhibit the proteolytic action of endogenous trypsin with negative consequences on protein digestibility and amino acid uptake by the animals. Exogenous proteases are commonly not inhibited by trypsin inhibitor and some even have the potential to degrade this compound. In a recent publication, where soluble protein was identified by proteomics in the jejunum of broilers fed soybean meal, it was seen that several of the soy proteins including trypsin inhibitor could not or could only partially be digested by endogenous proteases (Cowieson *et al.*, 2016a; Recoules, 2017).

Also, while most endogenous protease activity comes from specific proteases,

exogenous proteases with broader substrate specificity have the potential to aid further in protein degradation by increasing protein digestibility beyond that of endogenous proteases (Cowieson and Roos, 2014). With increased protein digestibility comes a range of positive effects: there will be a smaller fraction of protein left for the unbeneficial bacteria in the hindgut to feed on, which could have positive effects on gut health. Furthermore, the increased protein digestibility leads to less nitrogen in the excreta, having a positive effect on both animal welfare (fewer footpad lesions) and the environment (decreased nitrogen emissions).

As proteases hydrolyse protein and enzymes themselves are proteins, it is theoretically possible that the exogenous proteases could degrade other exogenous or endogenous enzymes. However, this is a statistically highly unlikely event as the proteases are mixed in minute amounts into a feed with high levels of protein, so the chance that a protease will encounter another enzyme and not just feed protein is very low. Trials both *in vitro* (Fig. 6.4) and *in vivo* (Cowieson *et al.*, 2019) have shown that the activity of other exogenous enzymes such as carbohydrases and phytases is not negatively affected by addition of exogenous protease in a feed mixture.

6.5 Protein and Amino Acid Digestion and the Potential of Exogenous Proteases

Protein digestion in non-ruminants is initiated in the gastric gut by the combined function of hydrochloric acid and pepsin and is then completed in the small intestine via sequential activity of several pancreatic and brush-border peptidases (Moran, 2016). Absorption of free amino acids, di- and tripeptides occurs via a suite of specific amino acid transport proteins in the enterocytes and further hydrolysis occurs after absorption by cytosolic peptidases (Sterchi and Woodley, 1980; Ganapathy *et al.*, 2000). Ingested amino acids are required for muscle synthesis but they also have a host of important functional effects such as immune

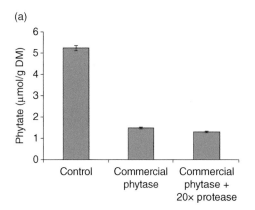
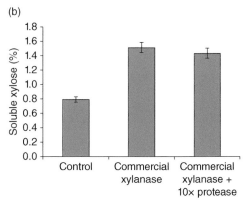

Fig. 6.4. *In vitro* data illustrating that exogenous protease does not degrade or negatively affect other exogenous enzymes. (a) Phytate release from a commercial phytase on a 70:30 mixture of maize:soybean meal is compared with control and a sample with both commercial phytase and 20× recommended dose of protease. (b) The amount of soluble xylose released by a commercial xylanase from a wheat bran-based diet compared with a control and a sample with both xylanase and 10× recommended dose of protease. In both cases, the addition of protease does not influence the effect of other exogenous enzymes. DM, dry matter. (Created by Novozymes 2021.)

function, contribution to intestinal energy budget, cell signalling, gene expression and others (Wu *et al.*, 2014). While some amino acids can be synthesized from various precursors, many are essential and must be supplied by the diet to avoid nutritional inadequacy. Alternative amino acids such as glycine and serine may be considered 'conditionally essential' as while they can be synthesized *de novo*, this process is not trivial and dietary supply is an advantage (Ospina-Rojas *et al.*, 2013).

During the process of protein digestion there is a considerable investment of energy and amino acids made by the host animal that is of sufficient magnitude to generate negative cephalic small intestinal amino acid digestibility values. Fuller and Reeds (1998) estimate that 1 g of endogenous protein is secreted into the gut for every 2 g of dietary protein that is ingested. Secretion of digestive enzymes, bile and mucins and turnover of intestinal cells demand constant replacement and consume significant quantities of energy, and these are only partially recovered by the terminal ileum. Duee *et al.* (1995) estimate that the intestinal tract consumes 20–25% of whole-body oxygen demand through the constant need for protein synthesis and cell turnover. Thus, during the normal digestive process the animal

must not only recover dietary protein of varying mechanical and chemical compatibility but also minimize the synthesis and loss of endogenous protein in order to conserve energy and maximize lifetime fecundity.

The digestibility of dietary protein varies depending on multiple factors including the type and balance of protein in the diet, the age of the animal, feed processing conditions, presence of antinutrients, the inclusion of various additives and others (Cowieson and Roos, 2016; Moran, 2016). In order to reduce variability in digestibility of amino acids and to reduce loss of endogenous amino acids, the use of exogenous proteases has become increasingly common in recent years.

Supplementation of production animal diets with exogenous protease was pioneered by Lewis *et al.* (1955) and Baker *et al.* (1956), and the initial focus was on the effect of supplemental pepsin and pancreatin on feed conversion. Since this early pioneering work many additional reports on the usefulness of exogenous proteases in animal nutrition have been published and suggest significant potential to improve performance across multiple diet types (Castanon and Marquardt, 1989; Huo *et al.*, 1993; Guenter *et al.*, 1995; Hessing *et al.*, 1996; Rooke *et al.*, 1998; Thorpe and Beal, 2001; Odetallah *et al.*, 2003, 2005; Angel *et al.*, 2010;

Freitas *et al.*, 2011; Barekatain *et al.*, 2013; Zuo *et al.*, 2015; Cowieson *et al.*, 2019). However, alternative work has shown that some variance may exist in the potential of exogenous protease to improve performance outcomes for livestock (Walk and Poernama, 2018; Walk *et al.*, 2019). Variability in the response to exogenous enzymes per se is not unexpected and this is likely to be associated with a range of factors such as inherent quality of the diets fed, limiting nutrients, duration experiments, substrate concentrations and others (Bedford, 2002). Similarly, in the case of exogenous protease, some variance in response is likely and this may be associated with the type of protease fed (pH optimum, source organism, substrate specificity), type of dietary protein, animal species and age, as well as several other factors (Cowieson and Roos, 2016). However, one important factor that drives the magnitude of the response to exogenous protease for ileal amino acid digestibility is the inherent digestibility of amino acids in the control feed (Cowieson and Roos, 2014). Indeed, Cowieson and Roos (2014) noted that this single factor explained about 47% of the variance in the biological effect of protease on amino acid digestibility in both pigs and poultry (Fig. 6.5). This implies that

exogenous protease may be a useful tool to reduce variance in amino acid digestibility as diets or animals that have an inherently low nutritional value may benefit more from supplemental protease. Evidence for significant variability in amino acid digestibility at the level of the individual broiler has recently been published and shows the potential for intervention with exogenous protease to improve population uniformity (Cowieson *et al.*, 2020).

Superficially, the beneficial effects of exogenous protease in non-ruminant animal diets are delivered by augmentation of endogenous protease architecture and improved retention of recalcitrant dietary amino acids. While this is true and a large meta-analysis of more than 800 observations across multiple diet types revealed a mean response in ileal amino acid digestibility of +3.74% (ranging from 2.7 to 5.4% depending on the amino acid) (Cowieson and Roos, 2014), substantial adjacent beneficial effects have been observed. Importantly, the addition of exogenous protease to animal diets appears to reduce the antinutritional effects of proteinaceous antinutrients such as trypsin inhibitors, lectins and antigenic proteins. For example, Cowieson *et al.* (2016b) noted that exogenous protease addition upregulated the

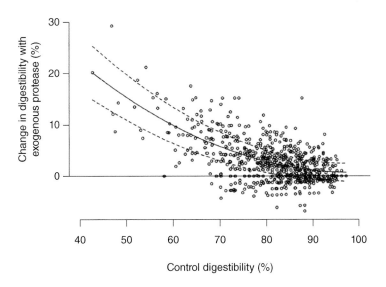

Fig. 6.5. Correlation between control digestibility (%) and the effect of a monocomponent exogenous protease. Mean response was +3.74%. (From Cowieson and Roos, 2014. Figure used with permission.)

expression of claudin-1 and various amino acid transporters in the intestine of broilers, suggesting beneficial effects on tight junction integrity and nutrient absorption. Similar beneficial effects of protease addition on peptide transport function have recently been reported (Cowieson *et al.*, 2018). Cowieson and Roos (2014) also noted that the pattern of response to supplemental protease across all amino acids reflected the amino acid profile of intestinal mucin, suggesting that some of the beneficial effects may originate from reduced synthesis and/or loss of mucin from the gut. This observation confirms a previous report where exogenous protease significantly increased the thickness of the adherent mucin layer in broilers (Peek *et al.*, 2009). Exogenous protease addition has also recently been shown to significantly increase dietary metabolizable and net energy in broiler chickens. Cowieson *et al.* (2018) reported that exogenous protease increased net energy by 107 kcal/kg in broiler chickens fed a maize–wheat-based diet that already contained both xylanase and phytase. Effects of exogenous protease on metabolizable and digestible energy have previously been reported. Fru-Nji *et al.* (2011) reported an increase in metabolizable energy with protease addition of 51–212 kcal/kg for broilers fed a maize–soy-based diet. Freitas *et al.* (2011) observed an increase in apparent metabolizable energy of up to 194 kcal/kg with protease addition to a maize–soy-based diet. Kalmendal and Tauson (2012) reported an increase in metabolizable energy of a wheat–soy-based diet of 114 kcal/kg. Olukosi *et al.* (2015) noted an increase in apparent metabolizable energy of 177 kcal/kg when protease was added to a maize–soy–canola–distillers-based diet. Finally, Cowieson *et al.* (2016b) observed an increase in metabolizable energy of 28–131 kcal/kg when protease was added to maize–soy- or maize–canola-based diets for broilers. Thus, the effects of protease are extensive and extend from primary effects on amino acid retention (some of which are delivered via reductions in endogenous amino acid loss) to improvements in tight junction integrity, mucin barrier function, peptide transport and energy metabolic efficiency.

6.6   Conclusions

Exogenous amylases and proteases have the potential to increase the digestibility of starch, energy and amino acids in the diets of pigs and poultry. However, more research is needed to fully explore the mode of action and the complementarity of effect with adjacent feed enzymes. A greater appreciation for factors that contribute to variation in the retention of starch and protein in farm animals will inform optimal use of these enzymes and enable their strategic deployment as part of enzyme admixtures. Future work should focus on a better understanding of starch and protein structure at the tertiary and quaternary level and how exogenous enzymes may augment the endogenous enzyme array. Furthermore, it is critical that endogenous energy and amino acid flow is more routinely considered in animal nutrition and separation made between effects generated by changes to both exogenous and endogenous nutrient retention. It is unlikely that all non-ruminant animal diets will require the simultaneous use of exogenous phytase, non-starch polysaccharide-degrading enzymes, protease and amylase. However, consideration of the growth stage of the animal in question, key limiting nutrients, substrate analysis and rapid ingredient quality prediction will enable the assembly of enzyme admixtures that will deliver consistent value creation. In the future it is likely that exogenous amylases and proteases will play a more significant role in the feed enzyme marketplace and complement incumbent enzymes to further enhance the sustainability of the food protein chain.

References

Angel, C.R., Saylor, W., Vieira, S.L. and Ward, N. (2010) Effects of a mono-component protease on performance and protein utilization in 7- to 22-day-old broiler chickens. *Poultry Science* 90, 2281–2286.

Baker, R.O., Lewis, C.J., Wilbur, R.W., Hartman, P.A., Speer, V.C., *et al.* (1956) Supplementation of baby pig diets with enzymes. *Journal of Animal Science* 15, 1245.

Barekatain, M.R., Antipatis, C., Choct, M. and Iji, P.A. (2013) Interaction between protease and xylanase in broiler chicken diets containing sorghum distillers' dried grains with solubles. *Animal Feed Science and Technology* 182, 71–81.

Barrett, A., Rawlings, N. and Woessner, F. (2012) *Handbook of Proteolytic Enzymes*, 2nd edn. Elsevier/Academic Press, London.

Bedford, M.R. (2002) The foundation of conducting feed enzyme research and the challenge of explaining the results. *Journal of Applied Poultry Research* 11, 464–470.

Bergmann, M. and Fruton, J.S. (1941) The specificity of proteinases. *Advances in Enzymology and Related Areas of Molecular Biology* 1, 63–98.

Bieth, J.G. (1978) Elastases: structure, function and pathological role. In: Robert, L., Cillin-Lapinet, G.M. and Bieth, J.G. (eds) *Frontiers of Matrix Biology*, vol. 6. Karger, Basel, Switzerland, pp. 1–82.

Castanon, J.I.R. and Marquardt, R.R. (1989) Effect of enzyme addition, autoclave treatment and fermenting on the nutritive value of field beans (*Vicia faba* L.). *Animal Feed Science and Technology* 26, 71–79.

Cowieson, A.J. (2005) Factors that affect the nutritional value of maize for broilers. *Animal Feed Science and Technology* 119, 293–305.

Cowieson, A.J. and Roos, F.F. (2014) Bioefficacy of a mono-component protease in the diets of pigs and poultry: a meta-analysis of effect on ileal amino acid digestibility. *Journal of Applied Animal Nutrition* 2, 1–8.

Cowieson, A.J. and Roos, F.F. (2016) Toward optimal value creation through the application of exogenous mono-component protease in the diets of non-ruminants. *Animal Feed Science and Technology* 221, 331–340.

Cowieson, A.J., Klausen, M., Pontoppidan, K., Umar-Faruk, M., Roos, F.F. and Giessing, A.M.B. (2016a) Identification of peptides in the terminal ileum of broiler chickens fed diets based on maize and soybean meal using proteomics. *Animal Production Science* 57, 1738–1750.

Cowieson, A.J., Lu, H., Ajuwon, K., Knap, I. and Adeola, O. (2016b) Interactive effects of dietary protein source and exogenous protease on growth performance, immune competence and jejunal health of broiler chickens. *Animal Production Science* 57, 252–261.

Cowieson, A.J., Toghyani, M., Kheravii, S.K., Wu, S.-B., Romero, L.F. and Choct, M. (2018) A mono-component protease improves performance, net energy, and digestibility of amino acids and starch, and upregulates jejunal expression of genes responsible for peptide transport in broilers fed corn/wheat-based diets supplemented with xylanase and phytase. *Poultry Science* 98, 1321–1332.

Cowieson, A.J., Smith, A., Sorbara, J.O.B., Pappenberger, G. and Olukosi, O.A. (2019) Efficacy of a mono-component exogenous protease in the presence of a high concentration of exogenous phytase on growth performance of broiler chickens. *Journal of Applied Poultry Research* 28, 638–646.

Cowieson, A.J., Bhuiyan, M.M., Sorbara, J.O.B., Pappenberger, G., Pedersen, M.B. and Choct, M. (2020) Contribution of individual broilers to variation in amino acid digestibility in soybean meal and the efficacy of an exogenous mono-component protease. *Poultry Science* 99, 1075–1083.

Croom, W.J., Brake, J., Coles, B.A., Havenstein, G.B., Christensen, V.L., *et al.* (1999) Is intestinal absorption capacity rate-limiting for performance in poultry? *Journal of Applied Poultry Research* 8, 242–252.

De Faria Castro, S., Bertechini, A.G., Costa Lima, E.M., Clemente, A.H.S., Ferreira, V.G.G. and de Carvalho, J.C.C. (2020) Effect of different levels of supplementary alpha-amylase in finishing broilers. *Acta Scientiarum: Animal Sciences* 42, 1–6.

Desnuelle, P. (1960) Chymotrypsin. In: Boyer, P.D., Lardy, H. and Myrback, K. (eds) *The Enzymes*, vol. 4. Academic Press, New York, pp. 93–118.

Duee, P.-H., Darcy-Vrillon, B., Blanchier, F. and Morel, M.-T. (1995) Fuel selection in intestinal cells. *Proceedings of the Nutrition Society* 54, 83–94.

Folk, J.E., Piez, K.A., Carroll, W.R. and Gladner, J.A. (1960) Carboxypeptidase B. IV. Purification and characterization of the porcine enzyme. *Journal of Biological Chemistry* 235, 2272–2277.

Freitas, D.M., Vieira, S.L., Angel, C.R., Favero, A. and Maiorka, A. (2011) Performance and nutrient utilization of broilers fed diets supplemented with a novel mono-component protease. *Journal of Applied Poultry Research* 20, 322–334.

Fru-Nji, F., Kluenter, A.-M., Fischer, M. and Pontoppidan, K. (2011) A feed serine protease improves broiler performance and increases protein and energy digestibility. *The Journal of Poultry Science* 48, 239–246.

Fruton, J.S. (1976) The mechanism of the catalytic action of pepsin and the related acid proteinases. *Advances in Enzymology and Related Areas of Molecular Biology* 44, 1–36.

Fuller, M.F. and Reeds, P.J. (1998) Nitrogen cycling in the gut. *Annual Review of Nutrition* 18, 385–411.

Ganapathy, V., Ganapathy, M.E. and Leibach, F.H. (2000) Intestinal transport of peptides and amino acids. In: Barrett, K.E. and Donowitz, M. (eds) *Current Topics in Membranes*, vol. 50. Academic Press, San Francisco, California, pp. 379–412.

Gibbon, B.C., Wang, X. and Larkins, B.A. (2003) Altered starch structure is associated with endosperm modification in quality protein maize. *Proceedings of the National Academy of Sciences USA* 100, 15239–15334.

Gracia, M.I., Araníbar, M.J., Lázaro, R., Medel, P. and Mateos, G.G. (2003) Alpha-amylase supplementation of broiler diets based on corn. *Poultry Science* 82, 436–442.

Guenter, W., Slominski, B.A., Simbaya, J., Morgan, A. and Campbell, L.D. (1995) Potential for improved utilization of canola meal using exogenous enzymes. In: *Proceedings of the 9th International Rapeseed Congress, Cambridge, UK, 4–7 July 1995*, vol. 1–2. Congress Organizing Committee, Cambridge, pp. 164–166.

Hessing, G.C., van Laarhoven, H., Rooke, J.A. and Morgan, A. (1996) Quality of soyabean meals (SBM) and effect of microbial enzymes in degrading soya antinutritional compounds (ANC). In: Buchanan, A. (ed.) *Proceedings of the 2nd International Soyabean Processing and Utilization Conference, Bangkok, Thailand, 8–12 January 1996*. Institute of Food Research and Product Development, Kasetsart University, Bangkok, pp. 8–13.

Horváthová, V., Janecek, S. and Sturdík, E. (2001) Amylolytic enzymes: molecular aspects of their properties. *General Physiology and Biophysics* 20, 7–32.

Huo, G.C., Fowler, V.R., Inborr, J. and Bedford, M.R. (1993) The use of enzymes to denature antinutritive factors in soyabean. In: Van Der Poel, A.F.B., Huisman, J. and Saini, H.S. (eds) *Recent Advances of Research in Antinutritional Factors in Legume Seeds: Analytical Methods, Animal Nutrition, Feed (Bio)Technology, Plant Breeding*. Wageningen Academic Publishers, Wageningen, the Netherlands, pp. 517–521.

Itani, K. and Svihus, B. (2019) Feed processing and structural components affect starch digestion dynamics in broiler chickens. *British Poultry Science* 60, 246–255.

Jiang, Z., Zhou, Y., Lu, F., Han, Z. and Wang, T. (2008) Effects of different levels of supplementary alpha-amylase on digestive enzyme activities and pancreatic amylase mRNA expression of young broilers. *Asian-Australasian Journal of Animal Science* 21, 97–102.

Kalmendal, R. and Tauson, R. (2012) Effects of a xylanase and protease, individually or in combination, and an ionophore coccidiostat on performance, nutrient utilization, and intestinal morphology in broiler chickens fed a wheat–soybean meal-based diet. *Poultry Science* 91, 1387–1393.

Krogdahl, A. and Sell, J.L. (1989) Influence of age on lipase, amylase and protease activities in pancreatic tissue and intestinal contents of young turkeys. *Poultry Science* 68, 1561–1568.

Lewis, C.J., Catron, D.V., Liu, C.H., Speer, V.C. and Ashton, G.C. (1955) Enzyme supplementation of baby pig diets. *Journal of Agricultural and Food Chemistry* 3, 1047–1050.

Lombard, V., Hemalatha, G.R., Drula, E., Coutinho, P.M. and Henrissat, B. (2014) The carbohydrate-active enzymes database (CAZy) in 2013. *Nucleic Acids Research* 42, 490–495.

Mahagna, M., Nir, I., Larbier, M. and Nitsan, Z. (1995) Effect of age and exogenous amylase and protease on development of the digestive tract, pancreatic enzyme activities and digestibility of nutrients in young meat-type chicks. *Reproduction, Nutrition, Development* 35, 201–212.

McDonald, P., Edwards, R.A., Greenhalgh, J.F.D., Morgan, C.A., Sinclair, L.A. and Wilkinson, R.G. (2010) Digestion. *Animal Nutrition*, 7th edn. Pearson, Harlow, UK, pp. 156–191.

Moran, E.T. (1982) Starch digestion in fowl. *Poultry Science* 61, 1257–1267.

Moran, E.T. (1985) Digestion and absorption of carbohydrates in fowl and events through perinatal development. *The Journal of Nutrition* 115, 665–674.

Moran, E.T. (2016) Gastric digestion of protein through pancreozyme action optimizes intestinal forms for absorption, mucin formation and villus integrity. *Animal Feed Science and Technology* 221, 284–303.

Odetallah, N.H., Wang, J.J., Garlich, J.D. and Shih, J.C. (2003) Keratinase in starter diets improves growth of broiler chicks. *Poultry Science* 82, 664–670.

Odetallah, N.H., Wang, J.J. and Garlich, J.D. (2005) Versazyme supplementation of broiler diets improves market growth performance. *Poultry Science* 84, 858–864.

Olukosi, O.A., Beeson, L.A., Englyst, K. and Romero, L.F. (2015) Effects of exogenous proteases without or with carbohydrases on nutrient digestibility and disappearance of non-starch polysaccharides in broiler chickens. *Poultry Science* 94, 2662–2669.

Onderci, M., Sahin, N., Sahin, K., Cikim, G., Aydin, A., *et al.* (2006) Efficacy of supplementation of alpha-amylase-producing bacterial culture on the performance, nutrient use, and gut morphology of broiler chickens fed a corn-based diet. *Poultry Science* 85, 505–510.

Ospina-Rojas, I.C., Murakami, A.E., Oliveira, C.A.L. and Guerra, A.F.Q.G. (2013) Supplemental glycine and threonine effects on performance, intestinal mucosa development, and nutrient utilization of growing broiler chickens. *Poultry Science* 92, 2724–2731.

Payen, A. and Persoz, J.-F. (1833) Mémoire sur la diastase, les principaux produits de ses réactions et leurs applications aux arts industriels. *Annales de Chimie et de Physique* 53, 73–92.

Peek, H.W., Van Der Klis, J.D., Vermeulen, B. and Landman, W.J.M. (2009) Dietary protease can alleviate negative effects of a coccidiosis infection on production performance in broiler chickens. *Animal Feed Science and Technology* 150, 151–159.

Recoules, E., Sabboh-Jourdan, H., Narcy, A., Lessire, M., Harichaux, G., *et al.* (2017) Exploring *in vivo* digestion of plant proteins in broiler chickens. *Poultry Science* 96, 1735–1747.

Ritz, C.W., Hulet, R.M., Self, B.B. and Denbow, D.M. (1995) Growth and intestinal morphology of male turkeys as influenced by dietary supplementation of amylase and xylanase. *Poultry Science* 74, 1329–1334.

Rooke, J.A., Slessor, M., Fraser, H. and Thomson, J.R. (1998) Growth performance and gut function of piglets weaned at four weeks of age and fed protease-treated soya-bean meal. *Animal Feed Science and Technology* 70, 175–190.

Stam, M.R., Danchin, E.G., Rancurel, C., Coutinho, P.M. and Henrissat, B. (2006) Dividing the large glycoside hydrolase family 13 into subfamilies: towards improved functional annotations of alpha-amylase-related proteins. *Protein Engineering, Design and Selection* 19, 555–562.

Stefanello, C., Vieira, S.L., Santiago, G.O., Kindlein, L., Sorbara, J.O.B. and Cowieson, A.J. (2015) Starch digestibility, energy utilization and growth performance of broilers fed corn–soybean basal diets supplemented with enzymes. *Poultry Science* 94, 2472–2479.

Stefanello, C., Vieira, S.L., Rios, H.V., Simoes, C.T., Ferzola, P.H., *et al.* (2017) Effects of energy, alpha-amylase and beta-xylanase on growth performance of broiler chickens. *Animal Feed Science and Technology* 225, 205–212.

Stefanello, C., Vieira, S.L., Soster, P., Dos Santos, B.M., Dalmoro, Y.K., *et al.* (2019) Utilization of corn-based diets supplemented with exogenous alpha-amylase for broilers. *Poultry Science* 98, 5862–5869.

Sterchi, E.E. and Woodley, J.F. (1980) Peptide hydrolases of the human small intestinal mucosa: distribution of activities between brush border membranes and cytosol. *Clinica Chimica Acta* 102, 49–56.

Svihus, B., Uhlen, A.K. and Harstad, O.M. (2005) Review: Effect of starch granule structure, associated components and processing on nutritive value of cereal starch. *Animal Feed Science and Technology* 122, 303–320.

Tan, A.K. and Eaton, D.L. (1995) Activation and characterization of procarboxypeptidase B from human plasma. *Biochemistry* 34, 5811–5816.

Tang, J. (1963) Specificity of pepsin and its dependence on a possible hydrophobic binding site. *Nature* 199, 1094–1095.

Tester, R.F., Karkalas, J. and Qi, X. (2004) Starch composition, fine structure and architecture. *Journal of Cereal Science* 39, 151–165.

Thorpe, J. and Beal, J.D. (2001) Vegetable protein meals and the effects of enzymes. In: Bedford, M.R. and Partridge, G.G. (eds) *Enzymes in Farm Animal Nutrition*, 1st edn. CAB International, Wallingford, UK, pp. 125–144.

Uni, Z., Ganot, S. and Sklan, D. (1998) Posthatch development of mucosal function in the broiler small intestine. *Poultry Science* 77, 75–82.

Vieira, S.L., Stefanello, C., Rios, H.V., Serafini, N.C., Hermes, R.G. and Sorbara, J.O.B. (2015) Efficacy and metabolizable energy equivalence of an α-amylase–β-glucanase complex for broilers. *Revista Brasileira de Ciencia Avicola* 17, 227–235.

Walk, C.L. and Poernama, F. (2018) Evaluation of phytase, xylanase and protease in reduced nutrient diets fed to broilers. *Journal of Applied Poultry Research* 28, 85–93.

Walk, C.L., Juntunen, K., Paloheimo, M. and Ledoux, D.R. (2019) Evaluation of novel protease enzymes on growth performance and nutrient digestibility of poultry: enzyme dose response. *Poultry Science* 98, 5525–5532.

Wiseman, J., Nicol, N.T. and Norton, G. (2000) Relationship between apparent metabolizable energy (AME) values and *in vivo/in vitro* starch digestibility of wheat for broilers. *World's Poultry Science Journal* 56, 305–318.

Wong, D.W.S. (1995) Amylolytic enzymes. *Food Enzymes: Structure and Mechanism*. Springer, Boston, Massachusetts, pp. 37–84.

Wu, G., Bazer, F.W., Dai, Z., Li, D., Wang, J. and Wu, J. (2014) Amino acid nutrition in animals: protein synthesis and beyond. *Annual Review of Animal Biosciences* 2, 387–417.

Yin, D., Yin, X., Wang, X., Lei, Z., Wang, M., *et al.* (2018) Supplementation of amylase combined with glucoamylase or protease changes intestinal microbiota diversity and benefits for broilers fed a diet of newly harvested corn. *Journal of Animal Science and Biotechnology* 9, 24–37.

Zuo, J., Ling, B., Long, L., Li, T., Lahaye, L., *et al.* (2015) Effect of dietary supplementation with protease on the growth performance, nutrient utilization, intestinal morphology, digestive enzymes and gene expression of weaned piglets. *Animal Nutrition* 1, 276–282.

7 Phytases: Biochemistry, Enzymology and Characteristics Relevant to Animal Feed Use

Daniel Menezes-Blackburn[1]*, Ralf Greiner[2] and Ursula Konietzny[3]

[1]*Sultan Qaboos University, Sultanate of Oman;* [2]*Federal Research Institute of Nutrition, and Food Institute of Food Technology and Bioprocess Engineering, Karlsruhe, Germany;* [3]*Dettenheim, Germany*

7.1 Introduction: Use of Phytases in Animal Nutrition

Phytases are a subgroup of phosphomonoesterases capable of initiating the stepwise dephosphorylation of phytate (*myo*-inositol (1,2,3,4,5,6)hexakisphosphate), the most abundant inositol phosphate found in nature. These enzymes have a huge diversity of biochemical properties and sources. Although microbial phytases represent the majority of the biochemically described phytases, many others have been identified in plants, and even in some animal tissues (Konietzny and Greiner, 2002). Extracellular microbial phytases are speculated to play an important role in nutrient cycling during decomposition of organic materials in a variety of ecosystems (Menezes-Blackburn *et al.*, 2013; Makoudi *et al.*, 2018). Intracellular microbial phytases, on the other hand, may not be involved in the dephosphorylation of extracellular phytate (Greiner, 2007). These enzymes are, in general, non-specific phosphatases that also exhibit phytate-degrading activity and, therefore, are best described as phytate-degrading enzymes (Konietzny and Greiner, 2002). Although fewer than 100 different species have been described expressing measurable phytase activity, it has been speculated that every cell should carry *myo*-inositol phosphatases given that *myo*-inositol phosphates are widespread molecular signalling metabolites (Menezes-Blackburn and Greiner, 2015).

Hydrolytic enzymes such as phytases are widely used as feed supplements in order to improve the digestion and absorption of poorly available nutrients from the animal diet (Menezes-Blackburn and Greiner, 2015). Phytate is especially abundant in grain-based diets and represents both an unavailable phosphorus source and an antinutrient that prevents the uptake of multivalent minerals and trace elements by pigs and poultry (Menezes-Blackburn and Greiner, 2015). Under normal feeding conditions, monogastric animals have only a very limited ability to hydrolyse phytate due to the lack of significant endogenous phytase activity and low microbial population in the upper part of the digestive tract (Iqbal *et al.*, 1994). Numerous animal studies have shown the effectiveness of supplemented microbial phytase in improving the utilization of phosphate from phytate and reducing the need for orthophosphate supplementation of the feed (Simons *et al.*, 1990; Augspurger *et al.*, 2003;

*Email: danielblac@squ.edu.om

©CAB International 2022. *Enzymes in Farm Animal Nutrition, 3rd Edition* (M. Bedford *et al.* eds)
DOI: 10.1079/9781789241563.0007

Adeola *et al.*, 2006; Vallejo *et al.*, 2018). As a result, excretion of phosphate in areas of livestock management can be reduced by as much as 50%, making phytase currently the most effective tool for the animal industry to comply with environmental regulations regarding land phosphorus application (Menezes-Blackburn *et al.*, 2013). In addition, there is experimental evidence suggesting that phytase supplementation in grain-based feed results in an unintended, yet beneficial increase in amino acid availability and energy utilization by monogastric animals (Selle and Ravindran, 2007; Vallejo *et al.*, 2018).

The first commercial phytase product (*Aspergillus niger*) was launched on to the market in 1991, followed by phytase products from other donor organisms (DOs). In general, their large-scale production is based on the use of recombinant strains of filamentous fungi and yeasts (Menezes-Blackburn and Greiner, 2015). The main phytase products on the market now are BASF Natuphos® (DO: *A. niger*), Novozymes/DSM Ronozyme® (DO: *Citrobacter braakii* or *Peniophora lycii*), AB Vista Quantum® (DO: *Escherichia coli*), Danisco Animal Nutrition/DuPont Phyzyme® (DO: *E. coli*) and Axtra PHY® (DO: *Buttiauxella* sp.) (Menezes-Blackburn and Greiner, 2015; Menezes-Blackburn *et al.*, 2015). BASF has also a new phytase product (Natuphos® E) which is an engineered hybrid enzyme from three DOs (*Hafnia* sp., *Yersinia mollaretii* and *Buttiauxella gaviniae*), conserving the active-site codon from the first (*Hafnia* sp.) (Rychen *et al.*, 2017). These phytases are either 3- or 6-histidine acid phytases and are active at acid pH values (see next section) (Menezes-Blackburn and Greiner, 2015; Menezes-Blackburn *et al.*, 2015). The phytase market volume was in the range of €350 million in 2016 and is projected to reach €520 million in 2021 (MRS, 2017). Even if potential applications of phytase in food processing or the production of pharmaceuticals were reported (Greiner and Konietzny, 2006), phytases have been mainly, if not solely, used as monogastric animal feed additives in diets largely for swine and poultry, and to a smaller extent for fish and ruminants (Dersjant-Li *et al.*, 2015).

7.2 Phytase Catalytic Mechanisms

Phytases are a diverse subgroup of phosphatase enzymes that encompass a range of sizes, structures and catalytic mechanisms. Based on the catalytic mechanism, phytases can be referred to as histidine acid phytases (HAPhy), β-propeller phytases (BPPhy), cysteine phytases (CPhy) or purple acid phytases (PAPhy) (Iqbal *et al.*, 1994; Mullaney and Ullah, 2003; Greiner and Konietzny, 2006). With regard to their pH value of maximum activity, phytases can be further classified into acid and alkaline phytases. Additionally, phytases can be categorized based on the carbon in the *myo*-inositol ring of phytate at which dephosphorylation is initiated into 1/3-phytases (EC 3.1.3.8), 4/6-phytases (EC 3.1.3.26) and 5-phytases (EC 3.1.3.72). In order to describe biochemical pathways correctly, *myo*-inositol phosphates are numbered counterclockwise (D configuration). Thus, for example, several phytases of plant origin generating D-Ins(1,2,3,5,6)P_5 (identical with L-Ins(1,2,3,4,5)P_5) as the first dephosphorylation product have to be classified as 4-phytases. This is exceptionally important to distinguish them from the phytases from *E. coli* and *Paramecium*, which generate D-Ins(1,2,3,4,5)P_5 (identical with L-Ins(1,2,3,5,6) P_5) as the major *myo*-inositol pentakisphosphate and have therefore to be classified as 6-phytases. All phytases currently used for animal feed application belong to the class of histidine acid phytases (Menezes-Blackburn *et al.*, 2015) and despite many studies proposing their use in different applications, no β-propeller, cysteine or purple acid phytases are currently marketed in animal feed.

7.2.1 Histidine acid phytases (HAPhy)

The majority of the phytases known to date, including all commercially sold as feed additives, belong to the subfamily of histidine acid phosphatases (HAPs). They have been identified in many microorganisms, but also in plants and animals (Wodzinski and Ullah, 1996; Mullaney *et al.*, 2000; Konietzny and Greiner, 2002; Lei and Porres, 2003). These enzymes do not need cofactors for optimal activity. The structures of histidine acid phosphatases contain a conserved α/β-domain and a variable α-domain (Kostrewa et al., 1997; Lim et al., 2000). The active site is located at the interface between the two domains. Differences in substrate binding have been attributed to differences in the α-domain. Histidine acid phosphatases share the highly conserved sequence motif RH(G/N)XRXP, considered to be the phosphate acceptor site near the N-terminus (Ostanin et al., 1992; Lindqvist et al., 1994). However, not all histidine acid phosphatases are able to catalyse phytate dephosphorylation. In addition, one alkaline phytase has been reported to contain the characteristic HAP amino acid motifs. This enzyme was identified in lily pollen and requires Ca^{2+} for full catalytic activity (Mehta et al., 2006). Other plant alkaline phytases whose activity is enhanced in the presence of Ca^{2+} were found in cat's tail (Typha latifolia L.) pollen (Hara et al., 1985) and a number of legumes (Scott, 1991). Unfortunately, none of the corresponding genes has been sequenced to confirm the presence of the signature HAP motifs.

7.2.2   β-Propeller phytases (BPPhy)

β-Propeller phytases have a unique six-bladed propeller folding architecture with six calcium-binding sites in each protein molecule (Shin et al., 2001). Binding of three Ca^{2+} to high-affinity calcium-binding sites results in a dramatic increase in thermal stability by joining loop segments remote in the amino acid sequence. Binding of three additional Ca^{2+} to low-affinity calcium-binding sites at the top of the molecule turns on the catalytic activity of the enzyme by converting the highly negatively charged cleft into a favourable environment for the binding of phytate. Kinetic studies have established that β-propeller phytases could hydrolyse calcium phytate between pH 7.0 and 8.0 (Oh et al., 2004). Initially, β-propeller phytases were reported and commonly found in Bacillus species (Kerovuo et al., 1998; Kim et al., 1998a; Choi et al., 2001; Tye et al., 2002). Later, β-propeller phytases were identified in other genera such as Enterobacter (Yoon et al., 1996), Pedobacter (Huang et al., 2009), Xanthomonas (Chatterjee et al., 2003),

Paenibacillus (Jorquera et al., 2010), Geobacillus (Jorquera et al., 2018), Pseudomonas (Jang et al., 2018), Janthinobacterium (Zhang et al., 2011b), Serratia (Zhang et al., 2011a), Sphingomonas (Sanangelantoni et al., 2018) and Shewanella (Cheng and Lim, 2006). Furthermore, protein and gene sequence identities suggest that β-propeller phytases are widespread both in aquatic and terrestrial environments (Cheng and Lim, 2006; Kumar et al., 2016, 2017). The amino acid sequences of β-propeller phytases exhibit no homology to the sequences of any other known phosphatase (Greiner and Konietzny, 2010; Kumar et al., 2017). In contrast to histidine acid phytases, β-propeller phytases do not show any reduction in activity in the presence of fluoride (Tye et al., 2002; Cheng and Lim, 2006). High thermostability, the need for Ca^{2+} for enzyme activation, high substrate specificity and activity at alkaline pH values are some of the main features of these enzymes (Kumar et al., 2017).

7.2.3   Cysteine phytases (CPhy)

Cysteine phytases, also commonly known as protein tyrosine phytases (PTPhy), are enzymes characteristically reported from anaerobic ruminal bacteria such as Selenomonas ruminantium (Nakashima et al., 2007). These enzymes do not need cofactors for enzymatic activity and share a common active-site motif HCXXGXXR(T/S) (Chu et al., 2004). The active site forms a P loop that functions as a substrate-binding pocket unique to protein tyrosine phosphatases. This pocket is wider and deeper in S. ruminantium phytase and therefore able to accommodate the fully phosphorylated inositol group of phytate (Chu et al., 2004). Besides Selenomonas, PTPhy-like phytases were reported to be present in anaerobic bacteria genera such as Megasphaera (Puhl et al., 2009), Clostridium and Mitsuokella (Huang et al., 2011). These types of phytase were believed to be exclusive to anaerobic bacteria (Greiner and Konietzny, 2010); nevertheless, similar enzymes have been recently found in obligate aerobes such as Bdellovibrio sp. (Gruninger et al., 2014) and facultative anaerobes such as Lactobacillus sp. (Sharma et al., 2018).

7.2.4   Purple acid phytases (PAPhy)

Purple acid phytases are the commonly found plant phytases (Konietzny and Greiner, 2002; Dionisio *et al.*, 2011). These are binuclear metal-containing enzymes with optimal catalytic activity in acidic environments. The genes encoding PAPhy have been sequenced, revealing that they contain motif characteristics of a broad group of purple acid phosphatases (Hegeman and Grabau, 2001). Purple acid phosphatases, independent of their activity towards phytate, have representatives in plants, mammals, fungi and bacteria and contain binuclear Fe(III)–Me(II) centres where Me is Fe, Mn or Zn (Schenk *et al.*, 2000). Purple acid phosphatases with phytase activity are reported to act on seed phytate during seed germination (Hegeman and Grabau, 2001), and also to be exuded by plant roots under soil phosphorus starvation conditions in order to improve soil organic phosphorus cycling and phosphorus uptake by the plant (Tran *et al.*, 2010; Menezes-Blackburn *et al.*, 2013; Liu *et al.*, 2018). Plant species with PAPhy activity are widely reported, such as: clover (*Medicago trunculata* L.) (Xiao *et al.*, 2005), soybean (*Glycine max*) (Hegeman and Grabau, 2001), stylo (*Stylosanthes guianensis*) (Liu *et al.*, 2018), tobacco (*Nicotiana tabacum*) (Lung *et al.*, 2008), wheat (*Triticum aestivum* L.), barley (*Hordeum vulgare* L.), maize (*Zea mays* L.) and rice (*Oryza sativa* L.) (Dionisio *et al.*, 2011). A rare PAPhy was found in an earthworm cast bacterium, *Sphingobium* sp. (Ghorbani Nasrabadi *et al.*, 2018), indicating that this class of enzymes is not exclusive to plants at all.

7.3   Phytase Properties Relevant for Their Performance during Feed Digestion

It is currently accepted that commercial phytase properties are still not optimal for feed supplement applications (Menezes-Blackburn *et al.*, 2015). The 'ideal' phytase for this purpose should fulfil a series of quality criteria: it should be effective in releasing phytate phosphate in the digestive tract, stable to resist inactivation by heat from feed processing and storage, as well as cheap to produce

(Menezes-Blackburn and Greiner, 2015). Although the ability of a phytase to hydrolyse phytate in the digestive tract is determined by its enzymatic properties, it is extremely challenging to conclude from *in vitro* measured enzyme biochemical properties its performance in dephosphorylating phytate from complex feed materials across a variety of extreme environments present in the digestive tracts of distinct animals (Menezes-Blackburn *et al.*, 2015). It is important to consider that the pH is very low in the forestomach (crop) of poultry (pH 4.0–5.0), the proventriculus of poultry and the stomach of pigs and fish (pH 2.0–5.0) (Simon and Igbasan, 2002). Poultry gizzard has also been recently shown to display strong pH fluctuations between 0.6 and 3.8 (Lee *et al.*, 2017). On the other hand, the small intestine of animals presents a neutral pH environment (pH 6.5–7.5). Therefore, the pH range of optimal activity as well as the resistance to abrupt pH changes are key variables in phytase performance (Menezes-Blackburn *et al.*, 2015). Enzymes used as feed additives must be highly active at very low pH values and be able to withstand strong and quick pH transitions without losing their activity. Alkaline phytases, such as most β-propeller enzymes, are therefore highly inappropriate for application as feed supplements (Konietzny and Greiner, 2002). Stomach environments of vertebrates are usually very high in pepsin and therefore 'ideal' phytases must also be resistant to proteolytic hydrolysis. The specific activity of the chosen phytase towards phytate and its degradation products are also important; a lower concentration of the enzyme (on a protein basis) can be supplemented if the phytase has a higher specific activity. Thermostability is also a highly desired feature for these enzymes due to the high temperature used during feed processing. Other features such as substrate specificity, inhibitors and route of catalysis may also play a minor role on phytase performance as a feed additive.

7.3.1   pH Dependence of activity profile and pH stability of phytases

With the exception of some bacterial phytases, especially those of the genera

Bacillus and *Enterobacter* as well as some plant phytases, all phytases reported to date exhibit a pH optimum in the range between 4.0 and 6.0 (Table 7.1) (Konietzny and Greiner, 2002). Even though many phytases show maximal activity in the same pH range, their pH–activity profiles may differ considerably. As an example, the commercial phytases from *A. niger* (BASF Natuphos®), *C. braakii* (Novozymes/DSM Ronozyme®), *Buttiauxella* sp. (DuPont Axtra®) and *E. coli* (AB Vista Quantum®) demonstrate how different the pH–activity profiles of marketed feed phytases are (Fig. 7.1a). Menezes-Blackburn *et al.* (2015) performed an in-depth analysis of the implications of feed phytase biochemical properties on their catalytic performance, including the pH dependency of activity. Because phytases are in general supplemented according to their activity determined at standard conditions (pH 5.5, 37°C, sodium phytate 5 mmol/l) (Engelen *et al.*, 1994), the recommended phytase dose will differ in its phytate-degrading activities at other pH conditions. The pH–activity dependency curves relative to the standard assay pH demonstrate how widely variable the applied activity of these enzymes may be if based on the standard assay (Fig. 7.1b). *Buttiauxella* sp. (DuPont Axtra®) phytase clearly has an advantage over other commercial microbial phytases at pH values below 4. Therefore, differences in pH–activity profiles may in part explain the difference in effectiveness of different phytases in diets for swine and poultry (Augspurger *et al.*, 2003; Menezes-Blackburn and Greiner, 2015; Menezes-Blackburn *et al.*, 2015). Consequently, choosing another pH value for standard phytase activity determination might lead to a completely different result in respect to ranking of phytases. If standard phytase activity determinations were conducted at pH 3.5, 37°C and sodium phytate 5 mmol/l, similar to the approximate stomach pH, it would give much fairer grounds for feed phytase dose recommendation. However, it must be remembered that bioefficacy is determined not only by the pH–activity profile of the phytase,

but also by its stability under the pH conditions of the stomach or crop, its susceptibility to pepsin degradation, the concentration and diffusion of soluble phytate and the electrostatic environment in the stomach or crop (MRS, 2017). It was, for example, shown that the pH–activity profiles of a fungal and a bacterial phytase could be modified by both the buffer type and ionic strength (Ullah *et al.*, 2008; Menezes-Blackburn *et al.*, 2015).

In general, microbial acid phytases exhibit considerable enzymatic activity below pH 3.5, whereas plant acid phytases are almost inactive (Lei and Porres, 2003; Menezes-Blackburn *et al.*, 2015; MRS, 2017). It is obvious that a broad phytate-degrading activity profile, covering the complete pH range of the targeted animal digestive tract, is advantageous for efficient feed phytate dephosphorylation. Some phytases, for example the phytase from *E. coli* (Greiner *et al.*, 1993), have a narrow bell-shaped pH–activity profile, whereas other phytases were identified as having a very broad pH–activity profile. It was shown, for instance, that the *Aspergillus fumigatus* phytase exerts activity between pH 2.5 and 8.5 and maintains 80% of its optimal activity within the pH range 4.0–7.3 (Wyss *et al.*, 1999). Similar broad pH–activity profiles were reported for phytases from *Thermomyces lanuginosus* (Berka *et al.*, 1998), *Aspergillus terreus* (Wyss *et al.*, 1999) and *Yersinia rohdei* (Huang *et al.*, 2008). In addition, pH stability of some microbial phytases below pH 3.0 and above pH 8.0 is remarkable, whereas the stability of most plant phytases decreases dramatically at pH values below 4 and above 7.5. The phytases from *E. coli* (Greiner *et al.*, 1993), *A. niger* 11T53A9 (Greiner *et al.*, 2009) and Malaysian wastewater bacterium (Greiner *et al.*, 2007a), for example, did not lose significant enzymatic activity even after exposure to pH 2.0 for several hours. On the other hand, phytases from rye (Greiner *et al.*, 1998), spelt (Konietzny *et al.*, 1994) and barley (Greiner *et al.*, 2000b), as well as many other plant phytases, are very sensitive to acid pH, losing most of their initial activity within 24 h at pH 2.5.

Table 7.1. Basic characteristics of selected phytases.

Phytase source	Optimal conditions pH	Optimal conditions Temperature (°C)	Specific activity at 37°C (U/mg)	Phytase classification	Reference
Aspergillus niger	5.0–5.5	55–58	50–133	3-phytase	Wyss *et al.* (1999)
Aspergillus terreus	5.0–5.5	70	142–196	3-phytase	Wyss *et al.* (1999)
Aspergillus fumigatus	5.0–6.0	60	23–28	3-phytase	Wyss *et al.* (1999); Rodriguez *et al.* (2000)
Thermomyces lanuginosus	6.0	65	110	–	Berka *et al.* (1998)
Penicillium simplicissimum	4.0	55	3	–	Tseng *et al.* (2000)
Peniophora lycii	5.5	58	1080	6-phytase	Lassen *et al.* (2001); Ullah *et al.* (2008)
Candida krusei	4.6	40	1210	–	Quan *et al.* (2002)
Debaryomyces castellii	4.0–4.5	55–60	–	3-phytase	Ragon *et al.* (2008)
Saccharomyces cerevisiae	4.5	45	135	3-phytase	Greiner *et al.* (2001a)
Neurospora crassa	5.5	60	125	3-phytase	Zhou *et al.* (2006)
Escherichia coli	4.5	55–60	750–811	6-phytase	Greiner *et al.* (1993); Golovan *et al.* (2000)
Selenomonas ruminantium	4.5–5.0	55	668	3-phytase	Puhl *et al.* (2007)
S. ruminantium subsp. *lactilytica*	4.5	55	16	5-phytase	Puhl *et al.* (2008b)
Selenomonas lacticifex	4.5	40	440	3-phytase	Puhl *et al.* (2008a)
Megasphaera elsdenii	5.0	60	269	3-phytase	Puhl *et al.* (2009)
Klebsiella terrigena	5.0	58	205	3-phytase	Greiner *et al.* (1997); Greiner and Carlsson (2006)
Pantoea agglomerans	4.5	60	23	3-phytase	Greiner (2004b)
Citrobacter braakii	4.0	50	3457	–	Kim *et al.* (2003)
Pseudomonas syringae	5.5	40	769	3-phytase	Cho *et al.* (2003)
Bacillus subtilis	6.5–7.5	55–60	9–15	3-phytase	Kerovuo *et al.* (1998); Greiner *et al.* (2007b)
Bacillus amyloliquefaciens	7.0–8.0	70	20	3-phytase	Kim *et al.* (1998b); Greiner *et al.* (2007b)
Wheat PHY1, PHY2	5.0–6.0	45–50	127–242	4-phytase	Nakano *et al.* (2000)
Spelt D21	6.0	45	262	4-phytase	Konietzny *et al.* (1994)
Rye	6.0	45	517	4-phytase	Greiner and Alamiger (2001)
Oat	5.0	38	307	4-phytase	Greiner and Alamiger (2001)
Barley P1, P2	5.0–6.0	45–55	43–117	4-phytase	Greiner *et al.* (2000b)
Faba bean	5.0	50	636	4-phytase	Greiner *et al.* (2001b)
Lupin L11, L12, L2	5.0	50	498–607	3-phytase	Greiner (2002)
Lily pollen	8.0	55	0.2	5-phytase	Mehta *et al.* (2006)

(a)

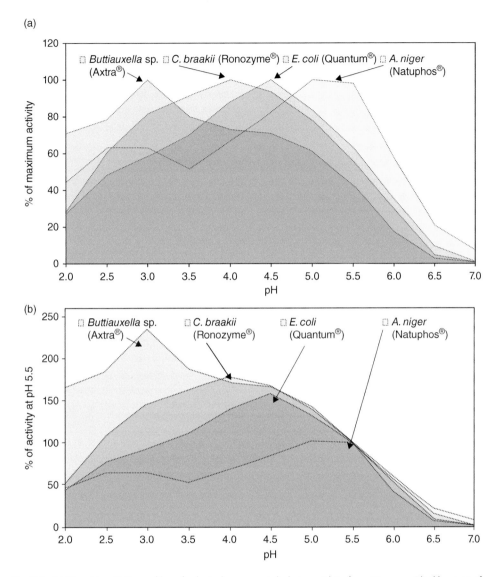

Fig. 7.1. (a) The pH–activity profiles of selected commercial phytases (data from Menezes-Blackburn *et al.*, 2015). The activity at optimal pH was taken as 100%. (b) The pH–activity profiles are shown as relative values compared with activity at pH 5.5 (100%). (Authors' own figures.)

7.3.2 Proteolytic stability

Since the digestive tract of different animals secretes large amounts of proteases to hydrolyse feed proteins, the effectiveness and limitations of feed supplementation with phytases may also depend on their susceptibility to proteolytic cleavage. The proteolytic stability is usually tested by incubating phytases with pepsin at pH 2.0 and pancreatin at pH 7.0. Differences in their ability to withstand degradation by these digestive proteases are observed through the loss of phytase activity during this incubation. Bacterial histidine acid phytases have been shown to exhibit a greater pepsin and pancreatin resistance than fungal acid phytases (Rodriguez *et al.*, 2000; Simon and Igbasan, 2002; Greiner *et al.*,

2007a; Huang *et al.*, 2008). The bacterial phytases (*E. coli*, *Klebsiella* spp. and Malaysian wastewater bacterium) are able to retain more than 80% of their initial activity after pepsin digestion, whereas phytases from *A. niger* and *P. lycii* can retain only 26–42% and 2–20%, respectively. After incubation with pancreatin, phytases from *E. coli* and *Klebsiella* spp. retained more than 90% of their initial activity, whereas the *A. niger* phytase retained only 23–34% and the *P. lycii* phytase was completely inactivated. The consensus phytase was the only fungal phytase that was reported to have a pepsin and pancreatin tolerance similar to that of bacterial histidine acid phytases (Simon and Igbasan, 2002). The *Bacillus subtilis* phytase possesses a high pancreatin resistance and a high susceptibility to pepsin digestion (Kerovuo *et al.*, 2000a). Furthermore, plant phytases are considered to be more susceptible to inactivation by gastrointestinal proteases (Greiner and Konietzny, 2010). It also has to be remembered that recombinant enzymes may differ in proteolytic resistance compared with their wild-type counterparts as reported for *E. coli* and *A. niger* phytases produced in *Pichia pastoris* (Rodriguez *et al.*, 2000).

In addition, the proteolytic stability of phytases has been studied in digesta supernatants from different gut segments of laying hens and broiler chickens, with similar results to those obtained during direct incubation with the corresponding proteases (Igbasan *et al.*, 2000; Simon and Igbasan, 2002). However, some phytases such as those of *B. subtilis*, *A. niger* and *P. lycii* show a much higher proteolytic stability in digesta supernatants when compared with direct incubation for the corresponding proteases (Greiner and Konietzny, 2010). The cause for this increase in stability is not known. However, it can be speculated that the greater tolerance might be due to the presence of additional proteins serving as substrates for the digestive proteases.

7.3.3 Thermostability

Thermostability is a particularly important feature of commercial phytases, since feed pelleting is commonly performed at temperatures between 60 and 95°C (Inborr and Bedford, 1994; Menezes-Blackburn and Greiner, 2015). Depending on the subsequent cooling system, the phytase is exposed to pelleting temperature for a time period in the range of seconds to minutes. Feed moisture content also greatly affects heat inactivation of enzymes during pelleting (Campbell and Bedford, 1992). If a given phytase is not thermostable, its inclusion into feed must be performed using a post-pellet spray apparatus for pelleted diets or chemical coating in order to bypass or overcome heat destruction of the enzyme (Greiner and Konietzny, 2010). The simplest and most practical solution is to use thermostable phytases as feed supplements. Likewise, an enzyme that can tolerate long-term storage or transport at ambient temperatures is undisputedly attractive. In purified form, most phytases from plants will have been irreversibly inactivated at temperatures above 70°C within minutes, whereas most corresponding microbial enzymes retain significant activity even after prolonged incubation.

The different phytases used as feed additives vary significantly in their thermostabilities (Inborr and Bedford, 1994; Menezes-Blackburn and Greiner, 2015). Menezes-Blackburn *et al.* (2015) measured the thermostability of seven commercial phytases; engineered *E. coli* (Quantum® Blue) was the best performing, being able to withstand 80°C for 30 min, followed by *Buttiauxella* sp. (Axtra®) and *P. lycii* (Ronozyme®) withstanding 70°C for 30 min without losing activity. All other phytases studied could not withstand temperatures over 60°C for 30 min without significant loss of enzymatic activity. Thermal stability of commercialized phytases was also previously determined by Simon and Igbasan (2002) at 70°C in aqueous solution. They reported the phytase from *A. niger* to be slightly more stable under the conditions applied than that from *P. lycii*, and the phytase from *E. coli* was shown to be even less stable than that from *P. lycii*. Among the phytases that are not on the market, the ones most resistant to high temperatures reported so far have been isolated from *Pichia anomala* (Vohra and Satyanarayana, 2002),

Schwanniomyces castellii (Segueilha *et al.*, 1992) and *Lactobacillus sanfranciscensis* (De Angelis *et al.*, 2003). Thermostability of the *B. subtilis* phytase is also due to its capacity to partially refold after heat treatment (Kerovuo *et al.*, 2000b). However, the stability of this enzyme is strongly dependent on the presence of Ca^{2+}.

7.3.4   Other forms of phytase activity inhibition

Besides pH, temperature and proteolytic activity, the presence of metals, high concentrations of inorganic phosphate and/or phytate as well as high ionic strength may negatively affect the activity of different phytases. The most potent inhibitors of histidine acid phytases were found to be Zn^{2+}, fluoride, molybdate, wolframate, vanadate and the hydrolysis product orthophosphate (Konietzny and Greiner, 2002). It is not clear whether metal ions modulate phytase activity by binding to the enzyme or by forming poorly soluble metal ion–phytate complexes (Greiner and Konietzny, 2010). The appearance of a precipitate while adding Fe^{2+} or Fe^{3+} to assay mixtures suggests that the observed reduction in dephosphorylation rate is due to a decrease in active substrate concentration by the formation of poorly soluble iron phytate (Konietzny *et al.*, 1994). The phytase from *A. niger* was shown to be completely unable to hydrolyse iron phytate while it showed a much lower activity towards calcium and aluminium phytate (Mezeli *et al.*, 2017). Moreover, calcium supplementation has been shown to decrease added phytase efficacy and cause phosphorus deficiency in poultry (Bedford and Rousseau, 2017). As with histidine acid phytases, enzymatic phytate dephosphorylation by *S. ruminantium* phytase is reduced in the presence of metal cations. The inhibitory effect of iron, copper, zinc and mercury cations was attributed to their ability to form complexes with phytate, but the stimulatory effect of lead cations remained unexplained (Yanke *et al.*, 1998). Fluoride, a well-known inhibitor of many

acid phosphatases, inhibits histidine acid phytases competitively, with inhibitor constants ranging from 0.1 to 0.5 mM.

The hydrolysis product orthophosphate and its structural analogues molybdate, wolframate and vanadate were recognized as competitive inhibitors of enzymatic phytate degradation. It has been suggested that these transition metal oxyanions exert their inhibitory effects by forming complexes that resemble the trigonal bipyramidal geometry of the transition state (Zhang *et al.*, 1997). Furthermore, the substrate phytate was also reported to act as an inhibitor of many acid phytases. The phytate concentration necessary to inhibit phytase activity ranges from 300 µM for the maize root enzyme (Hubel and Beck, 1996) up to 20 mM for the soybean enzyme (Gibson and Ullah, 1988). With high substrate concentrations, the charge due to phosphate groups may affect the local environment of the catalytic domain of the enzyme. This might inhibit conversion of the enzyme–substrate complex to enzyme and product, although inhibition due to the formation of poorly soluble phytase–phytate complexes cannot be ruled out. Substrate inhibition should be considered when determining phytase activity by the standard *in vitro* assay, because the activity of different phytases may be reduced to different degrees at the substrate concentration of the assay.

Last but not least, the ionic strength may affect phytase performance as well. The addition of up to 600 mM NaCl causes a strong inhibition of the activity of all commercial phytases, except for the phytase from *A. niger* (BASF Natuphos®) (Menezes-Blackburn *et al.*, 2015). The ionic strength of the medium regulates protein hydration and folding, leading to a decrease in activity at NaCl concentrations above only 100 mM.

7.3.5   Substrate specificity and end product of enzymatic phytate dephosphorylation

Substrate specificity may also have an effect on the *in vivo* performance of phytases. *In vitro* studies with purified phytases and sodium phytate as a substrate revealed that phytases hydrolyse phytate via a pathway of stepwise dephosphorylation resulting in the generation of orthophosphate and a series of partially phosphorylated *myo*-inositol phosphates (Konietzny and Greiner, 2002; Greiner and Konietzny, 2010). The partially phosphorylated inositol phosphates are released from the enzymes and serve as substrates for further hydrolysis. The different phosphate residues of phytate may be released at different rates and in different order for different phytases. In general, however, phytases do not have the capacity to dephosphorylate phytate completely. The phosphate residue at position C-2 in the *myo*-inositol ring was shown to be resistant to dephosphorylation by phytases. Independent of their bacterial, fungal or plant origin, the majority of histidine acid phytases release five of the six phosphate residues of phytate, and the final degradation product was identified as *myo*-inositol(2)phosphate (Greiner *et al.*, 2000a, 2001a, 2002, 2007a, 2009; Nakano *et al.*, 2000; Greiner and Alamiger, 2001; Greiner and Carlsson, 2006). Dephosphorylation of *myo*-inositol(2)phosphate occurs only in the presence of high enzyme concentration during prolonged incubation. After removal of the first phosphate residue from phytate, histidine acid phytases continue dephosphorylation adjacent to a free hydroxyl group. In addition, some glucose-1-phosphatases from the Enterobacteriaceae family are able to hydrolyse a single phosphate moiety at the D-3 position of phytate (Greiner, 2004a; Herter *et al.*, 2006). *Bacillus* alkaline phytases, as well as cat's tail and lily pollen phytases, can only hydrolyse three phosphate moieties of the phytate molecule yielding a *myo*-inositol trisphosphate as the final product of phytate dephosphorylation. In general, β-propeller phytases remove every second phosphate group on phytate, generating *myo*-inositol(2,4,6)trisphosphate as the final dephosphorylation product. Thus, histidine acid phytases are unable to dephosphorylate *myo*-inositol(2,4,6)trisphosphate, the final product of *Bacillus* phytase. The activity of phytases towards partially phosphorylated inositol phosphates is remarkably different, tending to increase towards the pentakis-phosphates (first product of dephosphorylation)

and decrease thereafter towards lower-order inositol phosphates (Greiner, 2017). These differences in kinetic parameters cause a decrease in the hydrolysis rate during phytate dephosphorylation by phytases.

In vitro feed experiments with microbial phytases suggest that enzymes with broad substrate specificity are better suited for animal nutrition purposes than enzymes with narrow substrate specificity (Wyss *et al.*, 1999). In general, phytases accept a variety of phosphorylated compounds as substrates, making them ideal phosphatases for application on complex substrates such as feeds (Konietzny and Greiner, 2002). Only a few phytases such as the β-propeller phytases from *Bacillus* species have high specificity towards phytate (Shimizu, 1992; Kim *et al.*, 1998b). Histidine acid phytases with broad substrate specificity readily dephosphorylate phytate to *myo*-inositol monophosphate, with no major accumulation of intermediates, whereas phytases with narrow substrate specificity result in *myo*-inositol tris- and bisphosphate accumulation during phytate dephosphorylation (Greiner and Konietzny, 2010).

High turnover numbers are expected to be a more desirable property for phytases used as feed additives than broad substrate specificity. The turnover numbers k_{cat} for hydrolysis of sodium phytate by phytases reported so far range from <10/s (Gibson and Ullah, 1988; Greiner *et al.*, 2000b) to 10,325/s (Huang *et al.*, 2006). High affinity for sodium phytate is expressed by a low Michaelis–Menten constant K_M, which represents the substrate concentration where half of the maximum turnover number is reached. K_M values of phytases studied range from <10 to 650 µM. Among the current commercial phytases, the lowest K_M values have been reported for *A. niger* (42 µM; BASF Natuphos®) whereas *C. braakii* showed the highest K_M (335 µM; Novozymes/DSM Ronozyme®) (Menezes-Blackburn *et al.*, 2015).

7.4 Specific Activity

Specific activity (activity per milligram of enzyme) is one of the key factors in the commercial exploitation of phytases. The higher the specific activity of a phytase, the higher the rate of phosphate release from phytate by a given mass of phytase. Nevertheless, phytases are supplemented according to their enzymatic activity and not according to their mass; therefore, if a given phytase has a low specific activity, a higher amount of phytase on a protein basis must be supplemented. Specific activity of commercial phytases is often confounded with the activity concentration of the produced enzyme (activity per milligram of proteins), since phytase products are often a complex mixture of proteins, not fully purified due to the high costs involved (Menezes-Blackburn *et al.*, 2015). Specific activities of phytases range from <10 U/mg (lily pollen, mung bean, soybean, maize, *Penicillium simplicissimum*) to >1000 U/mg (*C. braakii*, *Candida krusei*, *P. lycii*, *Yersinia* spp.) at 37°C and their individual optimum pH (Greiner and Konietzny, 2006, 2010). In general, microbial phytases seem to exhibit higher specific activities than their plant counterparts (Table 7.1). Commercially available phytases from *A. niger* and *E. coli* were reported to exhibit specific activities in the range of 50–133 and 750–811 U/mg, respectively (Wyss *et al.*, 1999; Golovan *et al.*, 2000; Konietzny and Greiner, 2002; Greiner *et al.*, 2009).

7.5   Phytases with More Advantageous Properties

Phytases with all the ideal properties for animal feed applications have not been found in nature to date. Naturally occurring phytases having the required level of thermostability for application in animal feeding have also not been identified in nature. The poor thermostability of phytases is therefore still a major concern in animal feed applications. Several strategies have been used to obtain an enzyme capable of withstanding higher temperatures. Thus, screening of different environments for phytases with more favourable properties for feed applications and engineering phytases in order to optimize their catalytic and stability features are suitable approaches to make better candidates

available for use as feed supplements (Ushasree *et al.*, 2017).

7.6   Screening Nature for Phytases

Screening microorganisms for phytase production is not a trivial exercise. The expression of phytases in microbial cells is often subject to complex regulation, but their formation is not triggered uniformly across classes (Konietzny and Greiner, 2004). A tight regulatory inhibition of the formation of phytases by phosphate levels is generally observed in microorganisms, including moulds, yeasts and bacteria. With the majority of microorganisms, however, it was demonstrated that phosphate concentration is not the only factor affecting phytase production. Depending on the microorganism under investigation, phytate dephosphorylation products, aeration/anaerobiosis, carbon starvation, glucose concentration, pH and temperature were all shown to modulate phytase synthesis in wild-type microbes (Powar and Jagannathan, 1982; Greiner *et al.*, 1993, 1997, 2009; Kerovuo *et al.*, 1998; Kim *et al.*, 1998a,b; De Angelis *et al.*, 2003; Greiner and Konietzny, 2010). Therefore, failure to detect phytase activity does not necessarily imply that the microorganism under investigation is not a phytase producer at all, but perhaps that the culture conditions are disadvantageous for its expression. In many cases the expressed phytase activity by a given microbe may be below the limit of detection of the assay used. In addition, fast and easy plate-screening methods depend upon the phytase being extracellularly secreted. However, most microorganisms produce only intracellular phytases. Extracellular phytase activity was observed almost exclusively in filamentous fungi and yeasts (Konietzny and Greiner, 2002). The only bacteria showing extracellular phytase activity were those of the genera *Bacillus* and *Enterobacter* (Yoon *et al.*, 1996; Kerovuo *et al.*, 1998; Menezes-Blackburn *et al.*, 2013).

Today, strategies such as (i) exploiting databases obtained from genome projects on microorganisms through a BLAST search using representative genes from the four classes of phytases (Cheng and Lim, 2006; Lim *et al.*, 2007) and (ii) identifying putative phytase-encoding genes by PCR using degenerate primers based on conserved amino acid sequences of each of the four classes of phytases (Huang *et al.*, 2009, 2010) are seen as an alternative to successfully identifying phytase-producing microorganisms. This exercise is nevertheless equally as laborious as screening nature by using the phytase activity itself for identifying new phytase-producing microbes, since: (i) many phytases share homology with other non-phytase phosphatases and if a putative phytase gene was identified in a 'collection microbe', the gene product may not accept phytate as a substrate; (ii) if the putative phytase gene encodes a phytase, in most cases the microbe will not express it in sufficient amounts to be detected by a phytase activity assay; therefore (iii) this phytase will need to be cloned and overexpressed in order to be characterized; and finally (iv) often degenerate primers show unspecific amplification, targeting other regions of the microbial genome that do not correspond to phytases. Additionally, the ultimate disadvantage of these strategies is that they will only identify phytases with the same catalytic mechanisms as the well-known and previously characterized phytases since the search depends upon known genetic sequences.

7.7 Engineering Phytases to Optimize their Catalytic and Stability Features

Tailor-made biocatalysts can be created from wild-type enzymes by either protein engineering or directed evolution techniques. The use of the term 'engineering' implies that there is some precise understanding of the system that is being modified. Thus, determinants for the property of an enzyme to be improved must be known and, therefore, rational enzyme design usually requires both the availability of the structure of the enzyme and knowledge about the relationships between sequence, structure and catalytic mechanism to make the desired changes.

Since site-directed mutagenesis techniques are well developed, the introduction of directed mutations is simple and relatively inexpensive. The major drawback in rational protein design is that detailed structural knowledge of an enzyme is often unavailable. Therefore, optimization of catalytic properties has been approached in the past mostly on a trial-and-error basis by random mutagenesis. However, rapid progress in solving protein structures by NMR spectroscopy (instead of by X-ray diffraction of crystals) and the enormously increasing number of sequences stored in public databases have significantly improved access to data and structures. Even if there are no structural data available, the structure of a homologous enzyme could be used as a model to select amino acid substitutions to increase selectivity, activity or stability of a given enzyme. Computer-aided molecular modelling seeks to identify the effect of amino acid alterations on enzyme folding and substrate recognition. However, it can be extremely difficult to predict the effects of a mutation, because even minor sequence changes by a single-point mutation may cause significant structural disturbance. Thus, even if one trait is successfully designed, it is virtually impossible to predict its effect on another trait.

One powerful tool for the development of biocatalysts with novel properties without any requirement for knowledge of enzyme structures or catalytic mechanisms is provided by a collection of methods mimicking the natural process of enzyme evolution in the test-tube by using modern molecular biology methods of mutation and recombination. This collection of methods has been termed 'directed evolution' (Chirumamilla *et al.*, 2001; Shivange and Schwaneberg, 2017). Furthermore, directed evolution provides the possibility of exploring enzyme functions never required in the natural environment and for which the molecular basis is poorly understood. Thus, this bottom-up design approach contrasts with the more conventional, previously mentioned top-down one in which proteins are tuned rationally using computer-based modelling and site-directed mutagenesis.

Protein engineering as well as direct evolution techniques have been applied to improve phytate hydrolysis at low pH values, enhance thermal tolerance of phytases and increase their specific activity in order to optimize phytases for animal feed applications.

Once amino acid sequence alignments and experimentally determined or homology-modelled three-dimensional structures have been used to identify active-site amino acids, site-directed mutagenesis can be used to alter this motif and shift phytase catalytic properties. The first site-directed mutagenesis experiments aimed to understand the effect of single amino acid substitutions on the enzyme catalytic properties such as pH optimum and specific activity (Tomschy et al., 2000; Mullaney et al., 2002) and its impact on phytase performance (Kim et al., 2006). There is still a need to improve our understanding of cooperative multiple substitutions (epistatic effects) on phytase properties (Shivange and Schwaneberg, 2017). In recent directed evolution studies, phytase thermostability has been the main target (Kim et al., 2008; Hesampour et al., 2015; Han et al., 2018; Tang et al., 2018; Ushasree et al., 2019) with significant improvements that have yet to reach the market (Menezes-Blackburn and Greiner, 2015; Menezes-Blackburn et al., 2015). Thermostability of bacterial phytases in particular can also be enhanced by taking advantage of post-translational modifications of a given phytase enzyme by its expression in eukaryotic hosts such as the yeast P. pastoris coupled with the introduction of glycosylation sites into the amino acid sequence by site-directed mutagenesis (Rodriguez et al., 2000). Gene site saturation mutagenesis technology was a further approach used to optimize thermostability and performance of phytases (Garrett et al., 2004; Shivange et al., 2014). In a random mutagenesis study the overall catalytic efficiency (k_{cat}/K_M) was improved by up to 152% and thermostability by 20%, showing that thermostability improvements are not necessarily to the detriment of catalytic efficiency (Kim and Lei, 2008).

Fully synthetic phytases have also been generated by using the consensus approach, which is based on the comparison of amino acid sequences of homologous proteins and subsequent calculation of a consensus amino acid sequence. This methodology has proven to be effective for improving phytase thermostability and performance as a feed additive (Lehmann et al., 2000, 2002; Gentile et al., 2003; Esteve-Garcia et al., 2005).

7.8   Combining Phytases with Complementary Properties

A combination of phytases with different initiation sites and/or complementary activities towards lower-order inositol phosphates could result in linearly additive responses or even synergistic effects in respect to phosphate release from feed material. A prerequisite for more efficient phosphate release from phytate is that reaction intermediates generated by one of the phytases are dephosphorylated faster than they are produced by the other phytase. However, different phytases may exhibit different phytate degradation pathways and therefore lead to the generation and accumulation of different myo-inositol phosphate intermediates (Fig. 7.2). It is unlikely that a particular phytase accepts all theoretically possible myo-inositol phosphate esters as a substrate. Therefore, some reaction intermediates generated by a certain phytase may be slowly dephosphorylated by a different phytase or may even act as a competitive inhibitor while binding to the active site without being hydrolysed. Thus, phytases that are planned to be used in combination have to be well tuned to achieve synergistic effects with respect to phosphate release from phytate in the gastrointestinal tract of an animal. Zimmermann et al. (2003) observed that intrinsic cereal phytase (rye, wheat) and supplemental A. niger phytase exhibit linear additivity in their response on apparent phosphorus absorption by pigs. This result implies that both types of phytase degrade phytate independently from each other. Synergistic effects have so far not been observed from the combination of various phytases. In addition, Greiner (2017) showed for the phytases from rye, A. niger and E. coli that reaction intermediates generated by

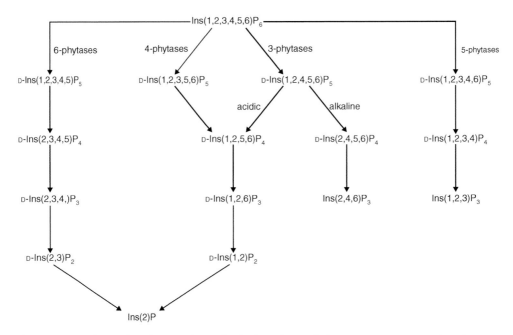

Fig. 7.2. Major phytate degradation pathways for the four classes of phytase. (From Greiner and Konietzny, 2010. Figure used with permission.)

one phytase are always dephosphorylated slower by a phytase with a different initiation site. If this observation is also applicable for phytases not included in that study, a combination of phytases with different initiation sites will never have any advantage compared with the use of a single phytase as a feed supplement. However, this needs to be experimentally verified.

7.9   Phytase Production Systems

A phytase product will not be competitive on the market if it cannot be produced at high yield and purity by a relatively inexpensive expression system. Wild-type organisms are not suitable for industrial applications because they tend to produce low levels of phytase activity, and the purification of these untagged enzymes is both tedious and cost-intensive. Therefore, highly efficient and cost-effective processes for phytase production by recombinant microorganisms have been massively applied for industrial enzymes in general. The fact that most of

the phytases characterized to date are monomeric proteins (Konietzny and Greiner, 2002) facilitates their overexpression in microbial and plant as well as in animal systems. The Novozymes/DSM Ronozyme® phytases are expressed and produced in *Aspergillus oryzae*, the AB Vista Quantum® and the Danisco Axtra® phytases are produced in *Trichoderma reesei*, the Danisco Phyzyme® phytase is produced in *Schizosaccharomyces pombe* while the BASF Natuphos® phytase is produced in *A. niger* (Menezes-Blackburn *et al.*, 2015).

Inclusion of phytase activity in the plant seed itself is an alternative strategy for improving nutrient management in animal production. Increased phytase activity in the plant seed can be achieved by heterologous expression of fungal and bacterial phytases. Only limited amounts of these transgenic seeds are required in compound feeds to ensure proper degradation of phytate (Pen *et al.*, 1993; Ponstein *et al.*, 2002; Chiera *et al.*, 2004; Bilyeu *et al.*, 2008). A different strategy to overcome the problems encountered in using phytase as a feed additive, such as cost, inactivation at the high temperatures required for pelleting feed and loss of activity during storage, might be to add those enzymes to the repertoire of digestive enzymes produced endogenously by swine and poultry. Transgenic swine expressing *E. coli* phytase in the saliva were shown to enable ample digestion of dietary phytate, removing the requirement for phosphate supplementation and reducing faecal phosphate output by up to 75% (Golovan *et al.*, 2001). This reduction even exceeded the 40% reduction reported for pigs fed phytase supplements at standard doses. These values can be exceeded if phytases are supplemented at very high doses.

7.10 Conclusions and Future Perspectives

Numerous feeding studies with poultry, swine and fish have demonstrated the efficacy of phytase supplementation for improving phosphorus and mineral availability. In particular, microbial histidine acid phytases offer technical and economic feasibility for their production and application. Microbial phytases show advantages compared with plant phytases in respect to properties favourable for animal feed applications, such as their pH–activity profiles, thermostabilities, protease tolerance and specific activity. However, it is important to realize that no single phytase is currently able to meet all the diverse needs of its commercial application. Thus, screening nature for phytases with more appropriate properties, coupled with engineering them for optimal catalytic and stability features, is a rational approach to deliver a phytase product more suited to animal feed applications. The quest for more effective phytases continues, with emphasis on thermal tolerance, a broad pH–activity profile and enhanced stability under the pH and proteolytic conditions of the digestive tract. Aside from the physicochemical properties of a supplementary phytase, its economic large-scale production is a further aspect that must be considered. Therefore, there is still interest in developing highly efficient and cost-effective processes for phytase production. Furthermore, combined supplementation of phytase with other feed enzymes such as carbohydrases and proteases should be exploited as a strategy to improve overall nutrient utilization of animal feeds.

References

Adeola, O., Olukosi, O., Jendza, J., Dilger, R. and Bedford, M. (2006) Response of growing pigs to *Peniophora lycii*- and *Escherichia coli*-derived phytases or varying ratios of calcium to total phosphorus. *Animal Science* 82, 637–644.

Augspurger, N., Webel, D., Lei, X. and Baker, D. (2003) Efficacy of an *E. coli* phytase expressed in yeast for releasing phytate-bound phosphorus in young chicks and pigs. *Journal of Animal Science* 81, 474–483.

Bedford, M. and Rousseau, X. (2017) Recent findings regarding calcium and phytase in poultry nutrition. *Animal Production Science* 57, 2311–2316.

Berka, R.M., Rey, M.W., Brown, K.M., Byun, T. and Klotz, A.V. (1998) Molecular characterization and expression of a phytase gene from the thermophilic fungus *Thermomyces lanuginosus*. *Applied and Environmental Microbiology* 64, 4423–4427.

Bilyeu, K.D., Zeng, P., Coello, P., Zhang, Z.J., Krishnan, H.B., *et al.* (2008) Quantitative conversion of phytate to inorganic phosphorus in soybean seeds expressing a bacterial phytase. *Plant Physiology* 146, 468–477.

Campbell, G. and Bedford, M. (1992) Enzyme applications for monogastric feeds: a review. *Canadian Journal of Animal Science* 72, 449–466.

Chatterjee, S., Sankaranarayanan, R. and Sonti, R. (2003) PhyA, a secreted protein of *Xanthomonas oryzae* pv. *oryzae*, is required for optimum virulence and growth on phytic acid as a sole phosphate source. *Molecular Plant–Microbe Interactions* 16, 973–982.

Cheng, C. and Lim, B. (2006) Beta-propeller phytases in the aquatic environment. *Archives of Microbiology* 185, 1–13.

Chiera, J.M., Finer, J.J. and Grabau, E.A. (2004) Ectopic expression of a soybean phytase in developing seeds of *Glycine max* to improve phosphorus availability. *Plant Molecular Biology* 56, 895–904.

Chirumamilla, R.R., Muralidhar, R., Marchant, R. and Nigam, P. (2001) Improving the quality of industrially important enzymes by directed evolution. *Molecular and Cellular Biochemistry* 224, 159–168.

Cho, J., Lee, C., Kang, S., Lee, J., Bok, J., *et al.* (2003) Purification and characterization of a phytase from *Pseudomonas syringae* MOK1. *Current Microbiology* 47, 290–294.

Choi, Y.M., Suh, H.J. and Kim, J.M. (2001) Purification and properties of extracellular phytase from *Bacillus* sp. KHU-10. *Journal of Protein Chemistry* 20, 287–292.

Chu, H.-M., Guo, R.-T., Lin, T.-W., Chou, C.-C., Shr, H.-L., *et al.* (2004) Structures of *Selenomonas ruminantium* phytase in complex with persulfated phytate: DSP phytase fold and mechanism for sequential substrate hydrolysis. *Structure* 12, 2015–2024.

De Angelis, M., Gallo, G., Corbo, M.R., McSweeney, P.L., Faccia, M., *et al.* (2003) Phytase activity in sourdough lactic acid bacteria: purification and characterization of a phytase from *Lactobacillus sanfranciscensis* CB1. *International Journal of Food Microbiology* 87, 259–270.

Dersjant-Li, Y., Awati, A., Schulze, H. and Partridge, G. (2015) Phytase in non-ruminant animal nutrition: a critical review on phytase activities in the gastrointestinal tract and influencing factors. *Journal of the Science of Food and Agriculture* 95, 878–896.

Dionisio, G., Madsen, C.K., Holm, P.B., Welinder, K.G., Jørgensen, M., *et al.* (2011) Cloning and characterization of purple acid phosphatase phytases from wheat, barley, maize and rice. *Plant Physiology* 156, 1087–1100.

Engelen, A.J., Randsdorp, P. and Smit, E. (1994) Simple and rapid determination of phytase activity. *Journal of AOAC International* 77, 760–764.

Esteve-Garcia, E., Perez-Vendrell, A.M. and Broz, J. (2005) Phosphorus equivalence of a consensus phytase produced by *Hansenula polymorpha* in diets for young turkeys. *Archives of Animal Nutrition* 59, 53–59.

Garrett, J.B., Kretz, K.A., O'Donoghue, E., Kerovuo, J., Kim, W., *et al.* (2004) Enhancing the thermal tolerance and gastric performance of a microbial phytase for use as a phosphate-mobilizing monogastric-feed supplement. *Applied and Environmental Microbiology* 70, 3041–3046.

Gentile, J., Roneker, K., Crowe, S., Pond, W. and Lei, X. (2003) Effectiveness of an experimental consensus phytase in improving dietary phytate-phosphorus utilization by weanling pigs. *Journal of Animal Science* 81, 2751–2757.

Ghorbani Nasrabadi, R., Greiner, R., Yamchi, A. and Nourzadeh Roshan, E. (2018) A novel purple acid phytase from an earthworm cast bacterium. *Journal of the Science of Food and Agriculture* 98, 3667–3674.

Gibson, D.M. and Ullah, A.H. (1988) Purification and characterization of phytase from cotyledons of germinating soybean seeds. *Archives of Biochemistry and Biophysics* 260, 503–513.

Golovan, S., Wang, G., Zhang, J. and Forsberg, C. (2000) Characterization and overproduction of the *Escherichia coli* appA encoded bifunctional enzyme that exhibits both phytase and acid phosphatase activities. *Canadian Journal of Microbiology* 46, 59–71.

Golovan, S.P., Meidinger, R.G., Ajakaiye, A., Cottrill, M., Wiederkehr, M.Z., *et al.* (2001) Pigs expressing salivary phytase produce low-phosphorus manure. *Nature Biotechnology* 19, 741–745.

Greiner, R. (2002) Purification and characterization of three phytases from germinated lupine seeds (*Lupinus albus* var. Amiga). *Journal of Agricultural and Food Chemistry* 50, 6858–6864.

Greiner, R. (2004a) Degradation of *myo*-inositol hexakisphosphate by a phytate-degrading enzyme from *Pantoea agglomerans*. *The Protein Journal* 23, 577–585.

Greiner, R. (2004b) Purification and properties of a phytate-degrading enzyme from *Pantoea agglomerans*. *The Protein Journal* 23, 567–576.

Greiner, R. (2007) Phytate-degrading enzymes: regulation of synthesis in microorganisms and plants. In: Turner, B., Richardson, A. and Mullaney, E. (eds) *Inositol Phosphates: Linking Agriculture and the Environment*. CAB International, Wallingford, UK, pp. 78–96.

Greiner, R. (2017) Activity of *Escherichia coli*, *Aspergillus niger*, and rye phytase toward partially phosphorylated *myo*-inositol phosphates. *Journal of Agricultural and Food Chemistry* 65, 9603–9607.

Greiner, R. and Alamiger, M. (2001) Stereospecificity of *myo*-inositol hexakisphosphate dephosphorylation by phytate-degrading enzymes of cereals. *Journal of Food Biochemistry* 25, 229–248.

Greiner, R. and Carlsson, N.-G. (2006) *myo*-Inositol phosphate isomers generated by the action of a phytate-degrading enzyme from *Klebsiella terrigena* on phytate. *Canadian Journal of Microbiology* 52, 759–768.

Greiner, R. and Konietzny, U. (2006) Phytase for food application. *Food Technology and Biotechnology* 44, 125–140.

Greiner, R. and Konietzny, U. (2010) Phytases: biochemistry, enzymology and characteristics relevant to animal feed use. In: Bedford, M.R and Partridge, G.G. (eds) *Enzymes in Farm Animal Nutrition*, 2nd edn. CAB International, Wallingford, UK, pp. 96–128.

Greiner, R., Konietzny, U. and Jany, K.-D. (1993) Purification and characterization of two phytases from *Escherichia coli*. *Archives of Biochemistry and Biophysics* 303, 107–113.

Greiner, R., Haller, E., Konietzny, U. and Jany, K.-D. (1997) Purification and characterization of a phytase from *Klebsiella terrigena*. *Archives of Biochemistry and Biophysics* 341, 201–206.

Greiner, R., Konietzny, U. and Jany, K. (1998) Purification and properties of a phytase from rye. *Journal of Food Biochemistry* 22, 143–161.

Greiner, R., Carlsson, N.-G. and Alminger, M.L. (2000a) Stereospecificity of *myo*-inositol hexakisphosphate dephosphorylation by a phytate-degrading enzyme of *Escherichia coli*. *Journal of Biotechnology* 84, 53–62.

Greiner, R., Jany, K.-D. and Alminger, M.L. (2000b) Identification and properties of *myo*-inositol hexakisphosphate phosphohydrolases (phytases) from barley (*Hordeum vulgare*). *Journal of Cereal Science* 31, 127–139.

Greiner, R., Alminger, M.L. and Carlsson, N.-G. (2001a) Stereospecificity of *myo*-inositol hexakisphosphate dephosphorylation by a phytate-degrading enzyme of baker's yeast. *Journal of Agricultural and Food Chemistry* 49, 2228–2233.

Greiner, R., Muzquiz, M., Burbano, C., Cuadrado, C., Pedrosa, M.M. and Goyoaga, C. (2001b) Purification and characterization of a phytate-degrading enzyme from germinated faba beans (*Vicia faba* var. Alameda). *Journal of Agricultural and Food Chemistry* 49, 2234–2240.

Greiner, R., Larsson Alminger, M., Carlsson, N.-G., Muzquiz, M., Burbano, C., *et al.* (2002) Pathway of dephosphorylation of *myo*-inositol hexakisphosphate by phytases of legume seeds. *Journal of Agricultural and Food Chemistry* 50, 6865–6870.

Greiner, R., Farouk, A.-E., Carlsson, N.-G. and Konietzny, U. (2007a) *myo*-Inositol phosphate isomers generated by the action of a phytase from a Malaysian waste-water bacterium. *The Protein Journal* 26, 577–584.

Greiner, R., Lim, B.L., Cheng, C.W. and Carlsson, N.G. (2007b) Pathway of phytate dephosphorylation by beta-propeller phytases of different origins. *Canadian Journal of Microbiology* 53, 488–495.

Greiner, R., Silva, L.G.D. and Couri, S. (2009) Purification and characterisation of an extracellular phytase from *Aspergillus niger* 11T53A9. *Brazilian Journal of Microbiology* 40, 795–807.

Gruninger, R.J., Thibault, J., Capeness, M.J., Till, R., Mosimann, S.C., *et al.* (2014) Structural and biochemical analysis of a unique phosphatase from *Bdellovibrio bacteriovorus* reveals its structural and functional relationship with the protein tyrosine phosphatase class of phytase. *PLoS ONE* 9, e94403.

Han, N., Miao, H., Yu, T., Xu, B., Yang, Y., *et al.* (2018) Enhancing thermal tolerance of *Aspergillus niger* PhyA phytase directed by structural comparison and computational simulation. *BMC Biotechnology* 18, 36.

Hara, A., Ebina, S., Kondo, A. and Funaguma, T. (1985) A new type of phytase from pollen of *Typha latifolia* L. *Agricultural and Biological Chemistry* 49, 3539–3544.

Hegeman, C.E. and Grabau, E.A. (2001) A novel phytase with sequence similarity to purple acid phosphatases is expressed in cotyledons of germinating soybean seedlings. *Plant Physiology* 126, 1598–1608.

Herter, T., Berezina, O., Zinin, N., Velikodvorskaya, G., Greiner, R. and Borriss, R. (2006) Glucose-1-phosphatase (AgpE) from *Enterobacter cloacae* displays enhanced phytase activity. *Applied Microbiology and Biotechnology* 70, 60–64.

Hesampour, A., Siadat, S.E.R., Malboobi, M.A., Mohandesi, N., Arab, S.S. and Ghahremanpour, M.M. (2015) Enhancement of thermostability and kinetic efficiency of *Aspergillus niger* PhyA phytase by site-directed mutagenesis. *Applied Biochemistry and Biotechnology* 175, 2528–2541.

Huang, H., Luo, H., Yang, P., Meng, K., Wang, Y., *et al.* (2006) A novel phytase with preferable characteristics from *Yersinia intermedia*. *Biochemical and Biophysical Research Communications* 350, 884–889.

Huang, H., Luo, H., Wang, Y., Fu, D., Shao, N., Wang, G., *et al.* (2008) A novel phytase from *Yersinia rohdei* with high phytate hydrolysis activity under low pH and strong pepsin conditions. *Applied Microbiology and Biotechnology* 80, 417.

Huang, H., Shao, N., Wang, Y., Luo, H., Yang, P., *et al.* (2009) A novel beta-propeller phytase from *Pedobacter nyackensis* MJ11 CGMCC 2503 with potential as an aquatic feed additive. *Applied Microbiology and Biotechnology* 83, 249–259.

Huang, H., Wang, G., Zhao, Y., Shi, P., Luo, H. and Yao, B. (2010) Direct and efficient cloning of full-length genes from environmental DNA by RT-qPCR and modified TAIL-PCR. *Applied Microbiology and Biotechnology* 87, 1141–1149.

Huang, H., Zhang, R., Fu, D., Luo, J., Li, Z., *et al.* (2011) Diversity, abundance and characterization of ruminal cysteine phytases suggest their important role in phytate degradation. *Environmental Microbiology* 13, 747–757.

Hubel, F. and Beck, E. (1996) Maize root phytase (purification, characterization, and localization of enzyme activity and its putative substrate). *Plant Physiology* 112, 1429–1436.

Igbasan, F., Männer, K., Miksch, G., Borriss, R., Farouk, A. and Simon, O. (2000) Comparative studies on the *in vitro* properties of phytases from various microbial origins. *Archives of Animal Nutrition* 53, 353–373.

Inborr, J. and Bedford, M. (1994) Stability of feed enzymes to steam pelleting during feed processing. *Animal Feed Science and Technology* 46, 179–196.

Iqbal, T., Lewis, K. and Cooper, B.J.G. (1994) Phytase activity in the human and rat small intestine. *Gut* 35, 1233–1236.

Jang, W.J., Lee, J.M., Park, H.D., Choi, Y.B. and Kong, I.-S. (2018) N-terminal domain of the beta-propeller phytase of *Pseudomonas* sp. FB15 plays a role for retention of low-temperature activity and catalytic efficiency. *Enzyme and Microbial Technology* 117, 84–90.

Jorquera, M.A., Crowley, D.E., Marschner, P., Greiner, R., Fernández, M.T., *et al.* (2010) Identification of β-propeller phytase-encoding genes in culturable *Paenibacillus* and *Bacillus* spp. from the rhizosphere of pasture plants on volcanic soils. *FEMS Microbiology Ecology* 75, 163–172.

Jorquera, M.A., Gabler, S., Inostroza, N.G., Acuña, J.J., Campos, M.A., *et al.* (2018) Screening and characterization of phytases from bacteria isolated from Chilean hydrothermal environments. *Microbial Ecology* 75, 387–399.

Kerovuo, J., Lauraeus, M., Nurminen, P., Kalkkinen, N. and Apajalahti, J. (1998) Isolation, characterization, molecular gene cloning, and sequencing of a novel phytase from *Bacillus subtilis*. *Applied and Environmental Microbiology* 64, 2079–2085.

Kerovuo, J., Lappalainen, I. and Reinikainen, T. (2000a) The metal dependence of *Bacillus subtilis* phytase. *Biochemical and Biophysical Research Communications* 268, 365–369.

Kerovuo, J., Rouvinen, J. and Hatzack, F. (2000b) Analysis of *myo*-inositol hexakisphosphate hydrolysis by *Bacillus* phytase: indication of a novel reaction mechanism. *Biochemical Journal* 352, 623–628.

Kim, H.-W., Kim, Y.-O., Lee, J.-H., Kim, K.-K. and Kim, Y.-J. (2003) Isolation and characterization of a phytase with improved properties from *Citrobacter braakii*. *Biotechnology Letters* 25, 1231–1234.

Kim, M.-S. and Lei, X.G. (2008) Enhancing thermostability of *Escherichia coli* phytase AppA2 by error-prone PCR. *Applied Microbiology and Biotechnology* 79, 69–75.

Kim, M.-S., Weaver, J.D. and Lei, X.G. (2008) Assembly of mutations for improving thermostability of *Escherichia coli* AppA2 phytase. *Applied Microbiology and Biotechnology* 79, 751–758.

Kim, T., Mullaney, E.J., Porres, J.M., Roneker, K.R., Crowe, S., *et al.* (2006) Shifting the pH profile of *Aspergillus niger* PhyA phytase to match the stomach pH enhances its effectiveness as an animal feed additive. *Applied and Environmental Microbiology* 72, 4397–4403.

Kim, Y.-O., Lee, J.-K., Kim, H.-K., Yu, J.-H. and Oh, T.-K. (1998a) Cloning of the thermostable phytase gene (*phy*) from *Bacillus* sp. DS11 and its overexpression in *Escherichia coli*. *FEMS Microbiology Letters* 162, 185–191.

Kim, Y.-O., Kim, H.-K., Bae, K.-S., Yu, J.-H. and Oh, T.-K. (1998b) Purification and properties of a thermostable phytase from *Bacillus* sp. DS11. *Enzyme and Microbial Technology* 22, 2–7.

Konietzny, U. and Greiner, R. (2002) Molecular and catalytic properties of phytate-degrading enzymes (phytases). *International Journal of Food Science & Technology* 37, 791–812.

Konietzny, U. and Greiner, R. (2004) Bacterial phytase: potential application, *in vivo* function and regulation of its synthesis. *Brazilian Journal of Microbiology* 35, 12–18.

Konietzny, U., Greiner, R. and Jany, K. (1994) Purification and characterization of a phytase from spelt. *Journal of Food Biochemistry* 18, 165–183.

Kostrewa, D., Grüninger-Leitch, F., D'Arcy, A., Broger, C. and Mitchell, D. (1997) Crystal structure of phytase from *Aspergillus ficuum* at 2.5 Å resolution. *Nature Structural and Molecular Biology* 4, 185–190.

Kumar, V., Yadav, A., Saxena, A., Sangwan, P. and Dhaliwal, H. (2016) Unravelling rhizospheric diversity and potential of phytase producing microbes. *SM Journal of Biology* 2, 1009.

Kumar, V., Yadav, A.N., Verma, P., Sangwan, P., Saxena, A., *et al.* (2017) β-Propeller phytases: diversity, catalytic attributes, current developments and potential biotechnological applications. *International Journal of Biological Macromolecules* 98, 595–609.

Lassen, S., Breinholt, J., Ostergaard, P., Brugger, R., Bischoff, A., *et al.* (2001) Expression, gene cloning, and characterization of five novel phytases from four basidiomycete fungi: *Peniophora lycii*, *Agrocybe pediades*, a *Ceriporia* sp., and *Trametes pubescens*. *Applied and Environmental Microbiology* 67, 4701–4707.

Lee, S., Dunne, J., Mottram, T. and Bedford, M. (2017) Effect of diet phase change, dietary Ca and P level and phytase on bird performance and real-time gizzard pH measurements. *British Poultry Science* 58, 290–297.

Lehmann, M., Kostrewa, D., Wyss, M., Brugger, R., D'Aarcy, A., *et al.* (2000) From DNA sequence to improved functionality: using protein sequence comparisons to rapidly design a thermostable consensus phytase. *Protein Engineering* 13, 49–57.

Lehmann, M., Loch, C., Middendorf, A., Studer, D., Lassen, S.F., *et al.* (2002) The consensus concept for thermostability engineering of proteins: further proof of concept. *Protein Engineering* 15, 403–411.

Lei, X.G. and Porres, J.M. (2003) Phytase enzymology, applications, and biotechnology. *Biotechnology Letters* 25, 1787–1794.

Lim, B.L., Yeung, P., Cheng, C. and Hill, J.E. (2007) Distribution and diversity of phytate-mineralizing bacteria. *The ISME Journal* 1, 321–330.

Lim, D., Golovan, S., Forsberg, C.W. and Jia, Z. (2000) Crystal structures of *Escherichia coli* phytase and its complex with phytate. *Nature Structural and Molecular Biology* 7, 108–113.

Lindqvist, Y., Schneider, G. and Vihko, P. (1994) Crystal structures of rat acid phosphatase complexed with the transition-state analogs vanadate and molybdate: implications for the reaction mechanism. *European Journal of Biochemistry* 221, 139–142.

Liu, P., Cai, Z., Chen, Z., Mo, X., Ding, X., *et al.* (2018) A root-associated purple acid phosphatase, SgPAP23, mediates extracellular phytate-P utilization in *Stylosanthes guianensis*. *Plant, Cell & Environment* 41, 2821–2834.

Lung, S.-C., Leung, A., Kuang, R., Wang, Y., Leung, P. and Lim, B.-L. (2008) Phytase activity in tobacco (*Nicotiana tabacum*) root exudates is exhibited by a purple acid phosphatase. *Phytochemistry* 69, 365–373.

Makoudi, B., Kabbadj, A., Mouradi, M., Amenc, L., Domergue, O., *et al.* (2018) Phosphorus deficiency increases nodule phytase activity of faba bean–rhizobia symbiosis. *Acta Physiologiae Plantarum* 40, 63.

Mehta, B.D., Jog, S.P., Johnson, S.C. and Murthy, P.P. (2006) Lily pollen alkaline phytase is a histidine phosphatase similar to mammalian multiple inositol polyphosphate phosphatase (MINPP). *Phytochemistry* 67, 1874–1886.

Menezes-Blackburn, D. and Greiner, R. (2015) Enzymes used in animal feed: leading technologies and forthcoming developments. In: Cirillo, G., Spizzirri, U.G. and Iemma, F. (eds) *Functional Polymers in Food Science: From Technology to Biology*, vol. 2: *Food Processing*. Wiley, Hoboken, New Jersey, pp. 47–73.

Menezes-Blackburn, D., Jorquera, M.A., Greiner, R., Gianfreda, L. and de la Luz Mora, M. (2013) Phytases and phytase-labile organic phosphorus in manures and soils. *Critical Reviews in Environmental Science and Technology* 43, 916–954.

Menezes-Blackburn, D., Gabler, S. and Greiner, R. (2015) Performance of seven commercial phytases in an *in vitro* simulation of poultry digestive tract. *Journal of Agricultural and Food Chemistry* 63, 6142–6149.

Mezeli, M.M., Menezes-Blackburn, D., George, T.S., Giles, C.D., Neilson, R. and Haygarth, P.M. (2017) Effect of citrate on *Aspergillus niger* phytase adsorption and catalytic activity in soil. *Geoderma* 305, 346–353.

MRS (Market Research Store) (2017) Global Phytases Market Report 2017. Document No. MRS-150562. BisReport p. 124. Available at: https://www.marketresearchstore.com/ (accessed 12 January 2019).

Mullaney, E.J. and Ullah, A.H. (2003) The term phytase comprises several different classes of enzymes. *Biochemical and Biophysical Research Communications* 312, 179–184.

Mullaney, E.J., Daly, C.B. and Ullah, A.H. (2000) Advances in phytase research. *Advances in Applied Microbiology* 47, 157–199.

Mullaney, E.J., Daly, C.B., Kim, T., Porres, J.M., Lei, X.G., *et al.* (2002) Site-directed mutagenesis of *Aspergillus niger* NRRL 3135 phytase at residue 300 to enhance catalysis at pH 4.0. *Biochemical and Biophysical Research Communications* 297, 1016–1020.

Nakano, T., Joh, T., Narita, K. and Hayakawa, T. (2000) The pathway of dephosphorylation of *myo*-inositol hexakisphosphate by phytases from wheat bran of *Triticum aestivum* L. cv. Nourin #61. *Bioscience, Biotechnology, and Biochemistry* 64, 995–1003.

Nakashima, B.A., McAllister, T.A., Sharma, R. and Selinger, L.B. (2007) Diversity of phytases in the rumen. *Microbial Ecology* 53, 82–88.

Oh, B.-C., Choi, W.-C., Park, S., Kim, Y.-O. and Oh, T.-K. (2004) Biochemical properties and substrate specificities of alkaline and histidine acid phytases. *Applied Microbiology and Biotechnology* 63, 362–372.

Ostanin, K., Harms, E.H., Stevis, P.E., Kuciel, R., Zhou, M.-M. and Van Etten, R. (1992) Overexpression, site-directed mutagenesis, and mechanism of *Escherichia coli* acid phosphatase. *Journal of Biological Chemistry* 267, 22830–22836.

Pen, J., Verwoerd, T.C., Van Paridon, P.A., Beudeker, R.F., Van Den Elzen, P.J., *et al.* (1993) Phytase-containing transgenic seeds as a novel feed additive for improved phosphorus utilization. *Bio/Technology* 11, 811–814.

Ponstein, A.S., Bade, J.B., Verwoerd, T.C., Molendijk, L., Storms, J., *et al.* (2002) Stable expression of phytase (phyA) in canola (*Brassica napus*) seeds: towards a commercial product. *Molecular Breeding* 10, 31–44.

Powar, V.K. and Jagannathan, V. (1982) Purification and properties of phytate-specific phosphatase from *Bacillus subtilis. Journal of Bacteriology* 151, 1102–1108.

Puhl, A.A., Gruninger, R.J., Greiner, R., Janzen, T.W., Mosimann, S.C. and Selinger, L.B. (2007) Kinetic and structural analysis of a bacterial protein tyrosine phosphatase-like *myo*-inositol polyphosphatase. *Protein Science* 16, 1368–1378.

Puhl, A.A., Greiner, R. and Selinger, L.B. (2008a) Kinetics, substrate specificity, and stereospecificity of two new protein tyrosine phosphatase-like inositol polyphosphatases from *Selenomonas lacticifex. Biochemistry and Cell Biology* 86, 322–330.

Puhl, A.A., Greiner, R. and Selinger, L.B. (2008b) A protein tyrosine phosphatase-like inositol polyphosphatase from *Selenomonas ruminantium* subsp. *lactilytica* has specificity for the 5-phosphate of *myo*-inositol hexakisphosphate. *The International Journal of Biochemistry & Cell Biology* 40, 2053–2064.

Puhl, A.A., Greiner, R. and Selinger, L.B. (2009) Stereospecificity of *myo*-inositol hexakisphosphate hydrolysis by a protein tyrosine phosphatase-like inositol polyphosphatase from *Megasphaera elsdenii. Applied Microbiology and Biotechnology* 82, 95–103.

Quan, C.S., Fan, S.D., Mang, L.H., Wang, Y.J. and Ohta, Y. (2002) Purification and properties of a phytase from *Candida krusei* WZ-001. *Journal of Bioscience and Bioengineering* 94, 419–425.

Ragon, M., Aumelas, A., Chemardin, P., Galvez, S., Moulin, G. and Boze, H. (2008) Complete hydrolysis of *myo*-inositol hexakisphosphate by a novel phytase from *Debaryomyces castellii* CBS 2923. *Applied Microbiology and Biotechnology* 78, 47–53.

Rodriguez, E., Mullaney, E. and Lei, X. (2000) Expression of the *Aspergillus fumigatus* phytase gene in *Pichia pastoris* and characterization of the recombinant enzyme. *Biochemical and Biophysical Research Communications* 268, 373–378.

Rychen, G., Aquilina, G., Azimonti, G., Bampidis, V., Bastos, M.D.L., *et al.* (2017) Safety and efficacy of Natuphos® E (6-phytase) as a feed additive for avian and porcine species. *EFSA Journal* 15, e05024.

Sanangelantoni, A.M., Malatrasi, M., Trivelloni, E., Visioli, G. and Agrimonti, C. (2018) A novel β-propeller phytase from the dioxin-degrading bacterium *Sphingomonas wittichii* RW-1. *Applied Microbiology and Biotechnology* 102, 8351–8358.

Schenk, G., Guddat, L., Ge, Y., Carrington, L., Hume, D., *et al.* (2000) Identification of mammalian-like purple acid phosphatases in a wide range of plants. *Gene* 250, 117–125.

Scott, J.J. (1991) Alkaline phytase activity in nonionic detergent extracts of legume seeds. *Plant Physiology* 95, 1298–1301.

Segueilha, L., Lambrechts, C., Boze, H., Moulin, G. and Galzy, P. (1992) Purification and properties of the phytase from *Schwanniomyces castellii. Journal of Fermentation Bioengineering* 74, 7–11.

Selle, P.H. and Ravindran, V. (2007) Microbial phytase in poultry nutrition. *Animal Feed Science and Technology* 135, 1–41.

Sharma, R., Kumar, P., Kaushal, V., Das, R. and Navani, N.K. (2018) A novel protein tyrosine phosphatase like phytase from *Lactobacillus fermentum* NKN51: cloning, characterization and application in mineral release for food technology applications. *Bioresource Technology* 249, 1000–1008.

Shimizu, M. (1992) Purification and characterization of phytase from *Bacillus subtilis* (*natto*) N-77. *Bioscience, Biotechnology, and Biochemistry* 56, 1266–1269.

Shin, S., Ha, N.-C., Oh, B.-C., Oh, T.-K. and Oh, B.-H. (2001) Enzyme mechanism and catalytic property of β propeller phytase. *Structure* 9, 851–858.

Shivange, A.V. and Schwaneberg, U. (2017) Recent advances in directed phytase evolution and rational phytase engineering. In: Alcalde, M. (ed.) *Directed Enzyme Evolution: Advances and Applications.* Springer, Cham, Switzerland, pp. 145–172.

Shivange, A.V., Dennig, A. and Schwaneberg, U. (2014) Multi-site saturation by OmniChange yields a pH- and thermally improved phytase. *Journal of Biotechnology* 170, 68–72.

Simon, O. and Igbasan, F. (2002) *In vitro* properties of phytases from various microbial origins. *International Journal of Food Science & Technology* 37, 813–822.

Simons, P., Versteegh, H.A., Jongbloed, A.W., Kemme, P., Slump, P., *et al.* (1990) Improvement of phosphorus availability by microbial phytase in broilers and pigs. *British Journal of Nutrition* 64, 525–540.

Tang, Z., Jin, W., Sun, R., Liao, Y., Zhen, T., *et al.* (2018) Improved thermostability and enzyme activity of a recombinant phyA mutant phytase from *Aspergillus niger* N25 by directed evolution and site-directed mutagenesis. *Enzyme and Microbial Technology* 108, 74–81.

Tomschy, A., Wyss, M., Kostrewa, D., Vogel, K., Tessier, M., *et al.* (2000) Active site residue 297 of *Aspergillus niger* phytase critically affects the catalytic properties. *FEBS Letters* 472, 169–172.

Tran, H.T., Hurley, B.A. and Plaxton, W.C. (2010) Feeding hungry plants: the role of purple acid phosphatases in phosphate nutrition. *Plant Science* 179, 14–27.

Tseng, Y., Fang, T. and Tseng, S. (2000) Isolation and characterization of a novel phytase from *Penicillium simplicissimum*. *Folia Microbiologica* 45, 121–127.

Tye, A., Siu, F., Leung, T. and Lim, B. (2002) Molecular cloning and the biochemical characterization of two novel phytases from *B. subtilis* 168 and *B. licheniformis*. *Applied Microbiology and Biotechnology* 59, 190–197.

Ullah, A.H., Sethumadhavan, K. and Mullaney, E.J. (2008) Salt effect on the pH profile and kinetic parameters of microbial phytases. *Journal of Agricultural and Food Chemistry* 56, 3398–3402.

Ushasree, M.V., Shyam, K., Vidya, J. and Pandey, A. (2017) Microbial phytase: impact of advances in genetic engineering in revolutionizing its properties and applications. *Bioresource Technology* 245, 1790–1799.

Ushasree, M.V., Jaiswal, A.K., Shyam, K. and Pandey, A. (2019) Thermostable phytase in feed and fuel industries. *Bioresource Technology* 278, 400–407.

Vallejo, L.H., Buendía, G., Elghandour, M.M., Menezes-Blackburn, D., Greiner, R. and Salem, A.Z. (2018) The effect of exogenous phytase supplementation on nutrient digestibility, ruminal fermentation and phosphorous bioavailability in Rambouillet sheep. *Journal of the Science of Food and Agriculture* 98, 5089–5094.

Vohra, A. and Satyanarayana, T. (2002) Purification and characterization of a thermostable and acid-stable phytase from *Pichia anomala*. *World Journal of Microbiology and Biotechnology* 18, 687–691.

Wodzinski, R.J. and Ullah, A. (1996) Phytase. *Advances in Applied Microbiology* 42, 263–302.

Wyss, M., Brugger, R., Kronenberger, A., Rémy, R., Fimbel, R., *et al.* (1999) Biochemical characterization of fungal phytases (*myo*-inositol hexakisphosphate phosphohydrolases): catalytic properties. *Applied and Environmental Microbiology* 65, 367–373.

Xiao, K., Harrison, M.J. and Wang, Z.-Y. (2005) Transgenic expression of a novel *M. truncatula* phytase gene results in improved acquisition of organic phosphorus by *Arabidopsis*. *Planta* 222, 27–36.

Yanke, L., Bae, H., Selinger, L. and Cheng, K. (1998) Phytase activity of anaerobic ruminal bacteria. *Microbiology* 144, 1565–1573.

Yoon, S.J., Choi, Y.J., Min, H.K., Cho, K.K., Kim, J.W., *et al.* (1996) Isolation and identification of phytase-producing bacterium, *Enterobacter* sp. 4, and enzymatic properties of phytase enzyme. *Enzyme and Microbial Technology* 18, 449–454.

Zhang, M., Zhou, M., Van Etten, R.L. and Stauffacher, C.V. (1997) Crystal structure of bovine low molecular weight phosphotyrosyl phosphatase complexed with the transition state analog vanadate. *Biochemistry* 36, 15–23.

Zhang, R., Yang, P., Huang, H., Shi, P., Yuan, T. and Yao, B. (2011a) Two types of phytases (histidine acid phytase and β-propeller phytase) in *Serratia* sp. TN49 from the gut of *Batocera horsfieldi* (Coleoptera) larvae. *Current Microbiology* 63, 408–415.

Zhang, R., Yang, P., Huang, H., Yuan, T., Shi, P., *et al.* (2011b) Molecular and biochemical characterization of a new alkaline β-propeller phytase from the insect symbiotic bacterium *Janthinobacterium* sp. TN115. *Applied Microbiology and Biotechnology* 92, 317–325.

Zhou, X.-L., Shen, W., Zhuge, J. and Wang, Z.-X. (2006) Biochemical properties of a thermostable phytase from *Neurospora crassa*. *FEMS Microbiology Letters* 258, 61–66.

Zimmermann, B., Lantzsch, H.-J., Mosenthin, R., Biesalski, H. and Drochner, W. (2003) Additivity of the effect of cereal and microbial phytases on apparent phosphorus absorption in growing pigs fed diets with marginal P supply. *Animal Feed Science and Technology* 104, 143–152.

8 Phytases: Potential and Limits of Phytate Destruction in the Digestive Tract of Pigs and Poultry

Markus Rodehutscord[1]*, Vera Sommerfeld[1], Imke Kühn[2] and Michael R. Bedford[3]
[1]*University of Hohenheim, Stuttgart, Germany; [2]AB Enzymes GmbH, Darmstadt, Germany; [3]AB Vista, Marlborough, UK*

8.1 Introduction

All living organisms depend upon a continuous supply of P for the formation of structural body components, such as bones, energy metabolism and other physiological mechanisms to function. From the total P supplied with the feed, only the part that is absorbed by intestinal epithelia can contribute to meeting the organism's requirement and is called digestible P. The P supply along the entire food chain currently is maintained by the uptake of P from soil, the application of fertilizer and the use of feed phosphates which are produced largely from rock phosphates. The global rock phosphate stores are limited and might face depletion within two centuries or less. This limitation, together with the reserves of these stores being present in only a few countries, is considered one of the greatest challenges for making food production more secure and sustainable (Gross, 2010; Neset and Cordell, 2012).

For the farm animal sector, two major approaches exist to address these challenges. One is the improved understanding of the requirement for digestible P and avoidance of P oversupply. The second is improving the P digestibility of plant P sources, especially in non-ruminants such as pigs and poultry. These challenges have initiated an increased volume of research regarding the presence and role of inositol phosphates in the gastrointestinal tract including the role of phytases for increasing P digestibility. Moreover, the complete degradation of the inositol phosphates yields *myo*-inositol, a nutrient which has been shown to elicit benefits in animal performance in its own right. This chapter provides an overview of findings from this research in poultry and pigs. Other animal species are addressed in other chapters of this book.

8.2 The Substrate and Its Implications in the Digestive Tract

Phytate is the target substrate. Phytate is any salt of phytic acid (*myo*-inositol(1,2,3,4,5,6) hexakis(dihydrogen phosphate); InsP$_6$). Pure InsP$_6$ has a molar mass of 660 g and the proportion of P in InsP$_6$ is 0.28. Phytate is the primary storage form of P in the plant kingdom and is found in plant seeds such as cereal and legume. In most cereal grains, legume grains and oilseeds, phytate is found

*Email: markus.rodehutscord@uni-hohenheim.de

©CAB International 2022. *Enzymes in Farm Animal Nutrition, 3rd Edition* (M. Bedford et al. eds)
DOI: 10.1079/9781789241563.0008

in globoids that are located in protein storage vacuoles. In cereal grains, a high proportion of the phytate-containing globoids are stored in the aleurone layer or pericarp. An exception is maize, which has most of the phytate associated with the germ. In oilseeds and legume grains, phytate is distributed throughout the whole kernel and often associated with proteins (Angel et al., 2002), but differences exist between plant species. In soybeans, phytate is evenly distributed in the protein storage vacuoles (Prattley and Stanley, 1982) whereas in rapeseed, phytate is stored in globoids that are surrounded by additional protein structures inside the protein storage vacuole (Gillespie et al., 2005).

Processing of plant seeds in the food and energy sectors delivers by-products enriched in phytate, such as bran, oilseed meal and dried distillers' grains with solubles. The utilization of both seeds and by-products in feed compounding makes phytate the most relevant source of P in plant-based diets for non-ruminants. The concentration of phytate-P in diets for non-ruminants is approximately 2.5 g/kg, although high variation is possible depending on feed raw materials used, which varies as a result of animal species and animal age. It is important to be aware of this variation and to know the phytate content of the actual feed when the effects of added phytase are considered in feed formulation.

The concentration of phytate is different between feed raw materials and also differs between batches of the same raw material (Eeckhout and De Paepe, 1994; Ravindran et al., 1994; Rodehutscord et al., 2016). For instance, the concentration of phytate-P in cereal grains is around 1.5–2.5 g/kg, while it can range from 3 to 5 g/kg in oilseed meals and from 5 to 16 g/kg in cereal-based bran. In most of the plant raw materials, one-half to two-thirds of total P is present in the form of phytate. However, this proportion is lower when the material has been exposed to a fermentation process, such as distillers' grains, moist ensiled maize-cob mix or fermented feed.

Assay specifications may affect the outcome of phytate analysis. Colorimetric assays measure orthophosphate release from any inositol phosphate upon application of phytase or other phosphatases. Chromatographic assays directly measure the inositol phosphates and advanced chromatographic assays distinguish between $InsP_6$ and other inositol phosphates with different degree of phosphorylation ($InsP_x$) and even between different positional isomers. Attempts have also been made to use near-infrared reflectance spectroscopy (NIRS) for rapid estimation of phytate or $InsP_6$ in feed raw materials (Tahir et al., 2012; Aureli et al., 2017) (see also Section 8.6.4). Hence, the term 'phytate' is not always used unambiguously in literature. Comparisons of data should be made with caution and consider the assays that were used.

Studies using chromatography assays indicate that inositol phosphates other than $InsP_6$ are negligible in most of the feed raw materials. However, in oilseed meals, especially rapeseed meal, up to one-third of total inositol phosphates has been found to be present as $InsP_5$ (Pontoppidan et al., 2007; Haese et al., 2017) and recently an even higher $InsP_5$ proportion was reported (up to 46%) (Olukosi et al., 2020). This indicates that initial phosphate release from $InsP_6$ may occur during harsh thermal processing. Extrusion cooking of cereal grains and grain milling may also cause an increase in the proportion of $InsP_5$ in total inositol phosphates (Kasim and Edwards, 1998; Pontoppidan et al., 2007).

Pure $InsP_6$ has 12 replaceable reactive acidic sites with six strong acid groups and six weak to very weak acidic groups (Angel et al., 2002). At the pH conditions prevailing in some parts of the digestive tract of animals, $InsP_6$ is negatively charged and forms complexes with bi- and trivalent cations or cationic amino acid residues of proteins (Selle et al., 2000; Angel et al., 2002; Morales et al., 2016). Phytate forms insoluble complexes with minerals in vitro. The strength of these complexes depends on the mineral, its concentration and specific pH value. At neutral pH, the ranking of the stability of the complexes formed with phytate was $Zn^{2+} > Cu^{2+} > Ni^{2+} > Co^{2+} > Mn^{2+} > Ca^{2+} > Fe^{2+}$ (Maenz et al., 1999). While these studies used free phytate in buffer solutions, phytate has also been shown to affect mineral bioavailability in animal studies. For instance, Zn supplementation of barley-based diets caused an increase in bone Zn content of broilers when the barley contained phytate at a conventional level but not at a low level (Linares *et al.*, 2007). This suggests that Zn is more available when less phytate is present in the grain and hence the bone was saturated with Zn under these conditions. This may also apply to other nutrients potentially binding to phytate.

With regard to plant storage proteins, *in vitro* studies have suggested that the amino acid composition of those proteins can influence the complexation of phytate, with higher proportions of basic amino acids leading to stronger binary complexes at low pH (Morales *et al.*, 2013). These authors found that added phytase had a greater effect on protein solubility in peas or faba beans, with convicilin, vicilin and legumin as the dominating protein fractions, than in soybeans (glycinin and β-conglycinin). Minor phytase effects were found in lupins (conglutin), wheat (gliadins and glutenins) and canola meal (oleosin and napin). The phytase effect was related to an increase in solubility of the respective protein fractions. However, another *in vitro* study found only low amounts of soluble phytate–protein complexes in maize, canola meal, sunflower seed meal and soybean meal (Kies *et al.*, 2006). In this work, insoluble complexes were found at a pH of 2, but not at a pH of 4 or higher. This suggests that such binary complexes do not exist in the plant itself but are built upon entering the acidic environment of the stomach.

The $InsP_x$ as intermediate products of $InsP_6$ degradation may also form complexes in the digestive tract. The binding capacity with minerals was similar for $InsP_6$, $InsP_5$, $InsP_4$ and $InsP_3$ when calculated per phosphate group (Persson *et al.*, 1998). However, the binding strength was reduced with reduction of phosphate groups bound to *myo*-inositol. Another *in vitro* study found a proportional decrease in binding strength from $InsP_6$ to $InsP_3$ towards Fe^{3+}. Complexation with soy protein and β-casein was strongest with $InsP_6$, significantly lower with $InsP_5$, and moreover there were differences between $InsP_5$ isomers, and negligible with $InsP_4$ to $InsP_1$ (Yu *et al.*, 2012). In that study, the activity of pepsin was still diminished by $InsP_3$ and $InsP_4$, but to a much lesser degree than by $InsP_5$ or $InsP_6$.

To summarize, phytate is a constituent of plant feedstuffs that makes a substantial contribution to the digestible P supply of animals if it is degraded in the digestive tract or during feed processing. Degradation of phytate also reduces or removes its antinutritional effects on the availability of other nutrients.

8.3 Phytate Degradation in the Digestive Tract without Added Phytase

Phosphate needs to be cleaved from the inositol ring before it can be utilized by the organism. Dephosphorylation of phytate needs phytases and other phosphatases. A comprehensive description of this group of enzymes and their properties is provided elsewhere in this book (see Menezes-Blackburn *et al.*, Chapter 7, this volume, 2022). It has been estimated that the phosphate released from phytate was almost completely absorbed in the small intestine of broiler chickens and available for the animal (Rodehutscord, 2016). Hence, the extent of dephosphorylation in the anterior part of the digestive tract is most relevant for allowing the animal to utilize plant-based P sources. In contrast, P released from inositol phosphates in the posterior sections of the digestive tract (caeca, large intestine) likely cannot be absorbed into the bloodstream and utilized by the animal. For this reason, pre-caecal and post-ileal phytate degradation are considered separately in the text that follows.

8.3.1 Pre-caecal phytate degradation

It has been proposed in the past, before the advent of exogenous phytases, that phytate-P was not or only to a minimal extent available for non-ruminants. This was believed to result from a lack of or insufficient activity of endogenous phytase provided by the intestinal tissues. More recent research indicates this paradigm needs to be revised since the efficiency of endogenous phytases can be significant in low-P low-Ca diets, especially in broiler chickens.

When results of several pig and broiler studies were compared, the mean disappearance of $InsP_6$ by the end of the ileum was 28% in pigs and 68% in broiler chickens when diets were mainly based on maize and soybean meal without a phytase supplement (Fig. 8.1). The variation among the studies within one animal species was high. Differences in the Ca concentration of the diets and some intrinsic phytase activity of maize, although very low overall, may be reasons for the variation as well as differences in the sampled region of the terminal small intestine. Of note, the values displayed in Fig. 8.1 were obtained when using diets that did not contain a mineral P supplement. This may be regarded as an artificial situation and not representative for practical-type diets for young birds. Nevertheless, it demonstrates the high biological potential the broiler chicken has to hydrolyse $InsP_6$ in the digestive tract.

Endogenous phytase and other phosphatases are involved in gastrointestinal

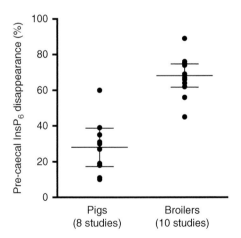

Fig. 8.1. Disappearance of $InsP_6$ determined at the end of the ileum when maize-based low-P diets were fed without a phytase supplement. The data are presented as means with 95% confidence intervals for studies in pigs and broilers. (Data from Jongbloed et al., 1992; Kemme et al., 1999, 2006; Rapp et al., 2001; Applegate et al., 2003; Tamim and Angel, 2003; Tamim et al., 2004; Baumgärtel et al., 2008; Leytem et al., 2008; Rutherfurd et al., 2014; Shastak et al., 2014; Zeng et al., 2014; Zeller et al., 2015a,c; Sommerfeld et al., 2018b; Ingelmann et al., 2019; Siegert et al., 2019b; Rosenfelder-Kuon et al., 2020a. Authors' own figure.)

$InsP_6$ degradation. These enzymes can be provided by epithelial cells of the animal or by bacteria and other microbes that are resident in the digestive tract, but the relative contributions of those sources have not been quantified yet. Nevertheless, pre-caecal $InsP_6$ disappearance was found to be 42% when studied in gnotobiotic broiler chickens (Sommerfeld et al., 2019). The authors assumed that phytase of microbial origin was not present in the digestive tract of those chickens and suggested that endogenous epithelial enzymes may be more important in $InsP_6$ degradation than microbial enzymes.

Studies that were conducted with broiler chickens and laying hens displayed some phytase activity when using purified brush-border membrane vesicles from different sections of the small intestine (Maenz and Classen, 1998; Onyango et al., 2006; Huber et al., 2015). Epithelial phytase was found highest in preparations of the duodenum and it decreased in the more posterior parts of the small intestine (Maenz and Classen, 1998). Epithelial phytase activity may be reduced at higher concentrations of inorganic phosphate in the intestinal lumen (Huber et al., 2015) and when Ca is supplemented to the diet (Applegate et al., 2003). Epithelial phytase and total phosphatase activities in the jejunum were found to be differently expressed in two commercial laying hen strains (Sommerfeld et al., 2020). In three experiments using different dietary Ca and vitamin D_3 combinations and different bird strains, a significant correlation between pre-caecal $InsP_6$ breakdown and V_{max} of phytase activity of the brush-border membrane vesicles was observed in one, but not in the other two experiments (Applegate et al., 2003). Hence, while brush-border membrane vesicles clearly show that substantial membrane-associated enzyme activity exists, its quantitative relevance for $InsP_6$ degradation in the complex situation of the digestive tract lumen is not well understood to date.

The microbiota colonizing the digestive tract may also provide phytase. In vitro studies have shown the $InsP_6$-degrading activity of various bacteria (Konietzny and Greiner, 2002; Vats and Banerjee, 2004). Lactic acid-producing bacteria isolated from the chicken intestine were identified as possible InsP$_6$-degrading candidates (Raghavendra and Halami, 2009). Among the bacteria in the small intestine of broiler chickens, lactobacilli are the most common (Rehman *et al.*, 2007; Witzig *et al.*, 2015). Interestingly, broiler chickens fed a diet supplemented with *Lactobacillus* species had increased P retention (Angel *et al.*, 2005), which suggests an increased InsP$_6$ degradation in the gut. Genes for InsP$_6$ phosphatases were also identified in *Bacteroides* spp., *Burkholderia* spp. and three species of the genus *Bifidobacterium*, which are all also present in the digestive tract of chickens (Tamayo-Ramos *et al.*, 2012; Stentz *et al.*, 2014). Supplementation of a coccidiostat largely affected the microbiota composition in crop and ileum contents, including lactobacillus strains, but pre-caecal InsP$_6$ disappearance was not affected (Künzel *et al.*, 2019b). This observation is not consistent with the suggestion that the ileal microbiome may play a role in InsP$_6$ degradation. Because of the complexity of factors affecting the identity and functionality of the gut microbiome, more work is needed that studies the gut microbiome and InsP$_6$ breakdown together in an attempt to evaluate relationships.

In contrast to added phytases, endogenous phytases have not been well characterized yet. Some indications can be provided by measurements of InsP$_6$ degradation products in the ileum. When feeding diets devoid of phytase, approximately half of the total InsP$_5$ present in the ileum was in the form of Ins(1,2,3,4,5)P$_5$, while the other half was similarly distributed between Ins(1,2,4,5,6)-P$_5$ and Ins(1,2,3,4,6)P$_5$ (Fig. 8.2). The enantiomers were not analytically separated and a differentiation between D- and/or L-forms will not be made herein for the sake of readability. The presence of different InsP$_5$ isomers in the ileum shows that the enzyme mix involved in InsP$_6$ degradation cannot be ascribed to any specific category (e.g. 6- or 3-phytase). The main activity seems to be that of a 6-phytase, with side activities also existing. Of note, the InsP$_5$ pattern found in the ileum likely is the result of mixed activities of mucosal and microbial phytases, and perhaps even residual plant intrinsic phytase activity. Often the intrinsic plant phytase levels are below the level of detection using standard assays; however, this does not discount their contribution to intestinal InsP$_6$ degradation as conditions of the assay and the intestine differ markedly. Some undegraded InsP$_5$ from the diet may also be present in the ileum. While the concentration of InsP$_5$ in the diets considered in Fig. 8.2 was low overall, about two-thirds of it were present as Ins(1,2,4,5,6)P$_5$ and the rest as

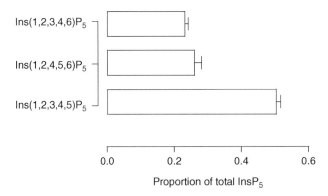

Fig. 8.2. Proportion of different InsP$_5$ isomers measured in the ileum of broiler chickens that were provided diets without added phytase. The bars show the mean and standard error of 22 diets from eight experiments. Other InsP$_5$ isomers were not detected in any of the experiments. (Data from Zeller *et al.*, 2015a,c; Sommerfeld *et al.*, 2018b, 2019; Künzel *et al.*, 2019b; Siegert *et al.*, 2019b. Authors' own figure.)

Ins(1,2,3,4,5)P$_5$. The presence of Ins(1,2,3,4,6)-P$_5$ in the ileum is difficult to explain at present. Initial InsP$_6$ dephosphorylation at the 5-position has been described for some bacteria (Puhl *et al.*, 2008; Haros *et al.*, 2009) but not for endogenous sources in the chicken gut. However, in gnotobiotic chickens, Ins(1,2,3,4,6)P$_5$ was found in the ileum after feeding a diet devoid of phytase as well as Ins(1,2,3,4,6)P$_5$. This indicates that mucosal phytases may in part belong to the group of 5-phytases.

Only a few studies investigated the InsP$_5$ pattern in the ileum of pigs. Here, the isomer with by far the highest proportion after feeding diets devoid of exogenous phytase was Ins(1,2,4,5,6)P$_5$, followed by Ins(1,2,3,4,5)P$_5$ (Lu *et al.*, 2020; Rosenfelder-Kuon *et al.*, 2020a). This is the opposite of that shown in Fig. 8.2 for broiler chickens. Because pre-caecal InsP$_6$ disappearance is much lower in pigs than broilers (Fig. 8.1), endogenous enzymes may not be very relevant in pigs and the InsP$_5$ pattern in the ileum mainly may reflect the InsP$_5$ pattern of the feed.

Other than in broiler chickens, studies on InsP$_6$ degradation in the gastrointestinal tract of turkeys and waterfowl are rare. However, an increasing number of studies indicates that differences in InsP$_6$ degradation exist between poultry species. In a comparative study that used P retention data, P utilization efficiency was higher in broiler chickens than turkeys and Pekin ducks when a plant-based basal diet was provided but lower for a mineral P supplemented to the same diet (Rodehutscord and Dieckmann, 2005). It can be speculated whether differences in the functionality of the crop among species contributed to the differences observed in the efficiency of plant-P utilization. P digestibility and P retention values of dried distillers' grains with solubles were higher in broiler chickens (94 and 92%) than in young turkeys (76 and 71%), respectively (Adebiyi and Olukosi, 2015). It is likely that differences in InsP$_6$ degradation in the digestive tract has contributed to these differences. Pre-caecal InsP$_6$ degradation by turkeys was 29% when fed a wheat–soybean meal-based diet without added phytase but increased to 45% upon addition of phytase 500 FTU/kg

(Ingelmann *et al.*, 2018). Nevertheless, this level of InsP$_6$ degradation was remarkably lower than that reported above from similar broiler studies. Consistently, pre-caecal InsP$_6$ degradation was much lower in a turkey trial compared with a broiler trial when maize-based diets were provided to the birds (Ingelmann *et al.*, 2019). Reasons for differences in InsP$_6$ degradation among poultry species are not well understood. They may be related to differences in endogenous enzyme activity, pH along the digestive tract, passage rate, microbiome or other factors.

Irrespective of the origin of endogenous phytase (epithelial or microbial), their activity on the substrate seems suppressed in the presence of feed phosphates. When mineral P sources were added to the diet, which is very common in the poultry industry, endogenous InsP$_6$ degradation by broilers was reduced by approximately 1.6 g (equivalent to 0.45 g of phytate-P) for each gram of mineral P that was supplemented (Fig 8.3). This effect was even more pronounced when Ca was also supplemented in addition to mineral P (Sommerfeld *et al.*, 2018b). This is an interesting phenomenon from the viewpoint of both biology and industry. When the broiler is challenged by insufficient quantities of digestible P in the feed, its InsP$_6$ degradation is high and a remarkable quantity of InsP$_6$-P becomes digestible. Digestible P supplied by other sources reduces the need for InsP$_6$ hydrolysis and the bird might therefore invest less resources into the corresponding pathways. A consequence for the industry is that supplements of a highly digestible mineral P source contribute less digestible P than assumed because the digestibility of InsP$_6$-P is concurrently reduced. These results from animal trials are consistent with earlier *in vitro* studies where P addition to the medium decreased synthesis of phosphatases including phytase by *Aspergillus ficuum* (Shieh *et al.*, 1969).

8.3.2 Post-ileal phytate degradation

Inositol phosphates that enter the large intestine or caeca can be dephosphorylated by the resident microbiota; however, phosphate

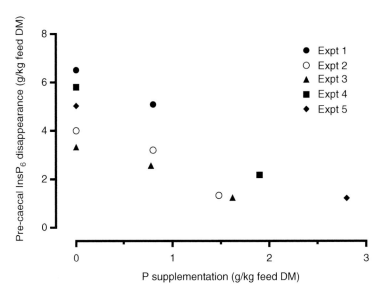

Fig. 8.3. Effects of mineral P supplements on the pre-caecal disappearance of $InsP_6$ in studies conducted with broiler chickens. The mean of estimated slopes of the linear regressions is –1.62. DM, dry matter. (Data from Shastak *et al.*, 2014; Zeller *et al.*, 2015c; Sommerfeld *et al.*, 2018b; Künzel *et al.*, 2019b. Authors' own figure.)

absorption in the post-ileal digestive tract is not known to exist and thus phosphate released here is excreted with the faeces and in other forms than bound to inositol.

As a consequence of low pre-caecal $InsP_6$ degradation in pigs (Fig. 8.1), the amount of $InsP_x$ entering the large intestine is high when diets without phytase are provided. However, irrespective of the amount of $InsP_6$ degraded pre-caecally, $InsP_6$ was barely found in faeces of growing-finishing pigs, indicating that post-ileal $InsP_6$ degradation was nearly complete (Sandberg *et al.*, 1993; Schlemmer *et al.*, 2001; Baumgärtel *et al.*, 2008; Rosenfelder-Kuon *et al.*, 2020a). In contrast, in a study that used weaner piglets, significant faecal $InsP_6$ excretion was found without added phytase. These differences were suggested to be due to the fermentative processes being less developed in piglets than in growing-finishing pigs (Lu *et al.*, 2020). It is not known whether epithelial phytases are active in the large intestine, and thus it is assumed that microbial fermentation is the main contributor to $InsP_6$ degradation. When total P digestibility was measured together with $InsP_6$ disappearance, differences between pre-caecal

and faecal $InsP_6$ disappearance were not reflected in incremental P digestibility values. This supports the view that P absorption in the large intestine of pigs is not relevant.

In poultry, substantial $InsP_6$ degradation occurs in the caeca. Concentrations of $InsP_6$ were markedly lower and those of some less phosphorylated inositol phosphates higher in caecal content of broiler chickens than in ileal content (Zeller *et al.*, 2015a). Such big differences were not observed in gnotobiotic broiler chickens (Sommerfeld *et al.*, 2019). In a comparative study, gnotobiotic broiler chickens had much higher $InsP_6$ levels in the caecal content than their conventional counterparts (Kerr *et al.*, 2000). In laying hens, the specific phytase activity in caecal content was higher by a factor of more than tenfold when compared with content from the crop, stomach and small intestine (Marounek *et al.*, 2010). The microbial population in the caeca has a very high diversity including bacteria known to be capable of $InsP_6$ breakdown (Rehman *et al.*, 2007; Witzig *et al.*, 2015). Correspondingly, phytase activity in the caecal content of laying hens was much higher than in the anterior sections of the digestive tract after feeding a maize–soybean meal-based diet (Marounek *et al.*, 2008). These data have indicated a high impact of micro-organisms to InsP$_6$ breakdown in the caeca. However, the relevance of caecal InsP$_6$ hydrolysis for P supply in poultry is still unclear. Based on the results of Son *et al.* (2002), it can be estimated that not more than one-quarter of ileal digesta enters the caeca for fermentation. As for other species, P absorption by caecal epithelia is unlikely to occur, hence P likely leaves the caeca largely in forms other than how it entered, for instance in microbial matter or as free phosphate. Some of this may be refluxed to the small intestine, as antiperistalsis is known in chickens (Svihus *et al.*, 2013), and become available for absorption. However, this has not been investigated yet.

8.3.3 Animal genetic effects

When different genetic strains of laying hens were supplied with the same feed, they excreted phytate in different amounts (Abudabos, 2012) and concentrations of InsP$_6$ in the digesta and activities of phosphatases in the epithelia of the jejunum differed (Sommerfeld *et al.*, 2020). The phenotypic variation in P utilization between individuals has been shown to be high in studies with pigs, laying hens, broiler chickens and Japanese quail (Düngelhoef *et al.*, 1994; Punna and Roland, 1999; Beck *et al.*, 2016; Sommerfeld *et al.*, 2020). The influence of genetics on this variation is of great interest. While InsP$_6$ degradation has rarely been looked at in this context, other traits with a relationship to P utilization have been investigated. In a pig study, the genomic heritabilities of the concentration of inorganic P and alkaline phosphatase activity in the plasma were 0.42 and 0.54, respectively (Reyer *et al.*, 2019). Broiler chickens exhibited a heritability of 0.10 for phytate P bioavailability and 0.22 for P utilization (Zhang *et al.*, 2003; De Verdal *et al.*, 2011). In a large crossing experiment with Japanese quail, estimated heritabilities were 0.14 for P utilization and 0.23–0.32 for bone ash traits

(Beck *et al.*, 2016; Künzel *et al.*, 2019a). The results from a gene mapping study revealed that P utilization is a polygenic trait, affected by many genes with small effects (Vollmar *et al.*, 2020a). In the same experiment, subgroups of animals with low and high P utilization showed distinct differences in the microbiota composition of the ileum (Borda-Molina *et al.*, 2020) and a microbiability of P utilization (i.e. the variation of P utilization explained by the microbiota) of 0.15 has been predicted (Vollmar *et al.*, 2020b). This shows that P utilization was affected by the genome of the animal and its intestinal microbiota composition. Different functional implications may exist. In a pilot study using quail selected for very low or very high P utilization, the ileal tissue was found to be a major driver of the differences in P utilization based on differential gene expression and microRNA analyses (Oster *et al.*, 2020; Ponsuksili *et al.*, 2020). However, with regard to InsP$_6$ degradation, the role of the genome is still underexplored. Nevertheless, P utilization and related traits have the potential to be included in revised breeding programmes.

8.4   Effects of Plant Intrinsic Phytase

Among cereal grains, intrinsic phytase activity is the highest in rye, followed by triticale, wheat and barley (Eeckhout and De Paepe, 1994; Rodehutscord *et al.*, 2016). Phytase activity is low in legume grains and hardly detectable in oat, maize and sorghum grains. Because plant intrinsic phytase is not particularly thermotolerant, feed that undergoes processes involving temperatures above 65°C, such as pelleting or extrusion, is virtually devoid of intrinsic phytase activity. However, plant intrinsic phytase can be active in the digestive tract of animals when unprocessed feed is offered, and under such conditions it is known to improve P digestibility. This is of specific relevance in production systems where the use of enzyme supplements produced by genetically modified organisms is not approved, such as in organic farming in the European

Union. However, the effects of plant intrinsic phytase on gastrointestinal $InsP_6$ degradation is different between pigs and poultry.

In pigs provided diets with high intrinsic phytase activity, phytase activity measured in the stomach was found to be reduced by 90% compared with the diet (Schlemmer *et al.*, 2001). Peptic digestion as well as an unfavourable pH for intrinsic plant phytases in the duodenum may result in only limited activities of plant phytase reaching the anterior small intestine (Yi and Kornegay, 1996). Consistently, Schlemmer *et al.* (2009) concluded that plant phytases might not be involved in a relevant hydrolysis of inositol phosphates in the small and large intestine while the stomach is the main location where the enzyme is active. Inactivation of the intrinsic phytase of a wheat–barley–soybean meal diet through steam pelleting at about 90°C resulted in pre-caecal $InsP_6$ degradation of 29% compared with 52% in the non-inactivated diet (Blaabjerg *et al.*, 2010). When comparing total tract P digestibility of raw materials in pigs using a standardized trial protocol, P digestibility was highest in wheat (high phytase activity) followed by barley (medium phytase activity) and maize or oilseed meals (low/no phytase activity) (Düngelhoef *et al.*, 1994; Rodehutscord *et al.*, 1996; Hovenjürgen *et al.*, 2003; Schemmer *et al.*, 2020). This demonstrates that intrinsic plant phytase is a relevant factor for P digestibility in the pig if not destroyed during feed processing.

In broiler chickens, plant intrinsic phytase would primarily be active in the crop prior to initiation of proteolysis in the gizzard. However, it is a matter of debate how relevant the intrinsic plant phytase activity can be for $InsP_6$ breakdown in broiler chickens. When wheat-based diets using different batches of wheat were used to measure P retention of broiler chickens, some positive relationship between intrinsic phytase activity of wheat and P retention were found (Barrier-Guillot *et al.*, 1996; Oloffs *et al.*, 2000). P retention in broiler chickens was also lower when extruded wheat was fed instead of non-extruded wheat (Oloffs *et al.*, 1998). Other studies that used different grains with different phytase activity did

not indicate a relationship between the intrinsic plant phytase activity and $InsP_6$ disappearance in broiler chickens (Juanpere *et al.*, 2004; Leytem *et al.*, 2008; Papp *et al.*, 2021). These divergent results have increased the interest in a better understanding of plant intrinsic phytase effects along the digestive tract. Following inclusion of microwave-treated wheat in the feed instead of untreated wheat, intrinsic phytase activity of the feed and $InsP_6$ disappearance in the crop of broiler chickens were markedly reduced (Zeller *et al.*, 2016). However, in the anterior small intestine, the differences in $InsP_6$ breakdown between the diets containing microwave-treated or untreated wheat disappeared, indicating that endogenous phytase sources had compensated for the lack of intrinsic plant phytase activity (Zeller *et al.*, 2015b). Other authors also concluded that intrinsic plant phytase contributes very little to pre-caecal $InsP_6$ degradation by broiler chickens and turkeys when compared with endogenous or added phytase (Leytem *et al.*, 2008; Shastak *et al.*, 2014; Ingelmann *et al.*, 2018).

8.5   Effects of Added Phytase

When phytase is added to the feed of non-ruminants, a remarkable increase in gastrointestinal $InsP_6$ degradation is achieved with related effects on P digestibility and other constituents of the feed.

8.5.1   Degradation of $InsP_6$ and phosphorus digestibility

The extent of effects of added phytase on degradation of $InsP_6$ depends on several factors such as animal species, $InsP_6$ content of the feed, amount of phytase added and diet composition.

In grower pigs, pre-caecal $InsP_6$ disappearance increased from 18 to 76% upon addition of 750 FTU/kg and up to 92% upon application of 1500 FTU/kg (Rosenfelder-Kuon *et al.*, 2020a). In weaner piglets, this increase was from 26 to 93% upon phytase supplementation at 1500 FTU/kg

(Lu *et al.*, 2020). In broiler chickens, pre-caecal InsP$_6$ disappearance of maize–soy-based diets reached values in the range of 76 to 93% when the feed contained 1200 FTU phytase/kg or more (Zeller *et al.*, 2015c; Sommerfeld *et al.*, 2018b; Künzel *et al.*, 2019b; Siegert *et al.*, 2019b; Krieg *et al.*, 2020). The response to increasing phytase dosages was non-linear (Fig. 8.4) and according to this data set, hardly any extra effect on InsP$_6$ degradation can be expected with dosages exceeding 1500 FTU/kg. However, a recent study found pre-caecal InsP6 disappearance of 98% when the feed contained 40,500 FTU/kg (Kriseldi *et al.*, 2021). Figure 8.4 also demonstrates that increasing phytase dosage can overcome most of the diminishing effects that mineral P and Ca supplements have on InsP$_6$ degradation in broiler chickens.

Only a few studies have investigated phytase effects on InsP$_6$ degradation in turkeys. In young turkeys, the supplementation of 500 FTU/kg feed increased pre-caecal InsP$_6$ disappearance to 45% in wheat-based diets (Ingelmann *et al.*, 2018) and to no more than 38% in maize-based diets (Ingelmann *et al.*, 2019), both values being distinctly lower

than that known to occur in broiler chickens fed similar diets. However, because endogenous InsP$_6$ degradation was much lower in turkeys, phytase supplementation caused greater InsP$_6$-P disappearance in turkeys than broilers (2.3 versus 1.4 g/kg feed dry matter) (Ingelmann *et al.*, 2019). When 3000 FTU/kg instead of 1500 or 500 FTU/kg was used, pre-caecal InsP$_6$ disappearance in turkeys was markedly increased (Olukosi *et al.*, 2020). Whether a level of pre-caecal InsP$_6$ disappearance of 90% or higher, such as has been shown in broiler chickens, can be achieved in turkeys at even higher levels of phytase supplementation has not been studied to date.

Pre-caecal InsP$_6$ disappearance values of 90% or higher have been consistently found in pigs and broiler chickens fed diets supplemented with very high dosages of phytase. This shows that the enzyme is very effective in the initial dephosphorylation of InsP$_6$. On closer inspection of the degradation products in the ileum, concentrations of InsP$_5$ were also reduced upon phytase supplementation. However, the enzyme is less effective on some of the lower InsP

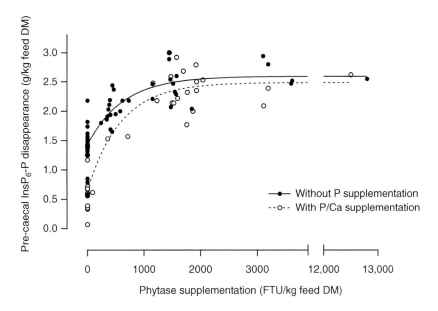

Fig. 8.4. Effects of phytase supplementation on pre-caecal InsP$_6$-P disappearance in broiler chickens in relation to the level of phytase supplementation. The data set is separated depending on whether mineral P was added or not. DM, dry matter. (Data from Zeller *et al.*, 2015a,b,c; Sommerfeld *et al.*, 2018a,b; Ingelmann *et al.*, 2019; Künzel *et al.*, 2019b, 2021; Siegert *et al.*, 2019b; Ajuwon *et al.*, 2020; Krieg *et al.*, 2020. Authors' own figure.)

isomers, which caused an increase in the concentrations of $InsP_4$, $InsP_3$ and $InsP_2$ in the ileum of pigs (Mesina *et al.*, 2019; Lu *et al.*, 2020; Rosenfelder-Kuon *et al.*, 2020a) and broiler chickens (Zeller *et al.*, 2015c; Sommerfeld *et al.*, 2018b). In pigs, this accumulation of lower InsP isomers tended to be less marked with higher phytase dosage; however, even at phytase dosages of 3000 FTU/kg feed there were still significant accumulations of these lower esters (Fig. 8.5). In broiler chickens, the relationship between $InsP_{3+4}$ accumulation and phytase dosage is less clear than in pigs. Specifically, accentuated accumulation of these lower isomers was found when diets containing rapeseed meal and sunflower meal were provided, which might have been caused by high $InsP_6$ concentrations of these meals.

As a consequence of accumulation of lower $InsP_x$ in the ileum, the increase in P digestibility upon phytase supplementation is not as high as the corresponding increase in pre-caecal $InsP_6$ disappearance. While pre-caecal $InsP_6$ disappearance with high phytase supplementation (≥ 1500 FTU/kg) in pigs can reach 85–95%, pre-caecal P digestibility did not exceed 62% (Lu *et al.*, 2020; Rosenfelder-Kuon *et al.*, 2020a).

Consistent with these data, total tract P digestibility in pigs reached an asymptotic value of 65% when estimated in a meta-analysis that used data from 88 digestibility experiments and included diets with phytase supplementation up to 2500 FTU/kg feed (Rosenfelder-Kuon *et al.*, 2020b). In broiler chickens, an analysis of data from several studies indicated that with increasing phytase supplementation, the predicted pre-caecal P digestibility was about 15 percentage units lower than predicted $InsP_6$ disappearance (Fig. 8.6). Reasons for this discrepancy in both pigs and poultry are not fully clear. While it is most likely that they reflect the limits of the dephosphorylating enzymes (exogenous and endogenous) and accumulation of lower $InsP_x$, it also is possible that phosphate absorption was limited. Alternatively, the P released may have precipitated in the small intestine with minerals such as Ca, explaining why phosphate cleaved from $InsP_x$ remained in the digesta. However, because P supply of the animals was marginal in most of the studies considered herein, a downregulation of phosphate absorption by the small intestinal epithelial tissues is not a likely reason for the discrepancy between $InsP_6$ disappearance and P digestibility.

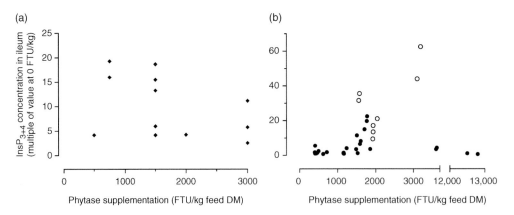

Fig. 8.5. Effects of phytase supplementation on the concentration of $InsP_3$ plus $InsP_4$ in the ileum. Concentrations are expressed as multiples of the concentrations measured for the respective diet without a phytase supplement for pigs (a) and broiler chickens (b). The open circles represent broiler diets with high inclusion levels (≥ 150 g/kg) of rapeseed meal or sunflower meal. DM, dry matter. (Pig data from Kühn *et al.*, 2016; Mesina *et al.*, 2019; Lu *et al.*, 2020; Rosenfelder-Kuon *et al.*, 2020a. Broiler data from Zeller *et al.*, 2015a,c; Sommerfeld *et al.*, 2018a,b; Ingelmann *et al.*, 2019; Künzel *et al.*, 2019b; Siegert *et al.*, 2019b; Krieg *et al.*, 2020. Authors' own figure.)

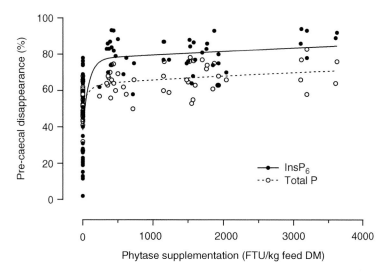

Fig. 8.6. Effects of phytase supplementation on the pre-caecal disappearance of InsP$_6$ and total P in broiler chickens. DM, dry matter. (Data from Zeller *et al.*, 2015a,b,c; Sommerfeld *et al.*, 2018a,b; Ingelmann *et al.*, 2019; Künzel *et al.*, 2019b; Siegert *et al.*, 2019b; Ajuwon *et al.*, 2020; Krieg *et al.*, 2020; Künzel *et al.*, 2021. Authors' own figure.)

8.5.2   Release of *myo*-inositol

The second end product of gastrointestinal InsP$_6$ degradation beside phosphate is *myo*-inositol. When the feed was not supplemented with phytase, the *myo*-inositol concentration in the ileum of broiler chickens was highly variable and reduced by supplements such as feed phosphates and limestone (Sommerfeld *et al.*, 2018b; Pirgozliev *et al.*, 2019; Ajuwon *et al.*, 2020). This shows that the endogenous enzymes can completely dephosphorylate some of the InsP$_6$ contained in the feed and this capacity is impaired by mineral supplements. When phytase is supplemented to the feed, the *myo*-inositol concentration in the ileum is distinctly increased in both pigs and broiler chickens, although with high variation between studies (Fig. 8.7). In young turkeys, the *myo*-inositol concentration in the ileum was significantly increased when the phytase supplementation of the feed was increased from 500 to 3000 FTU/kg (Olukosi *et al.*, 2020). This study did not involve a treatment without phytase supplementation. Concomitant with the incremental luminal concentrations of inositol with use of phytase is the increased expression of inositol transporter or cotransporter

genes in the intestine of broilers (Walk *et al.*, 2018) or pigs (Lu *et al.*, 2020).

Consistent with effects in the ileum, the *myo*-inositol concentration in blood increased with phytase supplementation in pigs and broiler chickens (Guggenbuhl *et al.*, 2016; Laird *et al.*, 2018; Sommerfeld *et al.*, 2018a; Ajuwon *et al.*, 2020; Lu *et al.*, 2020). The relevance of this increase for the metabolism of the animal is not well understood. *Myo*-inositol is involved in many cellular functions and its major role is as a constituent of phosphoinositides which are phosphorylated at different sites of the *myo*-inositol ring (Huber, 2016). *Myo*-inositol can be newly synthesized from glucose and as a result it is not possible to quantify the role of *myo*-inositol absorbed from the gut. Supplements of *myo*-inositol may increase the gain-to-feed ratio of broiler chickens (Sommerfeld *et al.*, 2018a) and cause metabolic responses such as increased plasma dopamine and serotonin levels (Gonzalez-Uarquin *et al.*, 2020a) or reduced fat content of the liver (Pirgozliev *et al.*, 2019). However, as reviewed elsewhere, the responses of animals to *myo*-inositol supplements overall are inconsistent (Gonzalez-Uarquin *et al.*, 2020b). To date it is not possible to distinguish

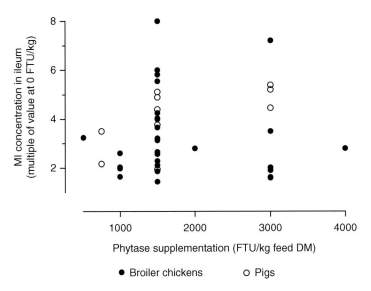

Fig. 8.7. Effects of phytase supplementation on the concentration of *myo*-inositol (MI) in the ileum of pigs and broiler chickens. Values are expressed as multiples of the control without phytase supplementation, which varied among studies from 0.5 to 5.9 μmol/g dried ileum content (pigs) and from 0.2 to 11.8 μmol/g dried ileum content (broilers). DM, dry matter. (Pig data from Mesina *et al.*, 2019; Lu *et al.*, 2020; Rosenfelder-Kuon *et al.*, 2020a. Broiler data from Sommerfeld *et al.*, 2018a,b; Künzel *et al.*, 2019b; Siegert *et al.*, 2019b; Walk and Olukosi, 2019; Ajuwon *et al.*, 2020; Krieg *et al.*, 2020. Authors' own figure.)

conditions when extra *myo*-inositol supply (in free form by phytase supplementation) has beneficial effects in pigs and poultry from those where such effects do not exist.

8.5.3 Amino acid digestibility

Besides release of phosphate and *myo*-inositol, phytase supplements may have indirect effects on other fractions in the digestive tract such as proteins and amino acids (see Section 8.2). Because InsP$_6$ can form binary or ternary complexes with proteins depending on the pH value in the digestive tract, those proteins may be less accessible for proteolysis and thus amino acid digestibility is impaired. InsP$_6$ degradation by phytases in the anterior sections of the digestive tract makes occurrence of those complexes less likely and hence increases amino acid digestibility. It appears from the literature that phytase supplements overall can increase amino acid digestibility, but effects were inconsistent among the studies.

While some studies showed significantly increased amino acid digestibility upon phytase supplementation, others did not.

In pigs, a meta-analysis of results from 34 publications found a significant increase of pre-caecal digestibility of all essential amino acids (Zouaoui *et al.*, 2018). In that analysis, the average increase of digestibility ranged from 0.9 percentage units for methionine to 1.5 percentage units for threonine when calculated for a supplementation level of 500 FTU/kg feed. In broiler chickens, recent studies reported an increase in pre-caecal amino acid digestibility overall in the range of 1.1–4.7 percentage units, although the effect was not statistically significant in all studies and for all amino acids (Sommerfeld *et al.*, 2018a,b; Borda-Molina *et al.*, 2019; Siegert *et al.*, 2019b; Walk and Olukosi, 2019; Ajuwon *et al.*, 2020; Babatunde *et al.*, 2020; Krieg *et al.*, 2020). Other studies found no or little or inconsistent phytase effects, perhaps because of lower dosages or other phytase products prevailing at the time they were conducted (Sebastian *et al.*, 1997; Adeola and Sands,

2003; Rodehutscord *et al.*, 2004). Digestibility of specific amino acids can be affected by phytase supplementation to a different extent and depending on the procedures of digestibility determination.

The variation of amino acid digestibility responses may be caused by factors such as level of phytase supplementation and ingredient composition of the diets. In regard to phytase dosage of broiler chicken feed, increasing from 500 to 1500 FTU/kg increased the average amino acid digestibility by an extra 1 percentage unit, but dosages higher than 1500 FTU/kg caused no further increase in amino acid digestibility (Sommerfeld *et al.*, 2018a; Siegert *et al.*, 2019b; Ajuwon *et al.*, 2020). Similarly, in dose–response studies (Ravindran *et al.*, 2006; Walters *et al.*, 2019; Babatunde *et al.*, 2020; Walk and Rama Rao, 2020), the biggest part of the response in amino acid digestibility was achieved at the lowest level of phytase supplementation (150–500 FTU/kg), while phytase added above this level did not consistently increase amino acid digestibility further, except in diets with very high phytate content from rice bran. This suggests that ingredient effects on amino acid digestibility responses may exist. When single ingredients (cereal grains and oilseed meals) were studied, phytase effects on amino acid digestibility were influenced by the ingredients used (Ravindran *et al.*, 1999). In a study that compared different oilseed meals in broiler chickens, phytase supplementation increased the pre-caecal amino acid digestibility by an average of 1 percentage unit in soybean meal, 3 percentage units in sunflower meal and 7 percentage units in rapeseed meal (Krieg *et al.*, 2020). Differences in amino acid digestibility between the oilseed meals became smaller as phytase supplementation increased but they still remained even at the highest supplementation level. However, the differences noted between these oilseed meals and their response to phytase supplementation with regard to amino acid digestibility were not detected when they were diluted in complete diets (Siegert *et al.*, 2019b; Krieg *et al.*, 2020). The underlying mechanism of ingredient-specific effects is not clear. Some authors suggested

that the phytate content of an ingredient explains the magnitude of responses in amino acid digestibility to phytase. However, a plethora of fractions other than phytate differ between ingredients and several of these may affect amino acid digestibility. In the meta-analysis of pig data (Zouaoui *et al.*, 2018), the dietary concentration of neutral detergent fibre (NDF), but not phytate, was found to negatively affect amino acid digestibility. Amino acid digestibility of rapeseed meal in laying hens was related to the content of neutral detergent insoluble nitrogen, which is associated with the NDF fraction (Rezvani *et al.*, 2012). It was argued that differences in protein–phytate complexes were unlikely to cause differences in phytase effects on amino acid digestibility of soybean meal, sunflower meal and rapeseed meal (Krieg *et al.*, 2020). It may thus be more appropriate to consider effects of feed ingredients per se rather than specific chemical fractions of the feed.

Added phytase may also influence amino acid digestibility by reducing endogenous protein secretion. Phytate can increase the endogenous secretion of proteins while passing through the digestive tract and thus increase amino acid losses of the animal. When fasted broilers were intubated with a dextrose solution, the excretion of crude mucin used as an indicator of endogenous protein and some amino acids were significantly increased when pure InsP$_6$ or a pure magnesium potassium phytate was added to the dextrose solution (Onyango *et al.*, 2009). Similarly, the flow of some amino acids at the terminal ileum of broiler chickens was increased when pure sodium phytate was supplemented to a synthetic diet and this effect could be compensated for by concurrent addition of phytase (Cowieson and Ravindran, 2007). These results prompted the hypothesis that phytase effects on amino acid digestibility can be explained in part by effects on endogenous protein secretion. However, it is not clear whether phytate contained in a complex feed matrix has the same or similar effects as pure phytate supplements in completely soluble or otherwise synthetic diets. A final answer is unlikely to be found because variation in phytate from ingredients cannot be achieved without confounding variation in other constituents of the feed. However, some studies tried to estimate the contribution of endogenous protein secretion by using different approaches. Sialic acid is a major constituent of secreted mucin. In pigs, the sialic acid content of ileal digesta was unaffected even though the $InsP_6$ content was largely reduced by phytase supplementation of an industry-type diet (Mesina *et al.*, 2019). In broilers, phytase supplementation reduced sialic acid excretion when precision feeding conditions and pure substrates were supplied (Cowieson *et al.*, 2004; Pirgozliev *et al.*, 2012), but not with industry-type diets and *ad libitum* access to the feed (Pirgozliev *et al.*, 2017). Phytase effects on amino acid digestibility in broiler chickens have also been studied using the regression approach. This approach allows for a discrimination of the effects of treatment on basal endogenous amino acid losses (Borda-Molina *et al.*, 2019; Siegert *et al.*, 2019b; Krieg *et al.*, 2020). Those studies suggested that endogenous amino acid losses were not a significant component of the effects of phytase on amino acid digestibility. Taken together, although pure phytate and phytase affected endogenous protein secretion in model studies, it may not be the case when complete diets are used.

Another reason for phytase influencing amino acid digestibility may relate to the supply of digestible P. Broiler studies often investigated the effects of phytase supplementation of a low-P diet on performance and amino acid digestibility and compared it with supplements of mineral P. In most of these studies, supplementing phytase led to an increase in pre-caecal amino acid digestibility, but the inclusion of mineral P also increased amino acid digestibility to the same or greater extent than phytase (Dilger *et al.*, 2004; Martinez-Amezcua *et al.*, 2006; Centeno *et al.*, 2007; Pieniazek *et al.*, 2017; Siegert *et al.*, 2019b; Babatunde *et al.*, 2020). It was hypothesized that the phytase effect on amino acid digestibility is not only a protein releasing effect, but also due to provision of P to an animal in a P-deficiency state (Martinez-Amezcua *et al.*, 2006). As P is

involved in the function of transporters in the intestine, for instance the Na–K–ATPase-dependent amino acid transporters, an increased provision of digestible P might increase amino acid uptake in the small intestine. Besides amino acid digestibility, feed intake was also increased by the supplementation of phytase or P in most of the studies. A lower feed and thus amino acid intake leads to an increased proportion of endogenous amino acids to total amino acids in the ileum and results in lower amino acid digestibility values in pigs and broiler chickens (Moter and Stein, 2004; Siegert *et al.*, 2019a). Thus, phytase effects on amino acid digestibility might be confounded by coexistence of effects on feed intake.

8.5.4 Minerals other than phosphorus

Phytate interacts with minerals other than P owing to the formation of $InsP_6$–mineral complexes as explained at the beginning of this chapter. Following passage through the stomach of the animal, the pH of the digesta increases and with it the formation of insoluble $InsP_6$–mineral complexes. Thus, $InsP_6$ degradation in the anterior part of the digestive tract by phytase is important because complexes are then less likely to be formed in the small intestine.

At a given Ca level in the diet, phytase may or may not increase pre-caecal Ca digestibility (Ravindran *et al.*, 2006; Olukosi *et al.*, 2013; Sommerfeld *et al.*, 2018b; Babatunde *et al.*, 2020). However, because the kidney is involved in Ca homeostasis, responses to phytase supplementation can be different between the pre-caecal and total excretion levels in birds (Olukosi *et al.*, 2013). Ca retention in the skeleton is tightly linked with P retention and thus the effects of added phytase on P release from $InsP_6$ in the digestive tract likely are the reason for effects observed on Ca retention. Supplements of Ca in the form of limestone or calcium formate reduced intrinsic $InsP_6$ degradation by broilers and the effects of added phytase (Sommerfeld *et al.*, 2018b; Krieg *et al.*, 2021).

Improvements in Zn bioavailability and Zn status with phytase supplementation were found for pigs and to a lesser extent for broilers (Schlegel et al., 2010). These authors suggested that Zn is used more efficiently by broilers due to the lower pH in the gizzard compared with that of the stomach in pigs, which serves to increase the solubility of Zn in the former. Results of a meta-analysis showed that bone Zn content of piglets decreased with increasing dietary phytate in the absence of phytase but increased upon phytase supplementation (Schlegel et al., 2013). Effects of supplemented Zn were independent of the Zn source and phytase effects on Zn-related traits were also independent of the Zn source in a study with weaner piglets (Revy et al., 2004). Pharmacological levels of Zn but not Cu in the diet of young pigs and broilers reduced the efficacy of a supplemented phytase, indicated by P release values and reduced bone ash (Augspurger et al., 2004), suggesting excess Zn can precipitate $InsP_6$ and make it intransigent to phytase hydrolysis.

Supplementation of high levels of Cu decreased P retention of broiler chickens in the presence and absence of phytase, the effect being more pronounced without phytase (Banks et al., 2004). In older broiler chickens, phytase supplementation increased tibia P concentration when no Cu was supplemented but not when Cu was also supplemented (Demirel et al., 2012). In weanling piglets, phytase supplementation increased Cu absorption, both with and without supplemented Cu (Adeola, 1995). Overall, studies investigating interaction effects of phytase and Cu are rare.

Strong binding to $InsP_6$ was also observed in vitro for Fe, whereby the binding strength decreased with increasing pH (Maenz et al., 1999). In vitro complexation with Fe^{3+} decreased proportionally from $InsP_6$ to $InsP_3$ and there was still some interaction with $InsP_2$ and $InsP_1$ (Yu et al., 2012). Trivalent cations may form stronger complexes with phytate than divalent cations (Maenz et al., 1999). Supportively, pre-caecal digestibility of P and Ca and tibia breaking strength were decreased in a broiler study with mid or high dietary Fe concentrations in the feed

when phytase was present (Akter et al., 2017), suggesting an increased complexation of Fe with phytate and probably Ca. This hypothesis is supported by in vitro findings where physiological concentrations of Ca and Mg were needed for the complexation of phytate and Fe (Sandberg et al., 1989). However, in young pigs, the dietary Fe level did not affect pre-caecal $InsP_6$ disappearance or bone ash weight in the presence of phytase (Laird et al., 2018), whereas higher Fe, Mn and Zn levels in the ribs of pigs (in addition to P and Ca) were found when phytase was added to a basal diet (Kühn et al., 2016), suggesting the interaction between Fe, Ca and phytate is not easily described.

Added phytase can also affect Na digestibility. Phytase supplements reduced the flow of Na at the distal ileum of broilers in some but not all experiments (Ravindran et al., 2006; Truong et al., 2017; Babatunde et al., 2020). In precision-fed broilers, phytase supplementation distinctly reduced Na excretion, especially when combined with $InsP_6$ supplementation (Cowieson et al., 2004; Pirgozliev et al., 2009). In contrast to other cations, Na^+ effects are likely related to endogenous secretion. It was suggested that phytate–protein complexes in the stomach trigger an increased secretion of pepsin and HCl in an attempt to maintain protein digestibility, thus provoking the need for greater secretion of sodium bicarbonate into the duodenum to buffer the excess acid exiting the gizzard (Selle et al., 2012). Phytase inclusion is presumed to reduce the formation of phytate–protein complexes and would thereby reduce the need for sodium bicarbonate secretion, thereby increasing Na digestibility.

8.6 From Mechanisms to Commercial Application of Phytase

The current commercial application of phytases is subject to the constraints laid down by the conditions under which they are used. The use of high doses and application of high matrices with them necessitate some methods of assurance that the enzyme will deliver the nutrients expected and as a result, feed compounders must not only be aware of how much enzyme is present in the feed, but also how much substrate and interfering minerals (such as Ca). If other enzymes or additives which claim similar nutrient matrices are present in the feed, then the interaction between them needs consideration. Regardless, the feed industry is recognizing additional benefits which accrue from the use of higher doses of phytase, such as relaxed constraints on maximal inclusion level of some ingredients and reduction of severity of some metabolic disorders. These observations and applications are discussed below.

8.6.1 Applicability of current matrix values and high phytase dosing

Improved understanding of how phytases function in destruction of $InsP_6$ and lower esters, as well as the effects of more complete dephosphorylation on animal performance, has not only had commercial benefits but also led to simultaneous reductions in nutrient excretion and thus pollution. While the use of phytase to enhance P utilization of plant origin is a well-established concept for more than 20 years, the additional benefits brought about by the reduction of concentrations of dietary phytate and its lower esters has led to a significant proportion of the industry using increased phytase application rates, which has been termed 'superdosing' (Cowieson *et al.*, 2011).

Current commercial use of phytase generally tends to fall into one of two groups. Standard application rates range from 250 to 750 FTU/kg feed where use of the P, Ca and Na matrix values are the most commonly employed with other nutrients such as amino acids and energy, if credited to the phytase, being attributed to the phytase in proportion to the P value suggested for any chosen dose. In this regard, the driver for phytase usage is purely economic although some pollution benefits will accrue. Higher dosages of about 1500 to 2500 FTU/kg feed are increasingly used whereby either a much larger matrix value is taken compared

with standard dosing, in which case even greater savings in feed costs are made, or a partial matrix is taken, which more than covers the cost of the enzyme and performance benefits are then captured due to the effect that higher dosages have on digestibility and efficiency of utilization of energy, amino acids and minerals (Cowieson *et al.*, 2011; Walk *et al.*, 2013, 2014). In addition to performance benefits, improved animal health associated with better bone formation (Kühn *et al.*, 2016) or well-being (Herwig *et al.*, 2019) has been observed; the latter may in part be due to the release of significant amounts of inositol (see Section 8.5.2).

The matrix value applied for any given dose of phytase is specific for the phytase source. This may be related to a combination of factors including differences in stability during the pelleting process and gastrointestinal tract, as well as differences in the efficiency of the phytase in degrading $InsP_6$ and each lower ester under the conditions of the gastrointestinal tract (Menezes-Blackburn *et al.*, 2015). Regardless, there is considerable variation in the matrix values estimated between trials which likely reflects the conditions of the assay employed. Most often these conditions are not the same as those under which the phytase is used commercially and as a result the ability of the enzyme to fulfil the matrix assigned might vary, which may result in significant 'safety margins' being applied. Thus, product characteristics such as heat stability and extent of phytate degradation under conditions more relevant to the commercial use of the enzyme need consideration by the end user if the application is to be successful. Ideally such information should be available to enable feed formulators to make relevant comparisons and arrive at a relevant decision given the intended application circumstances.

Commercial application of phytases often uses a nutrient matrix that is consistent across all animal species and age groups, which is not necessarily reflected in the literature data as outlined in the above sections. This could well be due to the divergence in the ingredient and nutrient contents of experimental diets compared with those in commercial practice as well as a commercial requirement for simple strategies. Often as not, such a 'one matrix' fits all approach goes hand in hand with a degree of caution in the matrix applied compared with that determined experimentally.

While integrators can benefit from the animal performance benefits derived from more complete phytate degradation, compound feed producers, who sell feed rather than meat, rely much more on the application of a matrix. Such matrix applications are currently applied only with lower phytase doses, thus knowledge of how to apply matrices which are robust when the target is maximal phytate destruction still needs to be researched further to widen this application across the whole industry.

8.6.2   Are matrix values of additives additive?

Commercial feed manufacturers routinely employ multiple additives, including phytase, in their diets, many of which may have a nutrient matrix associated with their use. The question of additivity of matrices from different additives in mixtures is often raised and clearly of great concern for the end user (Bedford and Cowieson, 2019). It is self-evident that each additive cannot continuously add more and more energy or digestible nutrient to the diet if there is an overlap in the mode of action. Consequently, it is essential for feed manufacturers to understand how each additive works so they can decide as to whether they should be combining matrices from different additives in a sub-additive, additive or even a synergistic manner. Certainly, much of the data for feed enzymes suggest that matrices are far from additive and should be considered at best sub-additive (Bedford and Cowieson, 2019). For example, phytases, xylanases and proteases may all have amino acid matrices associated with their use, but when all three are used in combination it is not a case of simply adding each individual matrix together (Lee *et al.*, 2018). Consequently, the end user must consider which products to use

first and discount the matrix of each subsequent addition. As noted above, it is not just enzymes that have matrices associated with their use and compounders must further consider the additivity of the matrix values they ascribe to products such as surfactants, probiotics, prebiotics and plant extracts, to name a few. While there are data in the literature to help end users consider how to combine enzyme matrices (Cowieson and Bedford, 2009; Cowieson *et al.*, 2010; Bedford and Cowieson, 2019), there is a paucity of data regarding the combination of enzyme matrices with other additives. This is mainly due to the almost infinite number of possible combinations as well as the variability of raw materials in use, which makes practical tests involving all possible combinations impossible.

8.6.3   Phytase use to increase usage levels of ingredients limited by their phytate content

In some situations, ingredient inclusion levels in diets have been restricted as a result of their phytate content (Pallauf and Rimbach, 1997; Ravindran *et al.*, 2000; Li *et al.*, 2001). If such restrictions are ignored, then the result is often growth depression of the animal. Such ingredients include cereal brans, some oilseed meals and also certain by-products with high variability might fall into this category (Ravindran *et al.*, 1994; Cossa *et al.*, 1999, 2000; Selle *et al.*, 2003) (also see Section 8.2). Several studies have shown that the constraints on the inclusion levels of these ingredients can be relaxed somewhat when phytase is included in the diet at elevated doses to ensure the degradation of phytate. Not only does this result in a cheaper diet, but it also makes use of local raw materials which can partially substitute imported ingredients (Wilcock and Walk, 2016). Ironically, these high-phytate ingredients are now viewed in some parts of the world as more desirable ingredients as their combination with high doses of phytase results in significant release of *myo*-inositol, which can bring benefits in terms of postabsorptive nutrient utilization (Lee and Bedford,

2016; Cowieson and Zhai, 2021) (also see Section 8.5.2).

8.6.4 Near-infrared reflectance spectroscopy as a tool to provide rapid estimate of dietary phytate content

While constraints on inclusion levels of phytate-rich ingredients can limit antinutritional effects, this approach may need to be reconsidered if a phytase is used. While InsP$_6$ is an antinutrient in the absence of a phytase, in its presence it is actually a substrate for P release and as such its concentration needs to be linked to the expected P matrix of the phytase (Morgan *et al.*, 2016). A major concern when higher doses of phytase are applied, and as a result a high P matrix is expected, is that there may not be enough phytate in the diet to provide the expected nutrient release. This is of particular importance when diets rich in animal by-products are employed, thus limiting inclusion levels of phytate-rich oilseed meals. Feed manufacturers routinely estimate the phytate-P content of their diets in order to ensure they do not overestimate the potential for P release. The use of NIRS is increasingly made by feed manufacturers to estimate the phytate content of their ingredients and thus provide an assumption of the dietary phytate-P content. Improvements in NIRS databases with regard to ingredient and dietary phytate estimates (Aureli *et al.*, 2017) can help the industry to use phytases more effectively as a result of enabling the matching of enzyme dose with substrate concentration. Analysis of multiple field samples has indicated that there is significant variability in phytate content of raw materials within and between ingredient types (also see Section 8.2). Moreover, regional differences in ingredient choice and usage rates for animal feeds further exacerbate the variation in phytate content of the diets noted around the world, as has been reported recently in aquafeeds (Fig. 8.8). This explains why ad hoc estimates of the phytate content of the ingredients employed is essential if phytase is to be used most efficiently.

8.6.5 Testing of phytase effects towards practical feeding conditions

Digestibility trials are often reported and are part of essential tools needed to understand

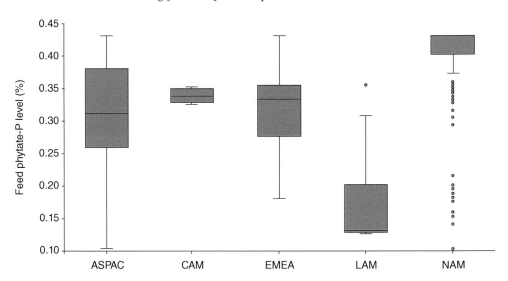

Fig. 8.8. Regional differences in the phytate-P level of feeds (%) for fish as determined by NIRS. The boxes show the upper and lower quartile and median, the lines show the extremes, and the dots show outliers and single data points. ASPAC, Asia Pacific; CAM, Central America; EMEA, Europe and Middle East; LAM, Latin America; NAM, North America (From Lee and Greenwood, 2020.)

the functionality of enzymes. Digestibility trials also appear to provide information of value with respect to provision of matrix values. However, commercial use of a phytase is usually under conditions that are more complex than those of the standardized trials which generated the digestibility data. Moreover, digestibility trials often fail to consider the effect that phytase application has on feed intake, which subsequently influences intake of digestible nutrients (Bedford, 2008; Walk and Bedford, 2020). As a result, digestibility data on their own are often not enough to derive matrix values that can be applied by commercial users. More often than not, full grow out trials to commercially relevant weights coupled with bone ash data are required in order to confirm that the proposed matrix for a phytase can be safely applied. The key concern for the industry is that digestibility data may overestimate the matrix of the phytase, resulting in the loss of not only animal live performance but more crucially bone development and strength. The latter of course is of great concern from a health and welfare aspect, which becomes even more important with the decreased use of mineral P in animal diets and the increase in performance of modern breeds.

8.6.6   Dietary calcium levels as a consideration for the industry

Ca levels in broiler diets continue to be a great concern for the industry as it is well established that excess Ca significantly reduces growth rates and efficacy of phytase, and deficiency results in bone defects and poor mineralization (Walk, 2016; Bedford and Rousseau, 2017; Momeneh et al., 2018; Sommerfeld et al., 2018b). In a recent study, most broiler rations contained significantly more Ca than intended (Walk, 2016), suggesting the industry works on the side of Ca excess rather than deficiency and that such a situation is likely to reduce the ability of an added phytase to degrade $InsP_6$ and its lower esters and hence to deliver the expected P matrix (Sommerfeld et al., 2018b; Krieg et al., 2021). Excess Ca has also been

shown to increase the incidence of wet litter (Bedford et al., 2007, 2012). As a direct impact, increased litter moisture results in significant foot quality issues (Farhadi et al., 2017), which has implications for animal health. As a result, the industry is taking a greater interest in the digestibility of different Ca sources in an attempt to formulate diets more accurately to the needs of the bird.

8.6.7   Phytase in the context of woody breast syndrome

Several studies have shown that the quantity of myo-inositol that is absorbed and transported from the intestine into the plasma and hence into tissues where it is used or stored (Kriseldi et al., 2018; Lu et al., 2019; Ajuwon et al., 2020) is directly proportional to the dose of phytase employed. A recent study has suggested that high phytase dosing is associated with higher erythrocytic content of $InsP_5$ and therefore their ability to release oxygen in tissues with low oxygen potential is presumably improved (Greene et al., 2019). Consistent with this relationship, high phytase dosing has recently been shown to be associated with reduced incidence of the most severe forms of woody breast, which is thought to be due to poor oxygenation of tissues and hence death and myopathy (Cauble et al., 2020). If this is the case, then other syndromes where hypoxia plays a role in their aetiology may benefit from very high doses of phytase which subsequently releases proportionately more inositol from phytate.

8.6.8   The importance of assay and heat stability in phytase efficacy

The most critical step the phytase must survive is that of feed manufacture due to the thermal effects of pelleting. The association of a particular response to a dose of phytase requires knowledge of the activity that is actually received by the animal and not simply that which was dosed into the mixer.

As a result, in-feed assays are essential if the matrix of the enzyme is to be accurately assessed. Unfortunately, the literature contains many papers where the in-feed activity of a phytase has not been determined (Rosen, 2002). As a consequence, it is very difficult to be certain of the dose received by the animal, which makes allocation of a matrix difficult to assess. Rapid in-feed assays are even more important for the end user to confirm correct dosage of the enzyme, preferably before the diet is fed. The conditions used by feed compounders for pelleting their feeds may be more aggressive than those used in pelleting feeds for experimental trials. Thus, the potential for losses in the commercial environment are far greater and hence the potential problems due to the loss of phytase activity are more likely. Some commercially used feed ingredients such as acids and pellet binders may inhibit enzyme recoveries in the feed. Therefore, the commercial user should regularly test the recovery of all enzyme products that go through the feed production process and especially for phytases. The consequence of significant losses of phytase activity are far more serious under commercial conditions where the stresses of high stocking densities and larger flocks create more likelihood of P-deficiency symptoms.

8.7 Outlook

Although phytase is in commercial application since more than 25 years, existing gaps of knowledge in both functionality of the enzyme and optimized dosing in animal feed require more research. Although supplemented phytase nowadays can increase pre-caecal $InsP_6$ disappearance to a level of 90%, some $InsP_6$ and lower inositol esters remain undegraded, which challenges research and enzyme development for further improvement of phytate-P utilization by pigs and poultry. Metabolic effects of degradation products such as *myo*-inositol and specific lower inositol phosphates are barely understood. Enzyme effects on digestibility of amino acids and minerals other than P are inconsistent in the literature. The reasons for this must be better understood in order to diversify and instil greater confidence in the matrix values used by the industry. The digestibility and requirements of antagonistic feed constituents such as Ca must be better elucidated in order to avoid excess inclusion in the feed. Precision application of phytase also requires precise values of the phytate content of feed raw materials actually in use. Future research in these areas may improve the sustainability of livestock production and maintain finite rock phosphate stores for the sake of future generations.

References

Abudabos, A.M. (2012) Phytate phosphorus utilization and intestinal phytase activity in laying hens. *Italian Journal of Animal Science* 11, 41–46.

Adebiyi, A. and Olukosi, O. (2015) Determination in broilers and turkeys of true phosphorus digestibility and retention in wheat distillers dried grains with solubles without or with phytase supplementation. *Animal Feed Science and Technology* 207, 112–119.

Adeola, O. (1995) Digestive utilization of minerals by weanling pigs fed copper- and phytase-supplemented diets. *Canadian Journal of Animal Science* 75, 603–610.

Adeola, O. and Sands, J.S. (2003) Does supplemental dietary microbial phytase improve amino acid utilization? A perspective that it does not. *Journal of Animal Science* 81, E78–E85.

Ajuwon, K.M., Sommerfeld, V., Paul, V., Däuber, M., Schollenberger, M., *et al.* (2020) Phytase dosing affects phytate degradation and Muc2 transporter gene expression in broiler starters. *Poultry Science* 99, 981–991.

Akter, M., Iji, P.A. and Graham, H. (2017) Increased iron level in phytase-supplemented diets reduces performance and nutrient utilisation in broiler chickens. *British Poultry Science* 58, 409–417.

Angel, R., Tamim, N.M., Applegate, T.J., Dhandu, A.S. and Ellestad, L.E. (2002) Phytic acid chemistry: influence on phytin-phosphorus availability and phytase efficacy. *Journal of Applied Poultry Research* 11, 471–480.

Angel, R., Dalloul, R.A. and Doerr, J. (2005) Performance of broiler chickens fed diets supplemented with a direct-fed microbial. *Poultry Science* 84, 1222–1231.

Applegate, T.J., Angel, R. and Classen, H.L. (2003) Effect of dietary calcium, 25-hydroxycholecalciferol, or bird strain on small intestinal phytase activity in broiler chickens. *Poultry Science* 82, 1140–1148.

Augspurger, N.R., Spencer, J.D., Webel, D.M. and Baker, D.H. (2004) Pharmacological zinc levels reduce the phosphorus-releasing efficacy of phytase in young pigs and chickens. *Journal of Animal Science* 82, 1732–1739.

Aureli, R., Ueberschlag, Q., Klein, F., Noël, C. and Guggenbuhl, P. (2017) Use of near infrared reflectance spectroscopy to predict phytate phosphorus, total phosphorus, and crude protein of common poultry feed ingredients. *Poultry Science* 96, 160–168.

Babatunde, O.O., Jendza, J.A., Ader, P., Xue, P., Adedokun, S.A., *et al.* (2020) Response of broiler chickens in the starter and finisher phases to 3 sources of microbial phytase. *Poultry Science* 99, 3997–4008.

Banks, K.M., Thompson, K.L., Jaynes, P. and Applegate, T.J. (2004) The effects of copper on the efficacy of phytase, growth, and phosphorus retention in broiler chicks. *Poultry Science* 83, 1335–1341.

Barrier-Guillot, B., Casado, P., Maupetit, P., Jondreville, C., Gatel, F., *et al.* (1996) Wheat phosphorus availability: 2 – *In vivo* study in broilers and pigs; relationship with endogenous phytasic activity and phytic phosphorus content in wheat. *Journal of the Science of Food and Agriculture* 70, 69–74.

Baumgärtel, T., Metzler, B.U., Mosenthin, R., Greiner, R. and Rodehutscord, M. (2008) Precaecal and postileal metabolism of P, Ca and N in pigs as affected by different carbohydrate sources fed at low level of P intake. *Archives of Animal Nutrition* 62, 169–181.

Beck, P., Piepho, H.-P., Rodehutscord, M. and Bennewitz, J. (2016) Inferring relationships between phosphorus utilization, feed per gain, and bodyweight gain in an F_2 cross of Japanese quail using recursive models. *Poultry Science* 95, 764–773.

Bedford, M.R. (2008) Pitfalls in digestibility techniques for evaluation of phytases. *Proceedings of the 13th Worlds Poultry Congress* 13, 76–85.

Bedford, M.R. and Cowieson, A.J. (2019) Matrix values for exogenous enzymes and their application in the real world. *Journal of Applied Poultry Research* 29, 15–22.

Bedford, M.R. and Rousseau, X. (2017) Recent findings regarding calcium and phytase in poultry nutrition. *Animal Production Science* 57, 2311–2316.

Bedford, M.R., Parr, T., Persia, M.E., Batal, A.B. and Wyatt, C.L. (2007) Influence of dietary calcium and phytase source on litter moisture and mineral content. *Poultry Science* 86(Suppl. 1), 673 (abstract).

Bedford, M.R., Walk, C.L. and Kuhn, I. (2012) Is phytase responsible for increasing water:feed intake ratio. *Poultry Science* 91(Suppl. 1), 18 (abstract).

Blaabjerg, K., Jørgensen, H., Tauson, A.H. and Poulsen, H.D. (2010) Heat-treatment, phytase and fermented liquid feeding affect the presence of inositol phosphates in ileal digesta and phosphorus digestibility in pigs fed a wheat and barley diet. *Animal* 4, 876–885.

Borda-Molina, D., Zuber, T., Siegert, W., Camarinha-Silva, A., Feuerstein, D., *et al.* (2019) Effects of protease and phytase supplements on small intestinal microbiota and amino acid digestibility in broiler chickens. *Poultry Science* 98, 2906–2918.

Borda-Molina, D., Roth, C., Hérnandez-Arriaga, A., Rissi, D., Vollmar, S., *et al.* (2020) Effects on the ileal microbiota of phosphorus and calcium utilization, bird performance, and gender in Japanese quail. *Animals* 10, 885.

Cauble, R.N., Greene, E.S., Orlowski, S., Walk, C., Bedford, M., *et al.* (2020) Research Note: Dietary phytase reduces broiler woody breast severity via potential modulation of breast muscle fatty acid profiles. *Poultry Science* 99, 4009–4015.

Centeno, C., Arija, I., Viveros, A. and Brenes, A. (2007) Effects of citric acid and microbial phytase on amino acid digestibility in broiler chickens. *British Poultry Science* 48, 469–479.

Cossa, J., Jeroch, H., Oloffs, K., Kluge, H., Drauschke, W., *et al.* (1999) Total phosphorus and phytate phosphorus content in grain maize (*Zea mays*). *Der Tropenlandwirt* 100, 181–188.

Cossa, J., Oloffs, K., Kluge, H., Drauschke, W. and Jeroch, H. (2000) Variabilities of total and phytate phosphorus contents as well as phytase activity in wheat. *Der Tropenlandwirt* 101, 119–126.

Cowieson, A.J. and Bedford, M.R. (2009) The effect of phytase and carbohydrase on ileal amino acid digestibility in monogastric diets: complimentary mode of action? *World's Poultry Science Journal* 65, 609–624.

Cowieson, A.J. and Ravindran, V. (2007) Effect of phytic acid and microbial phytase on the flow and amino acid composition of endogenous protein at the terminal ileum of growing broiler chickens. *British Journal of Nutrition* 98, 745–752.

Cowieson, A.J. and Zhai, H.-X. (2021) Research Note: The effect of sequential displacement of dietary dextrose with *myo*-inositol on broiler chicken growth performance, bone characteristics, ileal nutrient digestibility and total tract nutrient retention. *Poultry Science* 100, 993–997.

Cowieson, A.J., Acamovic, T. and Bedford, M.R. (2004) The effects of phytase and phytic acid on the loss of endogenous amino acids and minerals from broiler chickens. *British Poultry Science* 45, 101–108.

Cowieson, A.J., Bedford, M.R. and Ravindran, V. (2010) Interactions between xylanase and glucanase in maize–soy-based diets for broilers. *British Poultry Science* 51, 246–257.

Cowieson, A.J., Wilcock, P. and Bedford, M.R. (2011) Superdosing effects of phytase in poultry and other monogastrics. *World's Poultry Science Journal* 67, 225–235.

Demirel, G., Pekel, A.Y., Alp, M. and Kocabağlı, N. (2012) Effects of dietary supplementation of citric acid, copper, and microbial phytase on growth performance and mineral retention in broiler chickens fed a low available phosphorus diet. *Journal of Applied Poultry Research* 21, 335–347.

De Verdal, H., Narcy, A., Bastianelli, D., Chapuis, H., Meme, N., *et al.* (2011) Improving the efficiency of feed utilization in poultry by selection. 2. Genetic parameters of excretion traits and correlations with anatomy of the gastro-intestinal tract and digestive efficiency. *BMC Genetics* 12, 71.

Dilger, R.N., Onyango, E.M., Sands, J.S. and Adeola, O. (2004) Evaluation of microbial phytase in broiler diets. *Poultry Science* 83, 962–970.

Düngelhoef, M., Rodehutscord, M., Spiekers, H. and Pfeffer, E. (1994) Effects of supplemental microbial phytase on availability of phosphorus contained in maize, wheat and triticale to pigs. *Animal Feed Science and Technology* 49, 1–10.

Eeckhout, W. and De Paepe, M. (1994) Total phosphorus, phytate-phosphorus and phytase activity in plant feedstuffs. *Animal Feed Science and Technology* 47, 19–29.

Farhadi, D., Karimi, A., Sadeghi, G.H.A., Rostamzadeh, J. and Bedford, M.R. (2017) Effects of a high dose of microbial phytase and *myo*-inositol supplementation on growth performance, tibia mineralization, nutrient digestibility, litter moisture content, and foot problems in broiler chickens fed phosphorus-deficient diets. *Poultry Science* 96, 3664–3675.

Gillespie, J., Rogers, S.W., Deery, M., Dupree, P. and Rogers, J.C. (2005) A unique family of proteins associated with internalized membranes in protein storage vacuoles of the Brassicaceae. *The Plant Journal* 41, 429–441.

Gonzalez-Uarquin, F., Kenéz, Á., Rodehutscord, M. and Huber, K. (2020a) Dietary phytase and *myo*-inositol supplementation are associated with distinct plasma metabolome profile in broiler chickens. *Animal* 14, 549–559.

Gonzalez-Uarquin, F., Rodehutscord, M. and Huber, K. (2020b) *Myo*-inositol: its metabolism and potential implications for poultry nutrition – a review. *Poultry Science* 99, 893–905.

Greene, E., Flees, J., Dadgar, S., Mallmann, B., Orlowski, S., *et al.* (2019) Quantum Blue reduces the severity of woody breast myopathy via modulation of oxygen homeostasis-related genes in broiler chickens. *Frontiers in Physiology* 10, 1251.

Gross, M. (2010) Fears over phosphorus supplies. *Current Biology* 20, R386–R387.

Guggenbuhl, P., Calvo, E.P. and Fru, F. (2016) Effect of a bacterial 6-phytase on plasma *myo*-inositol concentrations and P and Ca utilization in swine. *Journal of Animal Science* 94, 243–245.

Haese, E., Möhring, J., Steingass, H., Schollenberger, M. and Rodehutscord, M. (2017) Effect of dietary mineral phosphorus and phytate on *in situ* ruminal phytate disappearance from different concentrates in dairy cows. *Journal of Dairy Science* 100, 3672–3684.

Haros, M., Carlsson, N.-G., Almgren, A., Larsson-Alminger, M., Sandberg, A.-S., *et al.* (2009) Phytate degradation by human gut isolated *Bifidobacterium pseudocatenulatum* ATCC27919 and its probiotic potential. *International Journal of Food Microbiology* 135, 7–14.

Herwig, E., Classen, H.L., Walk, C.L., Bedford, M.R. and Schwean-Lardner, K. (2019) Dietary inositol reduces fearfulness and avoidance in laying hens. *Animals* 9, 938.

Hovenjürgen, M., Rodehutscord, M. and Pfeffer, E. (2003) Effect of fertilization and variety on digestibility of phosphorus from plant feedstuffs in pigs. *Journal of Animal and Feed Sciences* 12, 83–93.

Huber, K. (2016) Cellular *myo*-inositol metabolism. In: Walk, C.L., Kühn, I., Stein, H.H., Kidd, M.T. and Rodehutscord, M. (eds) *Phytate Destruction – Consequences for Precision Animal Nutrition*. Wageningen Academic Publishers, Wageningen, the Netherlands, pp. 53–60.

Huber, K., Zeller, E. and Rodehutscord, M. (2015) Modulation of small intestinal phosphate transporter by dietary supplements of mineral phosphorus and phytase in broilers. *Poultry Science* 94, 1009–1017.

Ingelmann, C.-J., Witzig, M., Möhring, J., Schollenberger, M., Kühn, I., *et al.* (2018) Effect of supplemental phytase and xylanase in wheat-based diets on prececal phosphorus digestibility and phytate degradation in young turkeys. *Poultry Science* 97, 2011–2020.

Ingelmann, C.-J., Witzig, M., Möhring, J., Schollenberger, M., Kühn, I., *et al.* (2019) Phytate degradation and phosphorus digestibility in broilers and turkeys fed different corn sources with or without added phytase. *Poultry Science* 98, 912–922.

Jongbloed, A.W., Mroz, Z. and Kemme, P.A. (1992) The effect of supplementary *Aspergillus niger* phytase in diets for pigs on concentration and apparent digestibility of dry matter, total phosphorus, and phytic acid in different sections of the alimentary tract. *Journal of Animal Science* 70, 1159–1168.

Juanpere, J., Pérez-Vendrell, A.M. and Brufau, J. (2004) Effect of microbial phytase on broilers fed barley-based diets in the presence or not of endogenous phytase. *Animal Feed Science and Technology* 115, 265–279.

Kasim, A.B. and Edwards, H.M. Jr (1998) The analysis for inositol phosphate forms in feed ingredients. *Journal of the Science of Food and Agriculture* 76, 1–9.

Kemme, P.A., Jongbloed, A.W., Mroz, Z., Kogut, J. and Beynen, A.C. (1999) Digestibility of nutrients in growing-finishing pigs is affected by *Aspergillus niger* phytase, phytate and lactic acid levels. 2. Apparent total tract digestibility of phosphorus, calcium and magnesium and ileal degradation of phytic acid. *Livestock Production Science* 58, 119–127.

Kemme, P.A., Schlemmer, U., Mroz, Z. and Jongbloed, A.W. (2006) Monitoring the stepwise phytate degradation in the upper gastrointestinal tract of pigs. *Journal of the Science of Food and Agriculture* 86, 612–622.

Kerr, M.J., Classen, H.L. and Newkirk, R.W. (2000) The effects of gastrointestinal tract micro-flora and dietary phytase on inositol hexaphosphate hydrolysis in the chicken. *Poultry Science* 79(Suppl. 1), 11 (abstract).

Kies, A.K., De Jonge, L.H., Kemme, P.A. and Jongbloed, A.W. (2006) Interaction between protein, phytate, and microbial phytase. *In vitro* studies. *Journal of Agricultural and Food Chemistry* 54, 1753–1758.

Konietzny, U. and Greiner, R. (2002) Molecular and catalytic properties of phytate-degrading enzymes (phytases). *International Journal of Food Science & Technology* 37, 791–812.

Krieg, J., Siegert, W., Berghaus, D., Bock, J., Feuerstein, D., *et al.* (2020) Phytase supplementation effects on amino acid digestibility depend on the protein source in the diet but are not related to InsP$_6$ degradation in broiler chickens. *Poultry Science* 99, 3251–3265.

Krieg, J., Borda-Molina, D., Siegert, W., Sommerfeld, V., Chi, Y.P., *et al.* (2021) Effects of calcium level and source, acidification, and phytase on phytate degradation and the microbiota in the digestive tract of broiler chickens. *Animal Microbiome* 3, 23.

Kriseldi, R., Walk, C.L., Johnson, J., Bedford, M.R. and Dozier, W.A. (2018) Influence of phytase addition in diets fed to broilers on plasma inositol over time and inositol phosphate ester concentrations at 28 days of age. *Poultry Science* 97(Suppl. 1), 59 (abstract).

Kriseldi, R., Walk, C.L., Bedford, M.R. and Dozier, W.A. (2021) Inositol and gradient phytase supplementation in broiler diets during a 6-week production period: 2. Effects on phytate degradation and inositol liberation in gizzard and ileal digesta contents. *Poultry Science* 100, 100899.

Kühn, I., Schollenberger, M. and Männer, K. (2016) Effect of dietary phytase level on intestinal phytate degradation and bone mineralization in growing pigs. *Journal of Animal Science* 94, 264–267.

Künzel, S., Bennewitz, J. and Rodehutscord, M. (2019a) Genetic parameters for bone ash and phosphorus utilization in an F$_2$ cross of Japanese quail. *Poultry Science* 98, 4369–4372.

Künzel, S., Borda-Molina, D., Kraft, R., Sommerfeld, V., Kühn, I., *et al.* (2019b) Impact of coccidiostat and phytase supplementation on gut microbiota composition and phytate degradation in broiler chickens. *Animal Microbiome* 2, 1.

Künzel, S., Borda-Molina, D., Zuber, T., Hartung, J., Siegert, W., *et al.* (2021) Relative phytase efficacy values as affected by response traits, including ileal microbiota composition. *Poultry Science* 100, 101133.

Laird, S., Kühn, I. and Miller, H.M. (2018) Super-dosing phytase improves the growth performance of weaner pigs fed a low iron diet. *Animal Feed Science and Technology* 242, 150–160.

Lee, S. and Greenwood, W. (2020) Unlocking phytate potential through NIR technology. *Aquafeed* 12(1), 45–46. Available at: https://issuu.com/aquafeed.com/docs/aquafeed_0120_pr__no_bleed_/46 (accessed 17 September 2021).

Lee, S.A. and Bedford, M.R. (2016) Inositol – an effective growth promotor? *World's Poultry Science Journal* 72, 743–760.

Lee, S.A., Bedford, M.R. and Walk, C.L. (2018) Meta-analysis: explicit value of mono-component proteases in monogastric diets. *Poultry Science* 97, 2078–2085.

Leytem, A.B., Willing, B.P. and Thacker, P.A. (2008) Phytate utilization and phosphorus excretion by broiler chickens fed diets containing cereal grains varying in phytate and phytase content. *Animal Feed Science and Technology* 146, 160–168.

Li, Y.C., Ledoux, D.R., Veum, T.L., Raboy, V. and Zyla, K. (2001) Low phytic acid barley improves performance, bone mineralization, and phosphorus retention in turkey poults. *Journal of Applied Poultry Research* 10, 178–185.

Linares, L.B., Broomhead, J.N., Guaiume, E.A., Ledoux, D.R., Veum, T.L., *et al.* (2007) Effects of low phytate barley (*Hordeum vulgare* L.) on zinc utilization in young broiler chicks. *Poultry Science* 86, 299–308.

Lu, H., Kühn, I., Bedford, M.R., Whitfield, H., Brearley, C., *et al.* (2019) Effect of phytase on intestinal phytate breakdown, plasma inositol concentrations, and glucose transporter type 4 abundance in muscle membranes of weanling pigs. *Journal of Animal Science* 97, 3907–3919.

Lu, H., Shin, S., Kuehn, I., Bedford, M., Rodehutscord, M., *et al.* (2020) Effect of phytase on nutrient digestibility and expression of intestinal tight junction and nutrient transporter genes in pigs. *Journal of Animal Science* 98, 1–12.

Maenz, D.D. and Classen, H.L. (1998) Phytase activity in the small intestinal brush border membrane of the chicken. *Poultry Science* 77, 557–563.

Maenz, D.D., Engele-Schaan, C.M., Newkirk, R.W. and Classen, H.L. (1999) The effect of minerals and mineral chelators on the formation of phytase-resistant and phytase-susceptible forms of phytic acid in solution and in a slurry of canola meal. *Animal Feed Science and Technology* 81, 177–192.

Marounek, M., Skřivan, M., Dlouhá, G. and Břeňová, N. (2008) Availability of phytate phosphorus and endogenous phytase activity in the digestive tract of laying hens 20 and 47 weeks old. *Animal Feed Science and Technology* 146, 353–359.

Marounek, M., Skřivan, M., Rosero, O. and Rop, O. (2010) Intestinal and total tract phytate digestibility and phytase activity in the digestive tract of hens fed a wheat–maize–soyabean diet. *Journal of Animal and Feed Sciences* 19, 430–439.

Martinez-Amezcua, C., Parsons, C.M. and Baker, D.H. (2006) Effect of microbial phytase and citric acid on phosphorus bioavailability, apparent metabolizable energy, and amino acid digestibility in distillers dried grains with solubles in chicks. *Poultry Science* 85, 470–475.

Menezes-Blackburn, D., Gabler, S. and Greiner, R. (2015) Performance of seven commercial phytases in an *in vitro* simulation of poultry digestive tract. *Journal of Agricultural and Food Chemistry* 63, 6142–6149.

Menezes-Blackburn, D., Greiner, R. and Konietzny, U. (2022) Phytases: biochemistry, enzymology and characteristics relevant to animal feed use. In: Bedford, M.R., Partridge, G.G., Hruby, M. and Walk, C.L. (eds) *Enzymes in Farm Animal Nutrition*, 3rd edn. CAB International, Wallingford, UK, pp. 103–123.

Mesina, V.G.R., Lagos, L.V., Sulabo, R.C., Walk, C.L. and Stein, H.H. (2019) Effects of microbial phytase on mucin synthesis, gastric protein hydrolysis, and degradation of phytate along the gastrointestinal tract of growing pigs. *Journal of Animal Science* 97, 756–767.

Momeneh, T., Karimi, A., Sadeghi, G., Vaziry, A. and Bedford, M.R. (2018) Evaluation of dietary calcium level and source and phytase on growth performance, serum metabolites, and ileum mineral contents in broiler chicks fed adequate phosphorus diets from one to 28 days of age. *Poultry Science* 97, 1283–1289.

Morales, G.A., Rodrigañez, M.S.d., Márquez, L., Díaz, M. and Moyano, F.J. (2013) Solubilisation of protein fractions induced by *Escherichia coli* phytase and its effects on *in vitro* fish digestion of plant proteins. *Animal Feed Science and Technology* 181, 54–64.

Morales, G.A., Marquez, L., Hernández, A.J. and Moyano, F.J. (2016) Phytase effects on protein and phosphorus bioavailability in fish diets. In: Walk, C.L., Kühn, I., Stein, H.H., Kidd, M.T. and Rodehutscord, M. (eds) *Phytate Destruction – Consequences for Precision Animal Nutrition*. Wageningen Academic Publishers, Wageningen, the Netherlands, pp. 129–165.

Morgan, N.K., Walk, C.L., Bedford, M.R., Scholey, D.V. and Burton, E.J. (2016) Effect of feeding broilers diets differing in susceptible phytate content. *Animal Nutrition* 2, 33–39.

Moter, V. and Stein, H.H. (2004) Effect of feed intake on endogenous losses and amino acid and energy digestibility by growing pigs. *Journal of Animal Science* 82, 3518–3525.

Neset, T.-S.S. and Cordell, D. (2012) Global phosphorus scarcity: identifying synergies for a sustainable future. *Journal of the Science of Food and Agriculture* 92, 2–6.

Oloffs, K., Dolbusin, A. and Jeroch, H. (1998) Einfluß von mikrobieller und nativer Weizenphytase auf die Phosphor-Verwertung bei Broilern. *Archiv für Geflügelkunde* 62, 260–263.

Oloffs, K., Cossa, J. and Jeroch, H. (2000) Die Bedeutung der korneigenen (nativen) Phytaseaktivität im Weizen für die Phosphor-Verwertung bei Broilern und Legehennen. *Archiv für Geflügelkunde* 64, 157–161.

Olukosi, O.A., Kong, C., Fru-Nji, F., Ajuwon, K.M. and Adeola, O. (2013) Assessment of a bacterial 6-phytase in the diets of broiler chickens. *Poultry Science* 92, 2101–2108.

Olukosi, O.A., González-Ortiz, G., Whitfield, H. and Bedford, M.R. (2020) Comparative aspects of phytase and xylanase effects on performance, mineral digestibility, and ileal phytate degradation in broilers and turkeys. *Poultry Science* 99, 1528–1539.

Onyango, E.M., Asem, E.K. and Adeola, O. (2006) Dietary cholecalciferol and phosphorus influence intestinal mucosa phytase activity in broiler chicks. *British Poultry Science* 47, 632–639.

Onyango, E.M., Asem, E.K. and Adeola, O. (2009) Phytic acid increases mucin and endogenous amino acid losses from the gastrointestinal tract of chickens. *British Journal of Nutrition* 101, 836–842.

Oster, M., Reyer, H., Trakooljul, N., Weber, F.M., Xi, L., *et al.* (2020) Ileal transcriptome profiles of Japanese quail divergent in phosphorus utilization. *International Journal of Molecular Sciences* 21, 2762.

Pallauf, J. and Rimbach, G. (1997) Nutritional significance of phytic acid and phytase. *Archives of Animal Nutrition* 50, 301–319.

Papp, M., Sommerfeld, V., Schollenberger, M., Avenhaus, U. and Rodehutscord, M. (2021) Phytate degradation and phosphorus utilisation by broiler chickens fed diets containing wheat with increased phytase activity. *British Poultry Science*, in press. doi:/10.1080/00071668.2021.1966756

Persson, H., Türk, M., Nyman, M. and Sandberg, A.-S. (1998) Binding of Cu^{2+}, Zn^{2+}, and Cd^{2+} to inositol tri-, tetra-, penta-, and hexaphosphates. *Journal of Agricultural and Food Chemistry* 46, 3194–3200.

Pieniazek, J., Smith, K.A., Williams, M.P., Manangi, M.K., Vazquez-Anon, M., *et al.* (2017) Evaluation of increasing levels of a microbial phytase in phosphorus deficient broiler diets via live broiler performance, tibia bone ash, apparent metabolizable energy, and amino acid digestibility. *Poultry Science* 96, 370–382.

Pirgozliev, V., Acamovic, T. and Bedford, M.R. (2009) Previous exposure to dietary phytase reduces the endogenous energy losses from precision-fed chickens. *British Poultry Science* 50, 598–605.

Pirgozliev, V., Bedford, M.R., Oduguwa, O., Acamovic, T. and Allymehr, M. (2012) The effect of supplementary bacterial phytase on dietary metabolisable energy, nutrient retention and endogenous losses in precision fed broiler chickens. *Journal of Animal Physiology and Animal Nutrition* 96, 52–57.

Pirgozliev, V., Bedford, M.R., Rose, S.P., Whiting, I.M., Oluwatosin, O.O., *et al.* (2017) Phosphorus utilisation and growth performance of broiler chicken fed diets containing graded levels of supplementary *myo*-inositol with and without exogenous phytase. *Journal of World's Poultry Research* 7, 1–7.

Pirgozliev, V., Brearley, C.A., Rose, S.P. and Mansbridge, S.C. (2019) Manipulation of plasma *myo*-inositol in broiler chickens: effect on growth performance, dietary energy, nutrient availability, and hepatic function. *Poultry Science* 98, 260–268.

Ponsuksili, S., Reyer, H., Hadlich, F., Weber, F., Trakooljul, N., *et al.* (2020) Identification of the key molecular drivers of phosphorus utilization based on host miRNA–mRNA and gut microbiome interactions. *International Journal of Molecular Sciences* 21, 2818.

Pontoppidan, K., Pettersson, D. and Sandberg, A.-S. (2007) The type of thermal feed treatment influences the inositol phosphate composition. *Animal Feed Science and Technology* 132, 137–147.

Prattley, C.A. and Stanley, D.W. (1982) Protein–phytate interactions in soybeans. I. Localization of phytate in protein bodies and globoids. *Journal of Food Biochemistry* 6, 243–254.

Puhl, A.A., Greiner, R. and Selinger, L.B. (2008) A protein tyrosine phosphatase-like inositol polyphosphatase from *Selenomonas ruminantium* subsp. *lactilytica* has specificity for the 5-phosphate of *myo*-inositol hexakisphosphate. *The International Journal of Biochemistry & Cell Biology* 40, 2053–2064.

Punna, S. and Roland, D.A. (1999) Variation in phytate phosphorus utilization within the same broiler strain. *Journal of Applied Poultry Research* 8, 10–15.

Raghavendra, P. and Halami, P.M. (2009) Screening, selection and characterization of phytic acid degrading lactic acid bacteria from chicken intestine. *International Journal of Food Microbiology* 133, 129–134.

Rapp, C., Lantzsch, H.-J. and Drochner, W. (2001) Hydrolysis of phytic acid by intrinsic plant or supplemented microbial phytase (*Aspergillus niger*) in the stomach and small intestine of minipigs fitted with re-entrant cannulas. 3. Hydrolysis of phytic acid (IP_6) and occurrence of hydrolysis products (IP_5, IP_4, IP_3 and IP_2). *Journal of Animal Physiology and Animal Nutrition* 85, 420–430.

Ravindran, V., Ravindran, G. and Sivalogan, S. (1994) Total and phytate phosphorus contents of various foods and feedstuffs of plant origin. *Food Chemistry* 50, 133–136.

Ravindran, V., Cabahug, S., Ravindran, G. and Bryden, W.L. (1999) Influence of microbial phytase on apparent ileal amino acid digestibility of feedstuffs for broilers. *Poultry Science* 78, 699–706.

Ravindran, V., Cabahug, S., Ravindran, G., Selle, P.H. and Bryden, W.L. (2000) Response of broiler chickens to microbial phytase supplementation as influenced by dietary phytic acid and non-phytate phosphorous levels. II. Effects on apparent metabolisable energy, nutrient digestibility and nutrient retention. *British Poultry Science* 41, 193–200.

Ravindran, V., Morel, P.C., Partridge, G.G., Hruby, M. and Sands, J.S. (2006) Influence of an *Escherichia coli*-derived phytase on nutrient utilization in broiler starters fed diets containing varying concentrations of phytic acid. *Poultry Science* 85, 82–89.

Rehman, H.U., Vahjen, W., Awad, W.A. and Zentek, J. (2007) Indigenous bacteria and bacterial metabolic products in the gastrointestinal tract of broiler chickens. *Archives of Animal Nutrition* 61, 319–335.

Revy, P.S., Jondreville, C., Dourmad, J.Y. and Nys, Y. (2004) Effect of zinc supplemented as either an organic or an inorganic source and of microbial phytase on zinc and other minerals utilisation by weanling pigs. *Animal Feed Science and Technology* 116, 93–112.

Reyer, H., Oster, M., Wittenburg, D., Murani, E., Ponsuksili, S., *et al.* (2019) Genetic contribution to variation in blood calcium, phosphorus, and alkaline phosphatase activity in pigs. *Frontiers in Genetics* 10, 590.

Rezvani, M., Kluth, H., Bulang, M. and Rodehutscord, M. (2012) Variation in amino acid digestibility of rapeseed meal studied in caecectomised laying hens and relationship with chemical constituents. *British Poultry Science* 53, 665–674.

Rodehutscord, M. (2016) Interactions between minerals and phytate degradation in poultry – challenges for phosphorus digestibility assays. In: Walk, C.L., Kühn, I., Stein, H.H., Kidd, M.T. and Rodehutscord, M. (eds) *Phytate Destruction – Consequences for Precision Animal Nutrition*. Wageningen Academic Publishers, Wageningen, the Netherlands, pp. 167–177.

Rodehutscord, M. and Dieckmann, A. (2005) Comparative studies with three-week-old chickens, turkeys, ducks, and quails on the response in phosphorus utilization to a supplementation of monobasic calcium phosphate. *Poultry Science* 84, 1252–1260.

Rodehutscord, M., Faust, M. and Lorenz, H. (1996) Digestibility of phosphorus contained in soybean meal, barley, and different varieties of wheat, without and with supplemental phytase fed to pigs and additivity of digestibility in a wheat–soybean-meal diet. *Journal of Animal Physiology and Animal Nutrition* 75, 40–48.

Rodehutscord, M., Kapocius, M., Timmler, R. and Dieckmann, A. (2004) Linear regression approach to study amino acid digestibility in broiler chickens. *British Poultry Science* 45, 85–92.

Rodehutscord, M., Rückert, C., Maurer, H.P., Schenkel, H., Schipprack, W., *et al.* (2016) Variation in chemical composition and physical characteristics of cereal grains from different genotypes. *Archives of Animal Nutrition* 70, 87–107.

Rosen, G.D. (2002) Microbial phytase in broiler nutrition. In: Garnsworthy, P.C. and Wiseman, J. (eds) *Recent Advances in Animal Nutrition 2002*. Nottingham University Press, Nottingham, UK, pp. 105–118.

Rosenfelder-Kuon, P., Klein, N., Zegowitz, B., Schollenberger, M., Kühn, I., *et al.* (2020a) Phytate degradation cascade in pigs as affected by phytase supplementation and rapeseed cake inclusion in corn–soybean meal-based diets. *Journal of Animal Science* 98, 1–12.

Rosenfelder-Kuon, P., Siegert, W. and Rodehutscord, M. (2020b) Effect of microbial phytase supplementation on P digestibility in pigs: a meta-analysis. *Archives of Animal Nutrition* 74, 1–18.

Rutherfurd, S.M., Chung, T.K. and Moughan, P.J. (2014) Effect of microbial phytase on phytate P degradation and apparent digestibility of total P and Ca throughout the gastrointestinal tract of the growing pig. *Journal of Animal Science* 92, 189–197.

Sandberg, A.-S., Carlsson, N.-G. and Svanberg, U. (1989) Effects of inositol tri-, tetra-, penta-, and hexaphosphates on *in vitro* estimation of iron availability. *Journal of Food Science* 54, 159–161.

Sandberg, A.-S., Larsen, T. and Sandström, B. (1993) High dietary calcium level decreases colonic phytate degradation in pigs fed a rapeseed diet. *The Journal of Nutrition* 123, 559–566.

Schemmer, R., Spillner, C. and Südekum, K.-H. (2020) Phosphorus digestibility and metabolisable energy concentrations of contemporary wheat, barley, rye and triticale genotypes fed to growing pigs. *Archives of Animal Nutrition* 74, 429–444.

Schlegel, P., Nys, Y. and Jondreville, C. (2010) Zinc availability and digestive zinc solubility in piglets and broilers fed diets varying in their phytate contents, phytase activity and supplemented zinc source. *Animal* 4, 200–209.

Schlegel, P., Sauvant, D. and Jondreville, C. (2013) Bioavailability of zinc sources and their interaction with phytates in broilers and pigs. *Animal* 7, 47–59.

Schlemmer, U., Jany, K.-D., Berk, A., Schulz, E. and Rechkemmer, G. (2001) Degradation of phytate in the gut of pigs – pathway of gastro-intestinal inositol phosphate hydrolysis and enzymes involved. *Archives of Animal Nutrition* 55, 255–280.

Schlemmer, U., Frølich, W., Prieto, R.M. and Grases, F. (2009) Phytate in foods and significance for humans: food sources, intake, processing, bioavailability, protective role and analysis. *Molecular Nutrition & Food Research* 53, S330–S375.

Sebastian, S.T., Touchburn, S.P., Chavez, E.R. and Lague, P.C. (1997) Apparent digestibility of protein and amino acids in broiler chickens fed a corn–soybean diet supplemented with microbial phytase. *Poultry Science* 76, 1760–1769.

Selle, P.H., Ravindran, V., Caldwell, R.A. and Bryden, W.L. (2000) Phytate and phytase: consequences for protein utilisation. *Nutrition Research Reviews* 13, 255–278.

Selle, P.H., Bryden, W.L. and Walker, A.R. (2003) Total and phytate-phosphorus contents and phytase activity of Australian-sourced feed ingredients for pigs and poultry. *Australian Journal of Experimental Agriculture* 43, 475–479.

Selle, P.H., Cowieson, A.J., Cowieson, N.P. and Ravindran, V. (2012) Protein–phytate interactions in pig and poultry nutrition: a reappraisal. *Nutrition Research Reviews* 25, 1–17.

Shastak, Y., Zeller, E., Witzig, M., Schollenberger, M. and Rodehutscord, M. (2014) Effects of the composition of the basal diet on the evaluation of mineral phosphorus sources and interactions with phytate hydrolysis in broilers. *Poultry Science* 93, 2548–2559.

Shieh, T.R., Wodzinski, R.J. and Ware, J.H. (1969) Regulation of the formation of acid phosphatases by inorganic phosphate in *Aspergillus ficuum. Journal of Bacteriology* 100, 1161–1165.

Siegert, W., Ganzer, C., Kluth, H. and Rodehutscord, M. (2019a) Effect of amino acid deficiency on precaecal amino acid digestibility in broiler chickens. *Journal of Animal Physiology and Animal Nutrition* 103, 723–737.

Siegert, W., Zuber, T., Sommerfeld, V., Krieg, J., Feuerstein, D., *et al.* (2019b) Prececal amino acid digestibility and phytate degradation in broiler chickens when using different oilseed meals, phytase and protease supplements in the feed. *Poultry Science* 98, 5700–5713.

Sommerfeld, V., Künzel, S., Schollenberger, M., Kühn, I. and Rodehutscord, M. (2018a) Influence of phytase or *myo*-inositol supplements on performance and phytate degradation products in the crop, ileum, and blood of broiler chickens. *Poultry Science* 97, 920–929.

Sommerfeld, V., Schollenberger, M., Kühn, I. and Rodehutscord, M. (2018b) Interactive effects of phosphorus, calcium, and phytase supplements on products of phytate degradation in the digestive tract of broiler chickens. *Poultry Science* 97, 1177–1188.

Sommerfeld, V., Van Kessel, A.G., Classen, H.L., Schollenberger, M., Kühn, I., *et al.* (2019) Phytate degradation in gnotobiotic broiler chickens and effects of dietary supplements of phosphorus, calcium, and phytase. *Poultry Science* 98, 5562–5570.

Sommerfeld, V., Huber, K., Bennewitz, J., Camarinha-Silva, A., Hasselmann, M., *et al.* (2020) Phytate degradation, *myo*-inositol release, and utilization of phosphorus and calcium by two strains of laying hens in five production periods. *Poultry Science* 99, 6797–6808.

Son, J.H., Ragland, D. and Adeola, O. (2002) Quantification of digesta flow into the caeca. *British Poultry Science* 43, 322–324.

Stentz, R., Osborne, S., Horn, N., Li, A.W.H., Hautefort, I., *et al.* (2014) A bacterial homolog of a eukaryotic inositol phosphate signaling enzyme mediates cross-kingdom dialog in the mammalian gut. *Cell Reports* 6, 646–656.

Svihus, B., Choct, M. and Classen, H.L. (2013) Function and nutritional roles of the avian caeca: a review. *World's Poultry Science Journal* 69, 249–263.

Tahir, M., Shim, M.Y., Ward, N.E., Westerhaus, M.O. and Pesti, G.M. (2012) Evaluation of near-infrared reflectance spectroscopy (NIRS) techniques for total and phytate phosphorus of common poultry feed ingredients. *Poultry Science* 91, 2540–2547.

Tamayo-Ramos, J.A., Sanz-Penella, J.M., Yebra, M.J., Monedero, V. and Haros, M. (2012) Novel phytases from *Bifidobacterium pseudocatenulatum* ATCC 27919 and *Bifidobacterium longum* subsp. *infantis* ATCC 15697. *Applied and Environmental Microbiology* 78, 5013–5015.

Tamim, N.M. and Angel, R. (2003) Phytate phosphorus hydrolysis as influenced by dietary calcium and micro-mineral source in broiler diets. *Journal of Agricultural and Food Chemistry* 51, 4687–4693.

Tamim, N.M., Angel, R. and Christman, M. (2004) Influence of dietary calcium and phytase on phytate phosphorus hydrolysis in broiler chickens. *Poultry Science* 83, 1358–1367.

Truong, H.H., Yu, S., Moss, A.F., Partridge, G.G., Liu, S.Y., *et al.* (2017) Phytase inclusions of 500 and 2000 FTU/kg in maize-based broiler diets impact on growth performance, nutrient utilisation, digestive dynamics of starch, protein (N), sodium and IP_6 phytate degradation in the gizzard and four small intestinal segments. *Animal Feed Science and Technology* 223, 13–22.

Vats, P. and Banerjee, U.C. (2004) Production studies and catalytic properties of phytases (*myo*-inositolhexakisphosphate phosphohydrolases): an overview. *Enzyme and Microbial Technology* 35, 3–14.

Vollmar, S., Haas, V., Schmid, M., Preuß, S., Joshi, R., *et al.* (2020a) Mapping genes for phosphorus utilization and correlated traits using a 4k SNP linkage map in Japanese quail (*Coturnix japonica*). *Animal Genetics* 52, 90–98.

Vollmar, S., Wellmann, R., Borda-Molina, D., Rodehutscord, M., Camarinha-Silva, A., *et al.* (2020b) The gut microbial architecture of efficiency traits in the domestic poultry model species Japanese quail (*Coturnix japonica*) assessed by mixed linear models. *G3: Genes|Genomes|Genetics* 10, 2553–2562.

Walk, C.L. (2016) The influence of calcium on phytase efficacy in non-ruminant animals. *Animal Production Science* 56, 1345–1349.

Walk, C.L. and Bedford, M.R. (2020) Application of exogenous enzymes: is digestibility an appropriate response variable? *Animal Production Science* 60, 993–998.

Walk, C.L. and Olukosi, O.A. (2019) Influence of graded concentrations of phytase in high-phytate diets on growth performance, apparent ileal amino acid digestibility, and phytate concentration in broilers from hatch to 28 D post-hatch. *Poultry Science* 98, 3884–3893.

Walk, C.L. and Rama Rao, S.V. (2020) Increasing dietary phytate has a significant anti-nutrient effect on apparent ileal amino acid digestibility and digestible amino acid intake requiring increasing doses of phytase as evidenced by prediction equations in broilers. *Poultry Science* 99, 290–300.

Walk, C.L., Bedford, M.R., Santos, T.S., Paiva, D., Bradley, J.R., *et al.* (2013) Extra-phosphoric effects of superdoses of a novel microbial phytase. *Poultry Science* 92, 719–725.

Walk, C.L., Santos, T.T. and Bedford, M.R. (2014) Influence of superdoses of a novel microbial phytase on growth performance, tibia ash, and gizzard phytate and inositol in young broilers. *Poultry Science* 93, 1172–1177.

Walk, C.L., Bedford, M.R. and Olukosi, O.A. (2018) Effect of phytase on growth performance, phytate degradation and gene expression of *myo*-inositol transporters in the small intestine, liver and kidney of 21 day old broilers. *Poultry Science* 97, 1155–1162.

Walters, H.G., Coelho, M., Coufal, C.D. and Lee, J.T. (2019) Effects of increasing phytase inclusion levels on broiler performance, nutrient digestibility, and bone mineralization in low-phosphorus diets. *Journal of Applied Poultry Research* 28, 1210–1225.

Wilcock, P. and Walk, C.L. (2016) Low phytate nutrition – what is the pig and poultry industry doing to counter dietary phytate as an anti-nutrient and how is it being applied? In: Walk, C.L., Kühn, I., Stein, H.H., Kidd, M.T. and Rodehutscord, M. (eds) *Phytate Destruction – Consequences for Precision Animal Nutrition*. Wageningen Academic Publishers, Wageningen, the Netherlands, pp. 87–106.

Witzig, M., Camarinha-Silva, A., Green-Engert, R., Hoelzle, K., Zeller, E., *et al.* (2015) Spatial variation of the gut microbiota in broiler chickens as affected by dietary available phosphorus and assessed by T-RFLP analysis and 454 pyrosequencing. *PLoS ONE* 10, e0143442.

Yi, Z. and Kornegay, E.T. (1996) Sites of phytase activity in the gastrointestinal tract of young pigs. *Animal Feed Science and Technology* 61, 361–368.

Yu, S., Cowieson, A., Gilbert, C., Plumstead, P. and Dalsgaard, S. (2012) Interactions of phytate and *myo*-inositol phosphate esters (IP_{1-5}) including IP_5 isomers with dietary protein and iron and inhibition of pepsin. *Journal of Animal Science* 90, 1824–1832.

Zeller, E., Schollenberger, M., Kühn, I. and Rodehutscord, M. (2015a) Hydrolysis of phytate and formation of inositol phosphate isomers without or with supplemented phytases in different segments of the digestive tract of broilers. *Journal of Nutritional Science* 4, e1.

Zeller, E., Schollenberger, M., Kühn, I. and Rodehutscord, M. (2015b) Effect of diets containing enzyme supplements and microwave-treated or untreated wheat on inositol phosphates in the small intestine of broilers. *Animal Feed Science and Technology* 204, 42–51.

Zeller, E., Schollenberger, M., Witzig, M., Shastak, Y., Kühn, I., *et al.* (2015c) Interactions between supplemented mineral phosphorus and phytase on phytate hydrolysis and inositol phosphates in the small intestine of broilers. *Poultry Science* 94, 1018–1029.

Zeller, E., Schollenberger, M., Kühn, I. and Rodehutscord, M. (2016) Dietary effects on inositol phosphate breakdown in the crop of broilers. *Archives of Animal Nutrition* 70, 57–71.

Zeng, Z.K., Wang, D., Piao, X.S., Li, P.F., Zhang, H.Y., *et al.* (2014) Effects of adding super dose phytase to the phosphorus-deficient diets of young pigs on growth performance, bone quality, minerals and amino acids digestibilities. *Asian-Australasian Journal of Animal Science* 27, 237–246.

Zhang, W., Aggrey, S.E., Pesti, G.M., Edwards, H.M. and Bakalli, R.I. (2003) Genetics of phytate phosphorus bioavailability: heritability and genetic correlations with growth and feed utilization traits in a random-bred chicken population. *Poultry Science* 82, 1075–1079.

Zouaoui, M., Létourneau-Montminy, M.P. and Guay, F. (2018) Effect of phytase on amino acid digestibility in pig: a meta-analysis. *Animal Feed Science and Technology* 238, 18–28.

9 Current Knowledge and Future Opportunities for Ruminant Enzymes

Christine Rosser[1], Stephanie A. Terry[1], Ajay Badhan[1], Tim A. McAllister[1] and Karen A. Beauchemin[1]*
[1]*Lethbridge Research and Development Centre, Agriculture and Agri-Food Canada, Lethbridge, Alberta, Canada*

9.1 Introduction

Ruminants harbour a unique population of microbiota in the rumen that allow for the efficient conversion of lignocellulose into animal products (i.e. milk, meat, fibre). This microbial consortium produces an array of enzymes that allow for the degradation of complex plant polysaccharides that make up plant cell walls. However, less than 50% of the energy in low-quality forages is digested by ruminants (McCartney *et al.*, 2006). Supplementation of diets with exogenous enzymes has the potential to improve nutrient digestion while reducing feed costs and improving animal performance. Research has mainly targeted the use of fibrolytic enzymes that enhance the degradation of plant fibre in the rumen as forages are often the main component of ruminant diets (Mottet *et al.*, 2018), although a limited number of studies have examined the use of amylases (Noziere *et al.*, 2014) and proteases (Sucu *et al.*, 2014) that degrade starch and proteins, respectively, as a means of improving the digestibility of grains. With increasing pressure to improve the sustainability and intensity of ruminant production, exogenous enzymes have the potential to improve the utilization of ruminant feeds.

Consideration of the complexity of the rumen microbiome and its role in plant cell wall degradation is a key component of any strategy to target improving the efficacy of exogenous enzymes. Similarly, identification of limiting enzymes can allow for microbial synergy to ensure that exogenous enzymes are not redundant within the rumen. There are also pre-consumption, ruminal and post-ruminal considerations that can impact the activity of exogenous enzymes throughout the digestive tract. Although exogenous enzymes are a potential means of improving feed utilization, the observed variability in animal responses has limited their adoption. The variability in responses can be attributed to various factors including dosage, application method, product formulation, dietary composition and animal production status. Novel strategies to improve enzyme effectiveness include enzyme delivery and discovery utilizing 'omic' techniques (i.e. metagenomics, metatranscriptomics, metaproteomics and metabolomics). This chapter reviews the current understanding of enzyme technology and highlights their role in improving the efficiency of ruminant production.

*Email: karen.beauchemin@agr.gc.ca

Chapter 9 © Agriculture and Agri-Food Canada 2022.
DOI: 10.1079/9781789241563.0009

9.2   Ruminant Enzymes

There is an array of commercially available exogenous enzymes for ruminants, although many of these are optimized for the textile, pulp and paper industries or for monogastric diets and do not account for the unique environment of the rumen. Most ruminant enzyme formulations are extracts from fungal cultures usually derived from *Aspergillus* spp. and *Trichoderma* spp. (Ribeiro *et al.*, 2016). Whereas enzymes for monogastrics target the degradation of β-glucans and arabinoxylans within the endosperm cell wall of grains (Mottet *et al.*, 2017; Alagawany *et al.*, 2018), ruminant enzymes mainly target cellulose and hemicellulose within plant fibre.

In grazing and mixed beef cattle production systems, roughages represent more than 80% of the diet (Mottet *et al.*, 2018). Mastication during eating and rumination physically damages plant tissues releasing cellular content from plant cells and exposes surfaces that are more amendable to microbial colonization (Terry *et al.*, 2019). Despite the damage to plant tissues done by mastication, microbial colonization and degradation within the rumen are limited by the lignification of plant cell walls. The inclusion of exogenous enzymes in ruminant diets is postulated to increase bacterial attachment through breakage of the matrix of polysaccharides, lignin and phenolic compounds within the plant cell wall. More recently, focus has been placed on identifying enzymes that synergistically enhance the activity of carbohydrate-active enzymes (CAZymes) produced by rumen microbes (Terry *et al.*, 2019).

9.3   Cell Wall Polysaccharides and Limits to Feed Degradation

The structural polysaccharides that make up plant cell walls are critical to providing plant structural integrity and protection against plant pathogens in the field (Ribeiro *et al.*, 2016). The same chemical characteristics that promote the survival of the plant in the field also limit fibre degradation within the rumen. Cellulose, hemicellulose, lignin and pectin are the main constituents within the plant cell wall. Lignin and hemicellulose are matrixed around cellulose microfibrils and are regarded as the main contributors to plant cell wall recalcitrance (Terry *et al.*, 2019). The extent of cellulose crystallinity as well as the cross-linkages among hemicellulose, cellulose and lignin limit the attachment and access of rumen microbes (Terry *et al.*, 2019).

The xylan backbone of hemicellulose has side groups that vary depending on plant species and the frequency, type and orientation of these branches alter the degree that hydrogen bonds link to cellulose or hemicellulose (Ribeiro *et al.*, 2016). Limited enzyme access to substrates, the ratio of cellulases to hemicellulases within the rumen, the enzyme to substrate ratio and the concentration of cell wall cross-linkages to phenolic compounds and lignin can limit the ruminal degradation of forages (Pech-Cervantes *et al.*, 2019; Terry *et al.*, 2019).

Attachment, adhesion, penetration and consortia formation are required for microbial enzymatic degradation of fibre in the rumen (Varga and Kolver, 1997). The formation of ferulate–polysaccharide–lignin cross-links poses a major restriction to the rate and extent of plant cell wall degradation (Meale *et al.*, 2014). These complexes sterically inhibit the access of enzymes to targeted carbohydrate linkages. Similarly, lignin is not truly degraded in the rumen as this is an oxidative process that cannot occur within the anaerobic environment of the rumen. However, hydrolysis of the linkages between hemicellulose and lignin can solubilize lignin and enhance the access of microbes to cellulose and hemicellulose (Meale *et al.*, 2014).

The extent of plant cell wall degradation in the rumen is a function of the rate of degradation and residence time of feed within the rumen. Selection of exogenous enzymes for ruminants must also consider factors such as feed intake, the passage rate of liquid and solid digesta, and post-ruminal digestion of nutrients (Meale *et al.*, 2014). Most of the exogenous enzymes aimed at improving ruminal feed degradation target carbohydrates, especially those more recalcitrant substrates that remain undigested and are excreted in the faeces (Elliott *et al.*, 2018). Fibrolytic enzymes act to make hemicellulose and cellulose more accessible to rumen microbiota; however, these carbohydrates take longer to degrade than the non-fibrous carbohydrates and therefore they require longer residence within the rumen to be metabolized.

Several exogenous enzymes have been shown to successfully increase the rate of rumen degradation, rather than the extent of degradation (Hristov *et al.*, 1998a; Colombatto *et al.*, 2007; Ranilla *et al.*, 2008). An increase in rate of degradation may decrease rumen retention time of feed and result in increased intake, but total digestion in the gastrointestinal tract is typically not increased unless the extent of rumen degradation of fibre is also increased. Therefore, to address the approach of increasing the extent of ruminal degradation, enzyme technology should focus on breaking the linkages formed between the polysaccharides of the plant cell wall.

Low rumen pH typical of ruminants experiencing subacute ruminal acidosis and fluctuation of pH within the rumen (5.7 to 7.2) can pose major limitations to enzymatic activity of the rumen fibrolytic bacteria because enzyme function is compromised at pH below 6.2 (Wang and McAllister, 2002; Li *et al.*, 2017). Commercial enzymes need to have optimal activity within the normal pH range of the rumen. Some commercial enzymes are of limited effectiveness because they function at a pH outside the normal range of the rumen, while many enzymes produced from aerobic fungi have a pH optimum of 4.0 to 6.0, which can be advantageous for ruminants with low rumen pH.

Fungal communities have been shown to play an integral role in fibre degradation and are enriched in animals as the forage proportion of the diet increases (Kumar *et al.*, 2015). Similarly, fibrolytic bacteria including *Butyrivibrio*, *Ruminococcus* and *Fibrobacter* are vulnerable to low pH and decrease in abundance in animals fed high-grain diets (Fernando *et al.*, 2010; Petri *et al.*, 2014). Metatranscriptomic analysis has also revealed that species richness and evenness of the transcriptionally active microbial community were reduced in beef cattle experiencing rumen acidosis, as was the activity of *Fibrobacter succinogenes*, *Ruminococcus albus* and *Ruminococcus bicirculans* (Ogunade *et al.*, 2019). The ratio of structural to non-structural carbohydrates influences rumen pH, with high levels of non-structural carbohydrates lowering rumen pH and inhibiting the activity of fibrolytic bacteria.

The rate-limiting nature of some of the enzymes within the rumen poses another limit to plant cell wall degradation by rumen microbiota. Ferulic acid esterases and enzymes involved in hemicellulose side chain removal are currently identified as the rate-limiting enzymes produced within the rumen (Ribeiro *et al.*, 2016). Ferulic esterases cleave the ester bonds formed between arabinose side chains on the xylan backbone and ferulic and *p*-coumaric acids (Qi *et al.*, 2011). Metagenomic discovery has found that feruloyl esterases from the rumen exhibit a wide range of activities and substrate specificity, and synergistically enhance the activity of endoxylanases (glycoside hydrolase (GH) families GH10 and GH11) in the hydrolysis of mono- and di-ferulic acid (Wong *et al.*, 2019) linkages which ultimately link to xylan backbones. Similarly, synergy between cellulase, xylanase (derived from *Trichoderma reesei*) and feruloyl esterase (*Aspergillus niger*) was observed in the saccharification of exploded wheat straw (Tabka *et al.*, 2006). Esterified arabinoxylan and the associated enzymatic activity of ruminal arabinofuranosidase and acetyl xylan esterase have also been suggested to be a rate-limiting step in xylan hydrolysis within the rumen due to the rich concentration of esterified arabinoxylan as a component of total tract indigestible residues obtained from bovine faeces (Badhan *et al.*, 2015).

9.4 Microbial Synergy

Rumen microbes produce specific enzymatic arrays of functionally diverse GHs that degrade the fibrous components within feed (Terry *et al.*, 2019). Efficient degradation requires coordination of the various enzymes that work in synergy to degrade cellulose, hemicellulose and xylan. The hydrolysis of cellulose involves the synergistic activity of three classes of cellulolytic enzymes: (i) endo-β-1,4-glucanases that randomly hydrolyse cellulose chains to produce cellulose oligomers; (ii) cellobiohydrolases that hydrolyse the cellulose chain from the non-reducing end to produce cellobiose; and (iii) β-glucosidases that release glucose from cellobiose and hydrolyse short cellulose chains (Beauchemin and Holtshausen, 2010; Terry *et al.*, 2019). Hemicellulose has a variable structure and requires an array of enzymes with more diverse functions, including endo-β-1,4-xylanase and β-1,4-xylosidase that depolymerize the hemicellulose xylan backbone and yield short xylan chains and xylose, respectively (Bhat and Hazlewood, 2001); and arabinofuranosidases, acetyl xylan esterases, feruloyl esterases and α-glucuronidases that hydrolyse the side chains (Ribeiro *et al.*, 2016).

Limited penetration into the plant cell interior, insufficient rate-limiting enzymatic activity and insufficient retention time of feed are all constraints to lignocellulosic degradation within the rumen (Badhan *et al.*, 2018). Exogenous enzymes typically contain a broad spectrum of enzymes from bacterial or fungal origin, most of which are already naturally produced by rumen microbiota. Identification of rate-limiting enzyme activities that act in synergy with enzymes produced by the rumen microbiome could enable specific selection of enzyme combinations that efficiently increase ruminal fibre degradation (Terry *et al.*, 2019). Such an approach was employed where the commercially available enzyme, Viscozyme® (Sigma Aldrich; Oakville, Ontario, Canada), was fractionated and specific GHs (GH74 endoglucanase; GH71 α-1,3-glucanase; GH5 mannanase; GH7 cellobiohydrolase; GH28 pectinase, esterases) were identified to contribute to the enhanced saccharification of barley straw in a ruminal batch culture (Badhan *et al.*, 2018).

Metagenomic and metatranscriptomic studies have revealed a scarcity or absence of certain cellulases (GH6, GH7, GH44, GH45, GH48), hemicellulases (GH12, GH51, GH54, GH62) and oligosaccharide-degrading (GH52, GH94) enzymes in the rumen of various ruminants (Terry *et al.*, 2019). Using this information, it was found that supplementing mixed rumen enzymes with endoglucanase (GH7), arabinofuranosidase or acetyl xylan esterase activity enhanced cellulosic saccharification compared with rumen enzymes alone (Badhan *et al.*, 2014, 2015). Alternatively, the lack or scarcity of GH families may not mean that these GH families limit feed degradation; rather, it may indicate that their activity is not necessary within the rumen or other GH families possess the ability to carry out the function of these scarce GHs. There is evidence suggesting that the degradation of structural polysaccharides follows first-order kinetics, with the rate of degradation being limited by accessible surface area rather than the activity or abundance of the microbial community. For example, cellulose degradation by *F. succinogenes* strains was shown to follow first-order kinetics with rate of degradation limited by accessible cellulose for microbial attachment (Weimer *et al.*, 1991; Neumann *et al.*, 2018). The importance of accessible surface area has also been demonstrated *in situ* where a recombinant xylanase only increased rumen degradability of crop residues that had been pretreated with ammonia fibre expansion, a process that increases cell wall surface area.

Expansins and expansin-like proteins are non-hydrolytic proteins that are encoded by plants and bacteria, and fungi, respectively (Pech-Cervantes *et al.*, 2019). These proteins act to loosen and disrupt the hydrogen bonds within the plant cell wall during plant growth and elongation. This activity results in expanded cellulose microfibrils, enhancing their accessibility to cellulases and thus accelerating the disruption of the plant cell wall matrix (Adesogan *et al.*, 2019; Pech-Cervantes *et al.*, 2019). A greater synergy between hemicellulases and cellulases with expansin-like proteins that act in synergy to improve hydrolysis of lignocellulose has been reported (Liu *et al.*, 2015). However, expansin-like proteins possess no hydrolytic activity as they lack the catalytic domain found in GH45 proteins (Pech-Cervantes *et al.*, 2019). Expansins and expansin-like proteins have been shown to synergistically increase the rate and extent of sugar release from cellulose degradation (Liu *et al.*, 2015). A synergistic effect of an expansin-like protein from *Bacillus subtilis* (BsEXLX1) and a commercial fibrolytic enzyme was observed when reducing sugar yield was increased by 22 and 36% in whole-plant maize silage and bermudagrass silages, respectively, compared with the enzyme alone (Pech-Cervantes *et al.*, 2019). Aside from this study by Pech-Cervantes *et al.* (2019), most research on expansins and expansin-like proteins has been conducted to improve biofuel production. Total and cumulative gas production was improved in a batch culture as a result of increased neutral detergent fibre (NDF) and hemicellulose degradability when a total mixed ration was supplemented with an expansin-like protein in combination with a fibrolytic enzyme product (Pech-Cervantes *et al.*, 2019). The biggest restriction to expansin and expansin-like research is that only small quantities of expansin-like proteins are produced by microbes and therefore there is a lack of commercially available product (Adesogan *et al.*, 2019). As is the case for exogenous feed enzymes, the efficacy of expansin-like proteins is dependent on the composition of the diet. For example, the bacterial expansin-like protein from *B. subtilis* (BsEXLX1) synergistically worked with an exogenous feed enzyme to improve fibre hydrolysis of a total mixed ration, but not maize silage (Pech-Cervantes *et al.*, 2018).

Anaerobic fungi possess an extensive range of enzymes that function to degrade plant structural polymers (Huws *et al.*, 2018). Expansin-related proteins in fungi, called swollenins, are proteins that share a sequence similar to plant expansins, but differ from expansins as they possess endoglucanase activity (Adesogan *et al.*, 2019). Fungi swollenins are double the size of expansin-like proteins found in plants and exhibit similarities of action with endoglucanases and cellobiohydrolases (Santos *et al.*, 2017). Swollenins have weak hydrolytic activity against cellulosic substrates but synergistically improve the hydrolytic performance of cellulases and xylanases (Andberg *et al.*, 2015; Li *et al.*, 2019). The swollenin from *T. reesei* used in combination with a fibrolytic enzyme increased enzymatic hydrolysis or sugar release from xylan, microcrystalline cellulose, rice straw, wheat straw and maize stover (Li *et al.*, 2019). Similarly, *in vitro* dry matter (DM) disappearances of rice, wheat and maize straw were increased when purified swollenin was added to the incubated rumen fluid. Further research is required to assess the efficacy of supplementing expansins, expansin-like proteins and swollenins into ruminant diets alone or in combination with fibrolytic enzymes. Their stability within the proteolytic environment of the rumen and the diversity of ruminant diets have to be considered, and whether they work synergistically with the endogenous enzymes produced within the rumen needs to be evaluated.

9.5 Applying Enzymes to Feed

The application of some exogenous enzymes in a liquid form to feed has been shown to hydrolyse complex polymers prior to the consumption of the feed, thereby solubilizing neutral and acid detergent fibre components of the plant cell wall (Meale *et al.*, 2014). The initial hydrolysis increases attachment sites for primary colonizers, so the application method of feed enzymes before feeding can enhance the effectiveness of enzyme technology (Adesogan, 2005). Results can be inconsistent, however, as applying a recombinant xylanase to barley straw 24 h before feeding did not alter the chemical composition of the straw (Ran *et al.*, 2019). Application of exogenous enzymes on to dry ingredients prior to feeding may increase the stability of enzymes due to binding with substrate before entering the rumen and being exposed to microbial proteases (Wang and McAllister, 2002). Alternatively, application of enzymes to wet silage appears ineffective, indicating that ensiling fermentation end products may inhibit exogenous enzyme activity (Meale *et al.*, 2014). Although application of exogenous fibrolytic enzymes to barley straw increased rumen bacterial colonization and the availability of reducing sugars, when excessive hydrolysis occurred prior to incubation, colonization was decreased (Wang et al., 2012). Additionally, a long incubation time of enzyme applied to feed prior to feeding to animals can be undesirable. For example, Aboagye et al. (2015) applied an enzyme product with endoglucanase and xylanase activities to lucerne hay at baling and reported greater internal heating of the bales after 50 days compared with control bales, indicating an enhanced oxidative process by the enzyme product and inherent microbes of the hay.

9.6 Animal Responses to Enzyme Supplementation

Supplementation of exogenous enzymes to ruminant diets has yielded varied responses in diet digestibility and animal performance. Several meta-analysis studies have been conducted to identify sources of variability that may account for the inconsistencies in the efficacy of exogenous enzymes. Two meta-analysis studies (Arriola et al., 2017; Tirado-González et al., 2018) have proposed that the variability in animal responses is caused by a combination of factors, including enzyme formulation, target substrate, enzyme dose and animal production status.

9.6.1 Enzyme formulation

Enzymes employed in ruminant nutrition are usually manufactured for industrial processes where temperature and pH optima do not coincide with the conditions of the gastrointestinal tract (Adesogan et al., 2014). For example, Adesogan et al. (2014) found that of 18 exogenous feed enzymes, 61% of endoglucanases and 83% of xylanases exhibited optimal activities that were outside the range of temperature and pH normally encountered in the rumen. Utilizing enzymes that function at optimal activity within the conditions of the rumen will help improve the efficacy and efficiency of enzymes for ruminants.

Most enzymes formulated for ruminant use contain cellulases and xylanases to degrade cellulose and xylan, respectively. Typically, only the main GH activities are specified or measured, with the minor GH activities varying among enzyme formulations and between batches of the same formulation. Yet, to enzymatically degrade cellulose and xylan a diverse range of GHs is required, and it is likely that enzyme formulations must target a diverse range of enzymatic activities to degrade this range of substrates (Meale et al., 2014). The lack of control of all GH activities within enzyme formulations may contribute to the inconsistent responses between and within feed enzymes.

Some variation in the response of animals to exogenous enzymes is due to the ratio of cellulase to xylanase in the formulation, with the most effective ratio differing depending upon diet composition. A meta-analysis reported that adding exogenous enzymes with cellulase:xylanase of 1:4 to 1:1 to high-forage legume-based diets increased milk production of dairy cows, whereas enzymes with primarily xylanase activity increased milk production of cows fed high-forage diets containing grasses (Tirado-González et al., 2018). The difficulty of performing a meta-analysis to examine the effects of enzyme formulation on animal performance is the lack of in vivo studies in which exogenous enzymes and carbohydrate composition of diets have been extensively characterized. Additionally, grouping enzymes as cellulases and xylanases does not account for the large variety of GHs with diverse activities within each category. Detailed analysis of the carbohydrate composition of the feed and the GH profile of supplemented exogenous enzymes would be beneficial for identifying the most effective enzyme formulations needed within the rumen to aid in improving rumen degradability of plant cell walls.

9.6.2 Target substrates

Feedstuffs are structurally complex and differ in chemical and physical structure, which limit their enzymatic saccharification within the rumen (Colombatto *et al.*, 2003). For example, monocot plants possess an abundance of hemicellulose with glucuronoarabinoxylans and mixed-linkage glucans (Pattathil *et al.*, 2015). Dicots possess a greater abundance of xyloglucans as well as pectic polysaccharides and structural proteins. Legumes have lower NDF content than grasses, due to less hemicellulose, although grass fibre can be more digestible than that of legumes when harvested at an early stage of maturity (Buxton and Redfearn, 1997). Carbohydrate composition of forage substrates undoubtedly dictates the most effective enzyme formulations. As mentioned previously, a meta-analysis showed that cellulase–xylanase combinations were more effective at improving milk production of dairy cows fed legume forages, whereas xylanase alone was more effective for dairy cows fed grass forages (Tirado-González *et al.*, 2018).

Type of diet also appears to affect animal responses to exogenous enzymes. Tirado-González *et al.* (2018) reported that exogenous enzymes increased milk yield of cows fed a high-forage diet, with no increase observed when forage to concentrate ratio was less than 50%. Similarly, a fibrolytic enzyme applied to a total mixed ration containing maize silage and lucerne hay increased total tract fibre digestibility and feed efficiency (Arriola *et al.*, 2011). However, when this enzyme was applied to a total mixed ration containing bermudagrass silage, feed efficiency was unaffected (Bernard *et al.*, 2010). For a particular diet, exogenous enzymes appear to be more effective when applied to a total mixed ration as compared with either the forage or concentrate portion of the diet (Arriola *et al.*, 2017).

NDF degradability had 10 times more endoglucanase III, 17 times more acetyl xylan esterase with a cellulose-binding domain 1, 33 times more xylanase III, 25 times more β-xylosidase, 7.7 times more polysaccharide monooxygenase with a cellulose-binding domain 1, and 3 times more swollenin (Romero *et al.*, 2015). Interestingly, most of these proteins are associated with the enzymatic deconstruction of hemicellulose. A meta-analysis revealed that increasing exogenous enzyme application rate had no effect on dairy cow performance (Arriola *et al.*, 2017), although this analysis was confounded by the variation in enzyme type, activity and the dietary composition to which the enzymes were applied.

Many studies that have attempted to determine optimal enzyme dose rate *in vivo* have found non-linear responses, where the greatest enzyme dose did not necessarily result in maximum digestibility. Increasing doses of cellulase (6400 to 32,000 IU/g DM) and xylanase (12,800 to 44,800 IU/g DM) were applied to maize stover to determine optimal *in vitro* dose rate (Bhasker *et al.*, 2013). At the lowest cellulase concentration, *in vitro* DM degradability was greater with higher doses of xylanase. Alternatively, at higher doses of cellulase, DM degradability was greatest with lower versus higher xylanase doses. The decreased response to higher enzyme doses may be the result of excess exogenous enzymes attaching to feed, thereby blocking attachment sites for rumen microbes (Nsereko *et al.*, 2002), or competition between added enzymes for attachment sites.

9.6.3 Enzyme dose

The enzyme concentration applied to feed should consider both protein content and enzyme activity as both have been shown to impact efficacy. Examination of 12 exogenous fibrolytic enzymes found that, relative to the least effective enzyme evaluated, the most effective enzymes at improving *in vitro*

9.6.4 Animal variability

Whether feed enzyme use improves animal performance appears to be related to the energy requirements of the animal. Animals that have higher demands for energy, such as dairy cows in early lactation, or growing cattle in feedlots, have shown greater responses to enzyme supplementation compared with cattle on restricted feed intake, or fed at maintenance (Beauchemin *et al.*, 2003). Stage of lactation of dairy cattle also influences enzyme efficacy as cows in early lactation receiving enzymes had 10–30% improved feed conversion efficiency and 18–24% higher fat-corrected milk yield, with no effect of exogenous enzymes observed during mid-lactation (Beauchemin and Holtshausen, 2010). The variability in enzyme effectiveness is likely related to differences in intake levels and digesta passage rates from the rumen, where animals with greater intakes have faster passage rates compared with animals fed at maintenance. As passage rate of feed from the rumen increases, extent of rumen degradation of fibre decreases and a greater proportion of undegraded fibre escapes the rumen. Enzymes that increase the rate of degradation of fibre lower the proportion of undegraded feed that is passed from the rumen when passage rate is rapid.

Improvements in animal performance due to enzyme supplementation are not immediate because changes in dietary energy supply can take time before manifesting in terms of improved animal productivity. In a study by Romero *et al.* (2016), milk production was only increased 3 weeks post-enzyme supplementation. Therefore, short-term studies are not appropriate for evaluating the effects of enzymes on animal production. For example, using the same exogenous enzyme, Holtshausen *et al.* (2011) found increased feed efficiency in a 10-week study whereas Chung *et al.* (2012) reported no effect of enzyme in a 21-day Latin square design experiment. Similarly, meta-analysis showed that increasing experimental duration of enzyme application increased milk yield and protein content in response to enzyme application (Arriola *et al.*, 2017).

9.7   Enzyme Delivery

9.7.1   Ruminal enzyme delivery

For ruminant feed enzymes to be effective, they must resist the proteases that are produced by rumen microbiota and post-ruminally by the host. Enzyme stability can be improved through the formation of disulfide bridges or salt bridges, or by altering the interactions of amino acids within the enzyme (Eijsink *et al.*, 2004; Ding *et al.*, 2008). However, altering the structure of these proteins to improve stability can negatively impact activity and alter the temperature and pH optima of the enzyme.

Effectiveness of ruminal delivery of enzymes is highly dependent on retention time within the rumen. Exogenous enzyme activity in ruminal fluid decreases after supplementation due to both enzyme inactivation and flow of enzymes out of the rumen with the liquid phase of the rumen contents (Hristov *et al.*, 1998b). Therefore, enzymes supplemented in diets fed to animals with long rumen retention times (i.e. cattle on maintenance diets) may require an improvement in proteolytic stability if they are to improve the extent of fibre degradation.

9.7.2   Post-ruminal enzyme delivery

An alternative enzyme delivery method is to provide enzymes that are mainly active post-ruminally. Average total tract digestibility of NDF in dairy cattle is only 50.4% (White *et al.*, 2017), therefore a large amount of fibre leaves the rumen that could potentially be digested post-ruminally. However, for most enzymes to be delivered post-ruminally they would need to be protected from rumen proteolysis, as well as the low pH present in the abomasum. *In vitro* incubation of an exogenous enzyme product in simulated gastric fluid reduced cellulase, β-glucosidase and β-xylosidase activity although xylanase activity remained stable (Morgavi *et al.*, 2001). However, when the same enzyme product was incubated in simulated intestinal fluid, cellulase activity was initially (up to 20 min of incubation) increased, suggesting that partial hydrolysis of the enzyme may have actually increased activity (Morgavi *et al.*, 2001).

9.8 Future of Enzyme Supplementation in Ruminants

9.8.1 Novel enzyme discovery

Adopting an informed and specialized approach using modern cutting-edge technologies is critical for the development of new enzyme-based technologies (Fig. 9.1). The effectiveness of exogenous enzymes for ruminants could be potentially improved through the discovery and identification of novel enzymes using nucleic acid-based technologies. By evaluating the metagenomes and transcriptomes of microbiomes that have high levels of desirable enzyme activity, novel enzymes can be discovered (Ribeiro *et al.*, 2016). Developing improved understanding of microbial cell wall degradation and recalcitrance of cell wall moieties towards rumen enzymatic degradation is critical. Fourier transmission infrared spectroscopy (FTIR) is a low-cost, powerful and high-throughput tool that generates a fingerprint of a sample composition, with absorption peaks corresponding to the frequency of vibrations between the bonds of the atoms (Badhan *et al.*, 2015). FTIR was used to identify recalcitrant cell wall bonds that resisted ruminal microbial digestion. Recalcitrance of cross-linked esterified xylan in undigested residue was reported based on higher abundance of spectral peaks associated with the vibration from the C=O bond from xylan and the unconjugated C=O stretch in xylan from acetic acid ester and pectin. Likewise, high-resolution glycomics analysis based on monoclonal antibody toolkits has been extensively applied to characterize cell walls (Pattathil *et al.*, 2015). Glycome profiling allows insight into the linkages and associations of close to 200 cell wall glycan epitopes and their relative extractability using the high-throughput ELISA. The application of monoclonal antibody toolkits to understand plant cell wall architecture of native forage fibre and its residual fraction after rumen degradation can

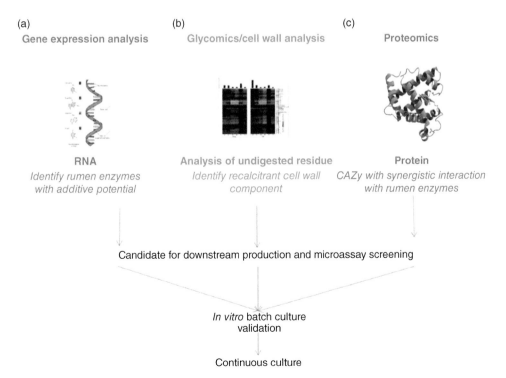

(a) Gene expression analysis

(b) Glycomics/cell wall analysis

(c) Proteomics

RNA
Identify rumen enzymes with additive potential

Analysis of undigested residue
Identify recalcitrant cell wall component

Protein
CAZy with synergistic interaction with rumen enzymes

Candidate for downstream production and microassay screening

In vitro batch culture validation

Continuous culture

Fig. 9.1. Application of 'omics' tools to study ruminal degradation of low-quality forage fibre. (Authors' own figure.)

provide useful insight to the progression of fibre degradation and recalcitrant cell wall components within indigestible residues. Similarly, linkages between the compositional nature of parental forage fibre and its ruminal indigestible residues as developed by glycosidic linkage analysis can lead to the identification of abundant resistant linkages. These resistant linkages can direct informed selection of enzyme activities that effectively degrade recalcitrant cell wall bonds and increase the extent of rumen microbial cell wall digestion.

A microassay described by Badhan *et al.* (2014) has shown promise for screening enzymes that complement the endogenous rumen enzymes produced by rumen microbiota. In brief, exogenous enzymes are combined with a mixture of rumen enzymes and their capability of improving *in vitro* degradability is compared with the mixture of rumen enzymes alone. Coupling microassay and proteomics techniques like blue native PAGE, liquid chromatography–mass spectrometry (LC–MS) and phylogenetic analysis, Badhan *et al.* (2018) developed an experimental pipeline to identify candidate enzyme activities within complex secretomes and commercial enzyme mixes

that act synergistically with rumen enzymes to enhance degradation (Fig. 9.2). Identification of effective enzyme activities within complex enzyme mixes is necessary as these mixes primarily contain redundant activities that are already expressed by microbiota within the rumen. Enzyme mixes that showed promising additive properties were fractionated using blue native PAGE. Fractions that synergistically enhanced saccharification yield of rumen enzymes were identified by the microarray. Enzyme activities within selected fractions were determined by LC–MS analysis and phylogenetic trees were generated to determine the substrate specificity of identified enzymes and its closest characterized CAZyme. Utilizing this technique, Ribeiro *et al.* (2018) screened 11 recombinant fibrolytic enzymes for their ability to improve the degradability of barley straw. They reported that compared with rumen enzymes alone, adding a recombinant xylanase improved 48 h NDF degradability by 2.5 and 1.6 percentage units in batch culture and artificial rumen experiments, respectively. However, the same recombinant xylanase had no effect on the extent of *in situ* fibre degradation of crop residues unless they

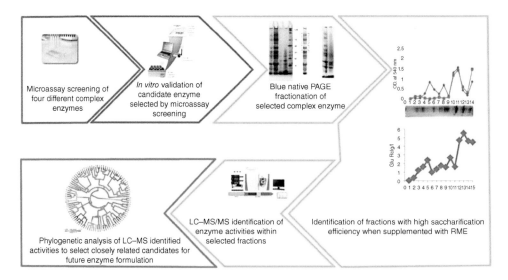

Fig. 9.2. Experimental pipeline to identify candidate enzyme activities within complex secretomes and commercial enzyme mixes that act synergistically with rumen microbial enzymes (RME) to enhance fibre degradation. (From Badhan *et al.*, 2018. Crown Copyright © 2018.)

were subject to ammonia fibre expansion to hydrolyse ester linkages (Beauchemin *et al.*, 2019). Ammonia fibre expansion treatment of cellulosic substrate partially solubilizes lignin, hydrolyses hemicellulose and increases cell wall surface area available for microbial attachment. The improvement in fibre degradation using enzymes in combination with forage pretreatments such as ammonia fibre expansion is a result of improved access of carbohydrases to the structural components of the plant cell wall.

9.8.2 Carbohydrate-active enzymes (CAZymes)

CAZymes are enzymes produced by microorganisms that play an important role in the degradation of complex carbohydrates (Terry *et al.*, 2019). Meta-omics studies suggest the majority of CAZymes that degrade fibre in the rumen have not been characterized (Hess *et al.*, 2011). Through meta-omics techniques researchers can further characterize and isolate CAZymes that are highly active within the rumen or find important CAZymes that are absent or rare within the rumen. While metagenomic sequencing provides insight into the abundance of genes present within the rumen, it does not necessarily reflect the degree of gene expression by microbiota (Terry *et al.*, 2019). For example, metagenomic studies have rarely found members of the cellulose-degrading GH48 family of CAZymes within the rumen (Zhang *et al.*, 2010), while metatranscriptomic studies have found an abundance of mRNA that corresponds to GH48 enzymes (Comtet-Marre *et al.*, 2017; Li and Guan, 2017). Fungi and ciliate protozoa have a substantial yet underestimated role in ruminal fibre degradation (Comtet-Marre *et al.*, 2017). Between 8.3 and 11.3% of the transcriptome of four major rumen fungi species that were cultured on different carbon sources encoded for CAZymes (Gruninger *et al.*, 2018). Similarly, anaerobic fungi and protozoa both contributed 9% to the relative proportion of cellulases in total non-ribosomal RNA, with small contributions to hemicellulases and oligosaccharide-degrading enzymes in a metatranscriptome analysis of rumen microbiota (Dai *et al.*, 2015; Terry *et al.*, 2019).

9.8.3 Cellulosome construction

Some ruminal bacteria and fungi produce cellulosomes that are highly organized complexes containing carbohydrate-binding modules (CBMs), scaffoldins and multiple enzymes (Artzi *et al.*, 2017). The CBMs help bind the cellulosome to the surface of the substrate, subsequently allowing the enzymes present on the scaffoldins to have close interactions with the substrate while reducing steric hindrance (Fierobe *et al.*, 2002). The multiple enzymes present in cellulosomes allow for enhanced synergy to degrade fibre more effectively (Terry *et al.*, 2019).

The majority of synthetic cellulosomes that have been constructed are for industrial purposes, such as ethanol production. For example, cellulose utilization systems for cellulosomal bacterium and cellulolytic fungi were constructed for *Saccharomyces cerevisiae* and the produced yeasts successfully co-fermented cellulose and galactose (Fan *et al.*, 2016). More recently, another yeast (*Kluyveromyces marxianus*) has been engineered to express a cellulosome that can accommodate up to 63 enzymes with the engineered enzyme exhibiting greater degradation efficiency of cellulosic substrates to release reducing sugars and ethanol (Anandharaj *et al.*, 2020). The application of this technology within the feed industry could significantly improve the effectiveness of exogenous enzymes.

9.8.4 Enzyme immobilization

Enzyme immobilization confines an enzyme to a matrix or support to improve the stability of the enzyme. Immobilization can be either irreversible (covalent binding, entrapment and cross-linking) or reversible (adsorption) (Brena *et al.*, 2013). The use of reversible immobilization of enzymes could slow the release of enzymes in the rumen or in the lower intestine. For enzyme immobilization to be used to stabilize enzymes used in ruminant feeds, the solid support must be safe to feed and stable in the gastrointestinal tract.

Immobilization of enzymes on to bacterial spores can improve enzyme stability, although it can alter the optimal activity conditions of the enzyme. An unbound amylase product had an optimal pH range of 4.5 to 7.0, but when the amylase product was immobilized on *B. subtilis* spores the optimal pH range increased to 5.0 to 10.0 (Gashtasbi *et al.*, 2014). Incubation of β-galactosidase immobilized on to *B. subtilis* spores at pH 4.0 for 24 h did not reduce enzyme activity, whereas the activity of the unbound β-galactosidase was reduced by 30% within 7 h of incubation (Sirec *et al.*, 2012). Antigen proteins that were adsorbed on to the surface of *B. subtilis* spores remained viable after passage through the murine gastrointestinal tract (Huang *et al.*, 2010), which suggests that this technique could be used to deliver active enzymes to the lower digestive tract of ruminants.

Immobilization is a reversible process, whereby changes in pH can result in the release of protein from the solid support. When immobilized proteins are incubated in buffers with the same pH as the isoelectric point of the bound particles, the proteins are released from the particle surface (Biehl *et al.*, 2018). Use of this information could allow for immobilization of enzymes to a solid support that would protect the enzymes from the proteolytic environment of the rumen, with their release upon contact with the low pH in the abomasum, increasing the flow of active enzymes to the small intestine.

9.8.5 Transgenics

There is some interest in supplementing ruminant diets with bacteria or fungi that have been genetically altered to overproduce cellulolytic enzymes. For transgenic

microbes to produce adequate amounts of enzymes in the rumen, the microbes would need to successfully colonize and compete against the natural microbiota within the rumen (Ribeiro *et al.*, 2016). Colonization of these exogenous microbes in the rumen has been limited, likely due to competition for resources from the already complex microbiome present in the rumen (McAllister *et al.*, 2011). Additionally, colonization of these microbes within the intestines is influenced by digesta passage rate, digesta acidity, concentration/hydrolytic activity of bile salts, ability to attach to intestinal mucosa and competition with host microbiota for resources (Bezkorovainy, 2001).

Transgenic bacteria have been designed to be enzyme delivery vehicles, by displaying enzymes on the surface of spores. This can be achieved by creating a fusion between genes coding for the enzyme protein and genes that code for specific surface proteins on the spore surface (Isticato *et al.*, 2001). Spore surface displayed enzymes were shown to be more heat stable and resistant to degradation at high and low pH (Kwon *et al.*, 2007) compared with free enzymes. Interestingly, Casula and Cutting (2002) found that *Bacillus* spores can germinate in the jejunum and ileum of mice and suggested this was initiated by acid-induced germination upon passage from the stomach. With the longer retention time and larger environmental changes in the ruminant digestive tract compared with that of mice, there is a potential that when fed to ruminants these spores could potentially germinate and re-sporulate multiple times throughout the entire gastrointestinal tract, dependent on diet.

Plants have been genetically engineered to produce cellulolytic enzymes within their biomass. While these plants have been developed primarily for use in the bioethanol industry, the use of this technology in ruminant feedstuffs has huge potential. Tobacco plants have been engineered to express endoglucanases, exoglucanases, β-glucosidase and xylanases in large quantities, and this approach can be more cost-effective than current commercial enzyme production methods (Verma *et al.*, 2010). Plastid transformation of

Nicotiana tabacum L. plants to produce xylanase and β-glucosidase enzymes allowed the plants to produce 1484 and 13,189 U/g leaf DM, respectively (Castiglia *et al.*, 2016). Similarly, transgenic rice plants edited to express exoglucanase showed increased enzymatic saccharification efficiencies correlated with cellulase activity in the transgenic plant (Furukawa *et al.*, 2014). Targeted gene editing may in the future provide a means to rapidly modify plant genomes to express enzymes as a way to supply ruminant enzymes.

The use of transgenic organisms as an enzyme delivery method appears to be effective in some circumstances. However, the use of transgenic organisms for food production has been highly contentious, and there has been consumer resistance to the use of transgenics in agriculture (Detmer and Glenting, 2006). Additionally, the regulatory process involved with getting approval for transgenic feed additives is extensive and costly, which can be prohibitive for feed companies to invest in this technology. However, the increasing social interest in reducing global carbon footprint may make the use of this technology more favourable in the future.

9.9 Conclusion

To optimize enzyme supplementation in ruminant diets, enzymes should have high activity and complement the endogenous enzyme activity present in the rumen. This includes focusing on supplementing diets with enzymes that have been identified as part of the rate-limiting step in fibre digestion, which varies depending upon diet composition. Exogenous enzymes should also have optimal activity at physiological temperatures and pH that are present within the ruminant gastrointestinal tract to improve their effectiveness. The use of novel enzyme discovery and delivery methods has the potential to reduce the variability in animal performance and improve the efficacy of enzyme supplementation in ruminant diets, subsequently increasing their utilization in commercial ruminant production systems.

References

Aboagye, I.A., Lynch, J.P., Church, J.S., Baah, J. and Beauchemin, K.A. (2015) Digestibility and growth performance of sheep fed alfalfa hay treated with fibrolytic enzymes and a ferulic acid esterase producing bacterial additive. *Animal Feed Science and Technology* 203, 53–66. doi: 10.1016/j.anifeedsci.2015.02.010

Adesogan, A. (2005) Improving forage quality and animal performance with fibrolytic enzymes. In: Proceedings of the 16th Annual Florida Ruminant Nutrition Symposium, Gainesville, Florida, pp. 91–109. Available at: https://animal.ifas.ufl.edu/apps/dairymedia/rns/2005/Adesogan.pdf (accessed 22 September 2021).

Adesogan, A.T., Ma, Z.X., Romero, J.J. and Arriola, K.G. (2014) Ruminant Nutrition Symposium: Improving cell wall digestion and animal performance with fibrolytic enzymes. *Journal of Animal Science* 92, 1317–1330. doi: 10.2527/jas.2013-7273

Adesogan, A.T., Arriola, K.G., Jiang, Y., Oyebade, A., Paula, E.M., *et al.* (2019) Symposium review: Technologies for improving fiber utilization. *Journal of Dairy Science* 102, 5726–5755. doi: 10.3168/jds.2018-15334

Alagawany, M., Elnesr, S.S. and Farag, M.R. (2018) The role of exogenous enzymes in promoting growth and improving nutrient digestibility in poultry. *Iranian Journal of Veterinary Research* 19, 157–164.

Anandharaj, M., Lin, Y.-J., Rani, R.P., Nadendla, E.K., Ho, M.-C., *et al.* (2020) Constructing a yeast to express the largest cellulosome complex on the cell surface. *Proceedings of the National Academy of Sciences USA* 117, 2385–2394. doi: 10.1073/pnas.1916529117

Andberg, M., Penttilä, M. and Saloheimo, M. (2015) Swollenin from *Trichoderma reesei* exhibits hydrolytic activity against cellulosic substrates with features of both endoglucanases and cellobiohydrolases. *Bioresource Technology* 181, 105–113. doi: 10.1016/j.biortech.2015.01.024

Arriola, K.G., Kim, S.C., Staples, C.R. and Adesogan, A.T. (2011) Effect of fibrolytic enzyme application to low- and high-concentrate diets on the performance of lactating dairy cattle. *Journal of Dairy Science* 94, 832–841. doi: 10.3168/jds.2010-3424

Arriola, K.G., Oliveira, A.S., Ma, Z.X., Lean, I.J., Giurcanu, M.C. and Adesogan, A.T. (2017) A meta-analysis on the effect of dietary application of exogenous fibrolytic enzymes on the performance of dairy cows. *Journal of Dairy Science* 100, 4513–4527. doi: 10.3168/jds.2016-12103

Artzi, L., Bayer, E.A. and Morais, S. (2017) Cellulosomes: bacterial nanomachines for dismantling plant polysaccharides. *Nature Reviews Microbiology* 15, 83–95. doi: 10.1038/nrmicro.2016.164

Badhan, A., Wang, Y., Gruninger, R., Patton, D., Powlowski, J., *et al.* (2014) Formulation of enzyme blends to maximize the hydrolysis of alkaline peroxide pretreated alfalfa hay and barley straw by rumen enzymes and commercial cellulases. *BMC Biotechnology* 14, 31. doi: 10.1186/1472-6750-14-31

Badhan, A., Wang, Y., Robert, G., Patton, D., Powlowski, J., *et al.* (2015) Improvement in saccharification yield of mixed rumen enzymes by identification of recalcitrant cell wall constituents using enzyme fingerprinting. *BioMed Research International* 2015, 562952. doi: 10.1155/2015/562952

Badhan, A., Ribeiro, G.O., Jones, D.R., Wang, Y., Abbott, D.W., *et al.* (2018) Identification of novel enzymes to enhance the ruminal digestion of barley straw. *Bioresource Technology* 260, 76–84. doi: 10.1016/j.biortech.2018.03.086

Beauchemin, K. and Holtshausen, L. (2010) Developments in enzyme usage in ruminants. In: Bedford, M.R. and Partridge, G.G. (eds) *Enzymes in Farm Animal Nutrition*, 2nd edn. CAB International, Wallingford, UK, pp. 206–230. doi: 10.1079/9781845936747.0001

Beauchemin, K.A., Colombatto, D., Morgavi, D.P. and Yang, W.Z. (2003) Use of exogenous fibrolytic enzymes to improve feed utilization by ruminants. *Journal of Animal Science* 81(14_suppl_2), E37–E47. doi: 10.2527/2003.8114_suppl_2E37x

Beauchemin, K.A., Ribeiro, G.O., Ran, T., Marami Milani, M.R., Yang, W., *et al.* (2019) Recombinant fibrolytic feed enzymes and ammonia fibre expansion (AFEX) pretreatment of crop residues to improve fibre degradability in cattle. *Animal Feed Science and Technology* 256, 114260. doi: 10.1016/j.anifeedsci.2019.114260

Bernard, J.K., Castro, J.J., Mullis, N.A., Adesogan, A.T., West, J.W. and Morantes, G. (2010) Effect of feeding alfalfa hay or Tifton 85 bermudagrass haylage with or without a cellulase enzyme on performance of Holstein cows. *Journal of Dairy Science* 93, 5280–5285. doi: 10.3168/jds.2010-3111

Bezkorovainy, A. (2001) Probiotics: determinants of survival and growth in the gut. *American Journal of Clinical Nutrition* 73(2 Suppl.), 399s–405s. doi: 10.1093/ajcn/73.2.399s

Bhasker, T.V., Nagalakshmi, D. and Rao, D.S. (2013) Development of appropriate fibrolytic enzyme combination for maize stover and its effect on rumen fermentation in sheep. *Asian-Australasian Journal of Animal Sciences* 26, 945–951. doi: 10.5713/ajas.2012.12590

Bhat, M.K. and Hazlewood, G.P. (2001) Enzymology and other characteristics of cellulases and xylanases. In: Bedford, M.R. and Partridge, G.G. (eds) *Enzymes in Farm Animal Nutrition*, 1st edn. CAB International, Wallingford, UK, pp. 11–60.

Biehl, P., von der Lühe, M. and Schacher, F.H. (2018) Reversible adsorption of methylene blue as cationic model cargo onto polyzwitterionic magnetic nanoparticles. *Macromolecular Rapid Communications* 39, 1800017. doi: 10.1002/marc.201800017

Brena, B., Gonzalez-Pombo, P. and Batista-Viera, F. (2013) Immobilization of enzymes: a literature survey. In: Guisan, J. (ed.) *Immobilization of Enzymes and Cells. Methods in Molecular Biology (Methods and Protocols)*, vol. 1051. Humana Press, Totowa, New Jersey, pp. 15–31. doi: 10.1007/978-1-62703-550-7_2

Buxton, D.R. and Redfearn, D.D. (1997) Plant limitations to fiber digestion and utilization. *The Journal of Nutrition* 127(5), 814S–818S. doi: 10.1093/jn/127.5.814S

Castiglia, D., Sannino, L., Marcolongo, L., Ionata, E., Tamburino, R., *et al.* (2016) High-level expression of thermostable cellulolytic enzymes in tobacco transplastomic plants and their use in hydrolysis of an industrially pretreated *Arundo donax* L. biomass. *Biotechnology for Biofuels* 9, 154. doi: 10.1186/s13068-016-0569-z

Casula, G. and Cutting, S.M. (2002) *Bacillus* probiotics: spore germination in the gastrointestinal tract. *Applied and Environmental Microbiology* 68, 2344–2352. doi: 10.1128/aem.68.5.2344-2352.2002

Chung, Y.H., Zhou, M., Holtshausen, L., Alexander, T.W., McAllister, T.A., *et al.* (2012) A fibrolytic enzyme additive for lactating Holstein cow diets: ruminal fermentation, rumen microbial populations, and enteric methane emissions. *Journal of Dairy Science* 95, 1419–1427. doi: 10.3168/jds.2011-4552

Colombatto, D., Morgavi, D.P., Furtado, A.F. and Beauchemin, K.A. (2003) Screening of exogenous enzymes for ruminant diets: relationship between biochemical characteristics and *in vitro* ruminal degradation. *Journal of Animal Science* 81, 2628–2638. doi: 10.2527/2003.81102628x

Colombatto, D., Mould, F.L., Bhat, M.K. and Owen, E. (2007) Influence of exogenous fibrolytic enzyme level and incubation pH on the *in vitro* ruminal fermentation of alfalfa stems. *Animal Feed Science and Technology* 137, 150–162. doi: 10.1016/j.anifeedsci.2006.10.001

Comtet-Marre, S., Parisot, N., Lepercq, P., Chaucheyras-Durand, F., Mosoni, P., *et al.* (2017) Metatranscriptomics reveals the active bacterial and eukaryotic fibrolytic communities in the rumen of dairy cows fed a mixed diet. *Frontiers in Microbiology* 8, 67. doi: 10.3389/fmicb.2017.00067

Dai, X., Tian, Y., Li, J., Su, X., Wang, X., *et al.* (2015) Metatranscriptomic analyses of plant cell wall polysaccharide degradation by microorganisms in the cow rumen. *Applied and Environmental Microbiology* 81, 1375–1386. doi: 10.1128/AEM.03682-14

Detmer, A. and Glenting, J. (2006) Live bacterial vaccines – a review and identification of potential hazards. *Microbial Cell Factories* 5, 23. doi: 10.1186/1475-2859-5-23

Ding, M., Teng, Y., Yin, Q., Zhao, J. and Zhao, F. (2008) The N-terminal cellulose-binding domain of EGXA increases thermal stability of xylanase and changes its specific activities on different substrates. *Acta Biochimica et Biophysica Sinica (Shanghai)* 40, 949–954. doi: 10.1111/j.1745-7270.2008.00481.x

Eijsink, V.G., Bjork, A., Gaseidnes, S., Sirevag, R., Synstad, B., *et al.* (2004) Rational engineering of enzyme stability. *Journal of Biotechnology* 113, 105–120. doi: 10.1016/j.jbiotec.2004.03.026

Elliott, C.L., Edwards, J.E., Wilkinson, T.J., Allison, G.G., McCaffrey, K., *et al.* (2018) Using 'omic' approaches to compare temporal bacterial colonization of *Lolium perenne, Lotus corniculatus,* and *Trifolium pratense* in the rumen. *Frontiers in Microbiology* 9, 2184. doi:10.3389/fmicb.2018.02184

Fan, L.-H., Zhang, Z.-J., Mei, S., Lu, Y.-Y., Li, M., *et al.* (2016) Engineering yeast with bifunctional minicellulosome and cellodextrin pathway for co-utilization of cellulose-mixed sugars. *Biotechnology for Biofuels* 9, 137. doi: 10.1186/s13068-016-0554-6

Fernando, S.C., Purvis, H.T. 2nd, Najar, F.Z., Sukharnikov, L.O., Krehbiel, C.R., *et al.* (2010) Rumen microbial population dynamics during adaptation to a high-grain diet. *Applied and Environmental Microbiology* 76, 7482–7490. doi: 10.1128/aem.00388-10

Fierobe, H.P., Bayer, E.A., Tardif, C., Czjzek, M., Mechaly, A., *et al.* (2002) Degradation of cellulose substrates by cellulosome chimeras. Substrate targeting versus proximity of enzyme components. *Journal of Biological Chemistry* 277, 49621–49630. doi: 10.1074/jbc.M207672200

Furukawa, K., Ichikawa, S., Nigorikawa, M., Sonoki, T. and Ito, Y. (2014) Enhanced production of reducing sugars from transgenic rice expressing exo-glucanase under the control of a senescence-inducible promoter. *Transgenic Research* 23, 531–537. doi: 10.1007/s11248-014-9786-z

Gashtasbi, F., Ahmadian, G. and Noghabi, K.A. (2014) New insights into the effectiveness of alpha-amylase enzyme presentation on the *Bacillus subtilis* spore surface by adsorption and covalent immobilization. *Enzyme and Microbial Technology* 64–65, 17–23. doi: 10.1016/j.enzmictec.2014.05.006

Gruninger, R.J., Nguyen, T.T.M., Reid, I.D., Yanke, J.L., Wang, P., *et al.* (2018) Application of transcriptomics to compare the carbohydrate active enzymes that are expressed by diverse genera of anaerobic fungi to degrade plant cell wall carbohydrates. *Frontiers in Microbiology* 9, 1581. doi: 10.3389/fmicb.2018.01581

Hess, M., Sczyrba, A., Egan, R., Kim, T.W., Chokhawala, H., *et al.* (2011) Metagenomic discovery of biomass-degrading genes and genomes from cow rumen. *Science* 331, 463–467. doi: 10.1126/science.1200387

Holtshausen, L., Beauchemin, K.A., Schwartzkopf-Genswein, K.S., González, L.A., McAllister, T.A. and Gibb, D.J. (2011) Performance, feeding behaviour and rumen pH profile of beef cattle fed corn silage in combination with barley grain, corn or wheat distillers' grain or wheat middlings. *Canadian Journal of Animal Science* 91, 703–710. doi: 10.4141/cjas2011-037

Hristov, A.N., McAllister, T.A. and Cheng, K.J. (1998a) Stability of exogenous polysaccharide-degrading enzymes in the rumen. *Animal Feed Science and Technology* 76, 161–168. doi: 10.1016/S0377-8401(98)00217-X

Hristov, A.N., McAllister, T.A. and Cheng, K.J. (1998b) Effect of dietary or abomasal supplementation of exogenous polysaccharide-degrading enzymes on rumen fermentation and nutrient digestibility. *Journal of Animal Science* 76, 3146–3156. doi: 10.2527/1998.76123146x

Huang, J.M., Hong, H.A., Van Tong, H., Hoang, T.H., Brisson, A. and Cutting, S.M. (2010) Mucosal delivery of antigens using adsorption to bacterial spores. *Vaccine* 28, 1021–1030. doi: 10.1016/j.vaccine.2009.10.127

Huws, S.A., Creevey, C.J., Oyama, L.B., Mizrahi, I., Denman, S.E., *et al.* (2018) Addressing global ruminant agricultural challenges through understanding the rumen microbiome: past, present, and future. *Frontiers in Microbiology* 9, 2161. doi: 10.3389/fmicb.2018.02161

Isticato, R., Cangiano, G., Tran, H.T., Ciabattini, A., Medaglini, D., *et al.* (2001) Surface display of recombinant proteins on *Bacillus subtilis* spores. *Journal of Bacteriology* 183, 6294–6301. doi: 10.1128/jb.183.21.6294-6301.2001

Kumar, S., Indugu, N., Vecchiarelli, B. and Pitta, D.W. (2015) Associative patterns among anaerobic fungi, methanogenic archaea, and bacterial communities in response to changes in diet and age in the rumen of dairy cows. *Frontiers in Microbiology* 6, 781. doi: 10.3389/fmicb.2015.00781

Kwon, S.J., Jung, H.C. and Pan, J.G. (2007) Transgalactosylation in a water–solvent biphasic reaction system with beta-galactosidase displayed on the surfaces of *Bacillus subtilis* spores. *Applied and Environmental Microbiology* 73, 2251–2256. doi: 10.1128/aem.01489-06

Li, F. and Guan, L.L. (2017) Metatranscriptomic profiling reveals linkages between the active rumen microbiome and feed efficiency in beef cattle. *Applied and Environmental Microbiology* 83, e00061-17. doi: 10.1128/AEM.00061-17

Li, F., Wang, Z., Dong, C., Li, F., Wang, W., *et al.* (2017) Rumen bacteria communities and performances of fattening lambs with a lower or greater subacute ruminal acidosis risk. *Frontiers in Microbiology* 8, 2506. doi: 10.3389/fmicb.2017.02506

Li, L., Qu, M., Liu, C., Xu, L., Pan, K., *et al.* (2019) Effects of recombinant swollenin on the enzymatic hydrolysis, rumen fermentation, and rumen microbiota during *in vitro* incubation of agricultural straws. *International Journal of Biological Macromolecules* 122, 348–358. doi: 10.1016/j.ijbiomac.2018.10.179

Liu, X., Ma, Y. and Zhang, M. (2015) Research advances in expansins and expansin-like proteins involved in lignocellulose degradation. *Biotechnology Letters* 37, 1541–1551. doi: 10.1007/s10529-015-1842-0

McAllister, T.A., Beauchemin, K.A., Alazzeh, A.Y., Baah, J., Teather, R.M. and Stanford, K. (2011) Review: The use of direct fed microbials to mitigate pathogens and enhance production in cattle. *Canadian Journal of Animal Science* 91, 193–211. doi: 10.4141/cjas10047

McCartney, D.H., Block, H.C., Dubeski, P.L. and Ohama, A.J. (2006) Review: The composition and availability of straw and chaff from small grain cereals for beef cattle in western Canada. *Canadian Journal of Animal Science* 86, 443–455. doi: 10.4141/A05-092

Meale, S.J., Beauchemin, K.A., Hristov, A.N., Chaves, A.V. and McAllister, T.A. (2014) Board-Invited Review: Opportunities and challenges in using exogenous enzymes to improve ruminant production. *Journal of Animal Science* 92, 427–442. doi: 10.2527/jas.2013-6869

Morgavi, D.P., Beauchemin, K.A., Nsereko, V.L., Rode, L.M., McAllister, T.A., *et al.* (2001) Resistance of feed enzymes to proteolytic inactivation by rumen microorganisms and gastrointestinal proteases. *Journal of Animal Science* 79, 1621–1630. doi: 10.2527/2001.7961621x

Mottet, A., de Haan, C., Falcucci, A., Tempio, G., Opio, C. and Gerber, P. (2017) Livestock: on our plates or eating at our table? A new analysis of the feed/food debate. *Global Food Security* 14, 1–8. doi: 10.1016/j.gfs.2017.01.001

Mottet, A., Teillard, F., Boettcher, P., De' Besi, G. and Besbes, B. (2018) Review: Domestic herbivores and food security: current contribution, trends and challenges for a sustainable development. *Animal* 12(Suppl. 2), s188–s198. doi: 10.1017/S1751731118002215

Neumann, A.P., Weimer, P.J. and Suen, G. (2018) A global analysis of gene expression in *Fibrobacter succinogenes* S85 grown on cellulose and soluble sugars at different growth rates. *Biotechnology for Biofuels* 11, 295. doi: 10.1186/s13068-018-1290-x

Noziere, P., Steinberg, W., Silberberg, M. and Morgavi, D.P. (2014) Amylase addition increases starch ruminal digestion in first-lactation cows fed high and low starch diets. *Journal of Dairy Science* 97, 2319–2328. doi: 10.3168/jds.2013-7095

Nsereko, V.L., Beauchemin, K.A., Morgavi, D.P., Rode, L.M., Furtado, A.F., *et al.* (2002) Effect of a fibrolytic enzyme preparation from *Trichoderma longibrachiatum* on the rumen microbial population of dairy cows. *Canadian Journal of Microbiology* 48, 14–20. doi: 10.1139/w01-131

Ogunade, I., Pech-Cervantes, A. and Schweickart, H. (2019) Metatranscriptomic analysis of sub-acute ruminal acidosis in beef cattle. *Animals* 9, 232. doi: 10.3390/ani9050232

Pattathil, S., Hahn, M.G., Dale, B.E. and Chundawat, S.P. (2015) Insights into plant cell wall structure, architecture, and integrity using glycome profiling of native and AFEX™-pre-treated biomass. *Journal of Experimental Botany* 66, 4279–4294. doi: 10.1093/jxb/erv107

Pech-Cervantes, A.A., Jiang, Y., Vyas, D., Arriola, K., Kim, D. and Adesogan, A. (2018) Effects of a recombinant bacterial expansin and an exogenous fibrolytic enzyme on pre-ingestive fiber hydrolysis, fermentation and digestibility of corn silage. *Journal of Dairy Science* 101(Suppl. 2), 354 (abstract).

Pech-Cervantes, A.A., Ogunade, I.M., Jiang, Y., Irfan, M., Arriola, K.G., *et al.* (2019) An expansin-like protein expands forage cell walls and synergistically increases hydrolysis, digestibility and fermentation of livestock feeds by fibrolytic enzymes. *PLoS ONE* 14, e0224381. doi: 10.1371/journal.pone.0224381

Petri, R.M., Schwaiger, T., Penner, G.B., Beauchemin, K.A., Forster, R.J., *et al.* (2014) Characterization of the core rumen microbiome in cattle during transition from forage to concentrate as well as during and after an acidotic challenge. *PLoS ONE* 8, e83424. doi: 10.1371/journal.pone.0083424

Qi, M., Wang, P., Selinger, L.B., Yanke, L.J., Forster, R.J. and McAllister, T.A. (2011) Isolation and characterization of a ferulic acid esterase (Fae1A) from the rumen fungus *Anaeromyces mucronatus*. *Journal of Applied Microbiology* 110, 1341–1350. doi: 10.1111/j.1365-2672.2011.04990.x

Ran, T., Saleem, A., Shen, Y., Ribeiro, G., Beauchemin, K., *et al.* (2019) Effects of a recombinant fibrolytic enzyme on fiber digestion, ruminal fermentation, nitrogen balance and total tract digestibility of heifers fed a high forage diet. *Journal of Animal Science* 97, 3578–3587. doi: 10.1093/jas/skz216

Ranilla, M.J., Tejido, M.L., Giraldo, L.A., Tricárico, J.M. and Carro, M.D. (2008) Effects of an exogenous fibrolytic enzyme preparation on *in vitro* ruminal fermentation of three forages and their isolated cell walls. *Animal Feed Science and Technology* 145, 109–121. doi: 10.1016/j.anifeedsci.2007.05.046

Ribeiro, G.O., Gruninger, R.J., Badhan, A. and McAllister, T.A. (2016) Mining the rumen for fibrolytic feed enzymes. *Animal Frontiers* 6(2), 20–26. doi: 10.2527/af.2016-0019

Ribeiro, G.O., Badhan, A., Huang, J., Beauchemin, K.A., Yang, W., *et al.* (2018) New recombinant fibrolytic enzymes for improved *in vitro* ruminal fiber degradability of barley straw. *Journal of Animal Science* 96, 3928–3942. doi: 10.1093/jas/sky251

Romero, J.J., Zarate, M.A., Arriola, K.G., Gonzalez, C.F., Silva-Sanchez, C., *et al.* (2015) Screening exogenous fibrolytic enzyme preparations for improved *in vitro* digestibility of bermudagrass haylage. *Journal of Dairy Science* 98, 2555–2567. doi: 10.3168/jds.2014-8059

Romero, J.J., Macias, E.G., Ma, Z.X., Martins, R.M., Staples, C.R., *et al.* (2016) Improving the performance of dairy cattle with a xylanase-rich exogenous enzyme preparation. *Journal of Dairy Science* 99, 3486–3496. doi: 10.3168/jds.2015-10082

Santos, C.A., Ferreira-Filho, J.A., O'Donovan, A., Gupta, V.K., Tuohy, M.G. and Souza, A.P. (2017) Production of a recombinant swollenin from *Trichoderma harzianum* in *Escherichia coli* and its potential synergistic role in biomass degradation. *Microbial Cell Factories* 16, 83. doi: 10.1186/s12934-017-0697-6

Sirec, T., Strazzulli, A., Isticato, R., De Felice, M., Moracci, M. and Ricca, E. (2012) Adsorption of beta-galactosidase of *Alicyclobacillus acidocaldarius* on wild type and mutants spores of *Bacillus subtilis*. *Microbial Cell Factories* 11, 100. doi: 10.1186/1475-2859-11-100

Sucu, E., Nayeri, A., Sanz-Fernandez, M.V., Upah, N.C. and Baumgard, L.H. (2014) The effects of supplemental protease enzymes on production variables in lactating Holstein cows. *Italian Journal of Animal Science* 13, 3186. doi: 10.4081/ijas.2014.3186

Tabka, M.G., Gimbert, I., Monod, F., Asther, M. and Sigoillot, J.-C. (2006) Enzymatic saccharification of wheat straw for bioethanol production by a combined cellulase xylanase and feruloyl esterase treatment. *Enzyme and Microbial Technology* 39, 897–902. doi: 10.1016/j.enzmictec.2006.01.021

Terry, S.A., Badhan, A., Wang, Y., Chaves, A.V. and McAllister, T.A. (2019) Fibre digestion by rumen microbiota – a review of recent metagenomic and metatranscriptomic studies. *Canadian Journal of Animal Science* 99, 678–692. doi: 10.1139/CJAS-2019-0024

Tirado-González, D.N., Miranda-Romero, L.A., Ruíz-Flores, A., Medina-Cuéllar, S.E., Ramírez-Valverde, R. and Tirado-Estrada, G. (2018) Meta-analysis: effects of exogenous fibrolytic enzymes in ruminant diets. *Journal of Applied Animal Research* 46, 771–783. doi: 10.1080/09712119.2017.1399135

Varga, G.A. and Kolver, E.S. (1997) Microbial and animal limitations to fiber digestion and utilization. *The Journal of Nutrition* 127(5), 819S–823S. doi: 10.1093/jn/127.5.819S

Verma, D., Kanagaraj, A., Jin, S., Singh, N.D., Kolattukudy, P.E. and Daniell, H. (2010) Chloroplast-derived enzyme cocktails hydrolyse lignocellulosic biomass and release fermentable sugars. *Plant Biotechnology Journal* 8, 332–350. doi: 10.1111/j.1467-7652.2009.00486.x

Wang, Y. and McAllister, T. (2002) Rumen microbes, enzymes and feed digestion – a review. *Asian-Australasian Journal of Animal Sciences* 15, 1659–1676. doi: 10.5713/ajas.2002.1659

Wang, Y., Ramirez-Bribiesca, J.E., Yanke, L.J., Tsang, A. and McAllister, T.A. (2012) Effect of exogenous fibrolytic enzyme application on the microbial attachment and digestion of barley straw *in vitro*. *Asian-Australasian Journal of Animal Sciences* 25, 66–74. doi: 10.5713/ajas.2011.11158

Weimer, P.J., French, A.D. and Calamari, T.A. (1991) Differential fermentation of cellulose allomorphs by ruminal cellulolytic bacteria. *Applied and Environmental Microbiology* 57, 3101–3106.

White, R.R., Roman-Garcia, Y., Firkins, J.L., VandeHaar, M.J., Armentano, L.E., *et al.* (2017) Evaluation of the National Research Council (2001) dairy model and derivation of new prediction equations. 1. Digestibility of fiber, fat, protein, and nonfiber carbohydrate. *Journal of Dairy Science* 100, 3591–3610. doi: 10.3168/jds.2015-10800

Wong, D.W.S., Chan, V.J. and Liao, H. (2019) Metagenomic discovery of feruloyl esterases from rumen microflora. *Applied Microbiology and Biotechnology* 103, 8449–8457. doi: 10.1007/s00253-019-10102-y

Zhang, X.Z., Zhang, Z., Zhu, Z., Sathitsuksanoh, N., Yang, Y. and Zhang, Y.H. (2010) The noncellulosomal family 48 cellobiohydrolase from *Clostridium phytofermentans* ISDg: heterologous expression, characterization, and processivity. *Applied Microbiology and Biotechnology* 86, 525–533. doi: 10.1007/s00253-009-2231-1

10   Enzyme Use in Aquaculture

**Gabriel A. Morales[1,2]*, Lorenzo Márquez[3], Adrian J. Hernández[4]
and Francisco J. Moyano[3]**

[1]*INPA-CONICET, Buenos Aires, Argentina;* [2]*Universidad de Buenos Aires, Buenos Aires,
Argentina;* [3]*Universidad de Almería, Almería, Spain;* [4]*Universidad Católica de Temuco,
Temuco, Chile*

10.1   Introduction

Global aquaculture production in 2016 was 80 million metric tonnes (MMT) of food fish (US$231.6 billion) and 30.1 MMT of aquatic plants (US$11.7 billion). The production of fisheries has been stagnant since the late 1980s and aquaculture has supported the bulk of the increase in the supply of fish for human nutrition worldwide (FAO, 2018). Worldwide, aquaculture showed significant growth of fed species farming; therefore, the global demand for ingredients with high protein content to produce aquafeeds represents a complex issue that requires innovative solutions for the future.

The development of the aquaculture industry in the last decades has been dependent on fishmeal as the main dietary protein ingredient in aquafeeds due to its high protein digestibility, well-balanced amino acid profile and absence of antinutritional factors (ANFs) (Gatlin *et al.*, 2007). Nevertheless, the rising price of fishmeal led to a global trend to reduce its inclusion in formulations. Market prices of fishmeal are steadily increasing and the use of alternative, cheaper protein ingredients has become a worldwide challenge. For this reason, the incorporation of plant-derived ingredients in fish feeds to replace fishmeal has received increasing attention by aquaculture nutritionists (Hardy, 2010). Currently, aquafeeds contain a high content of different plant ingredients such as soybean meal, rapeseed, lupin, sunflower, wheat and maize, among other cereals and legumes. These feedstuffs contain a wide variety of ANFs that may reduce feed intake and nutrient digestibility, also affecting the functionality of internal organs and reducing disease resistance in fish (Krogdahl *et al.*, 2010). The content in ANFs may be partially reduced by selective breeding and genetic modification of the plant species or by different physical-chemical treatments of the meals (e.g. alcohol extraction, heat, acidification, fermentation, etc.). However, in most cases the ANFs are still present in significant amounts in the final product and there is a general consensus about the adverse effects of the presence of these ANFs in the feed (Francis *et al.*, 2001; Gatlin *et al.*, 2007; Krogdahl *et al.*, 2010; NRC, 2011). Therefore, research on feed additives that may counteract the negative effects of ANFs and allow inclusion of high levels of plant ingredients in aquafeeds is imperative.

*Email: moralesg@agro.uba.ar

©CAB International 2022. *Enzymes in Farm Animal Nutrition, 3rd Edition* (M. Bedford et al. eds)
DOI: 10.1079/9781789241563.0010

Some ANFs, such as trypsin inhibitor, glycosylates and hemagglutinin, are thermolabile and can be partially inactivated by heating during feed production. However, other ANFs are thermally resistant and remain in the raw material. This is the case for non-digestible carbohydrates, saponins, gossypol, allergenic storage proteins, non-starch polysaccharides (NSPs) and phytic acid (InsP$_6$), among others (Francis *et al.*, 2001). Among the thermostable ANFs present in plant-based raw materials used for aquafeeds, NSPs and InsP$_6$ are the most relevant. If the negative effects of these ANFs are not properly reduced, they represent a high cost in terms of reduced animal performance and increased environmental impact (Castillo and Gatlin, 2015; Morales *et al.*, 2016). As pointed by Arbige *et al.* (2019), feed enzymes such as phytases, xylanases, amylases and proteases increase feed utilization efficiency and improve overall sustainability through the reduction of P and N in runoff.

For this chapter, the main consequences of NSPs and inositol phosphate isomers (InsPs) on nutrient digestibility, absorption, fish performance, health and the environment are discussed, as well as how the use of enzymes in aquaculture contributes to more efficient and eco-friendly fish production.

10.2   Non-Starch Polysaccharides (NSPs) and NSP-Degrading Enzymes

10.2.1   NSPs in fish feeds

Fish can obtain energy from starch (α-glucan), a complex polymer composed entirely of glucose monomers linked by α-glycosidic bonds. Starch can be hydrolysed by endogenous α-amylase (1,4-α-ᴅ-glucan glucanohydrolase), α-glucosidase (1,4-α-glucosidase) and oligo-1-6-glucosidase. The activity of these enzymes is highly variable depending on the species of fish and their feeding habits. In general, the relative importance of these endogenous digestive enzymes can be listed in the following order: herbivorous > omnivorous > carnivorous fish species (Krogdahl *et al.*, 2005).

The fibre present in grains and plant-based aquafeeds is formed by lignin and NSPs (NRC, 2011). Bach Knudsen (1997) and Sinha *et al.* (2011) have described the NSP content of the main ingredients used in fish feeds and the differences in the type of NSPs between cereals and legumes in great detail. The NSPs can be classified into three groups: cellulose, non-cellulosic polymers (arabinoxylans, mixed-linked β-glucans, mannans and xyloglucan) and pectic polysaccharides (arabinans, galactans and arabinogalactans) (Bailey, 1973). In general, β-glucans, arabinoxylans and cellulose are present at higher concentrations in cereal grains, whereas pectic polysaccharides are the main NSPs present in the legumes.

Cellulose is a straight-chain polymer composed of β-1,4-glucose monomers that are present in most cereals and legumes, mainly forming part of the cell walls of the seeds. Depending on plant species, variety and physical/chemical transformations of the grains, the feedstuff produced can vary largely in cellulose content.

Non-cellulosic polymers are a heterogeneous group of polysaccharide molecules composed of monomers of hexoses and pentoses (galactose, glucose, arabinose, xylose and mannose) and linked by β-glycosidic bonds (van Barneveld, 1999). Arabinoxylans are composed predominantly of arabinose and xylose, forming a polymer with β-1,4-linked xylose units to which substituents are attached through O-2 and O-3 atoms of the xylosyl residues (Perlin, 1951). Between 60 and 70% of the cell wall of the endosperm and the aleurone layer in most cereals used in aquafeeds consists of arabinoxylans. Arabinoxylans in cereal grains are predominantly insoluble in water (Mares and Stone, 1973). However, the arabinoxylans not bound to the cell walls form highly viscous solutions that can absorb up to ten times their weight of water (Sinha *et al.*, 2011).

Mixed-linked β-glucans are unique to the cereal grains and are known as cereal β-glucans. They form part of the sub-aleurone and endospermic cell wall and are associated with cellulose microfibrils (Ebringerová, 2006). β-Glucans consist of a linear chain of glucose units joined by both β-1,3 and β-1,4 linkages (Bengtsson *et al.*, 1990) and are considered a functional bioactive component for animal and human nutrition because of their ability to activate the immune system.

Mannans are linear chains of β-1,4-linked mannose units and can be divided into two groups: galactomannans and glucomannans. Galactomannans are reserve polysaccharides in the seed endosperm of some leguminous plants, such as in guar gum (often used as a pelleting binder in aquafeeds), they are water-soluble with water-holding proprieties, whereas glucomannans are present as a minor component in cereal grains (Sinha *et al.*, 2011). Pectins, also called 'pectic polysaccharides', are formed by α-1,4-linked D-galacturonic acid, which can interact with divalent cations, particularly Ca^{2+}, through their carboxyl groups resulting in particular properties with respect to viscosity, solubility and gelation (Thakur *et al.*, 1997).

In monogastric animals, it is generally assumed that NSPs enter the large intestine without having been digested, and it is in the caecum and/or colon that they are fermented by the intestinal microbiota (Montagne *et al.*, 2003). Although Haidar *et al.* (2016) reported that tilapia fed on a diet containing wheat dried distillers grains with solubles digested NSPs by more than 56% and that 17% of the total digested energy originated from these NSPs, most fish species are not able to hydrolyse the β-glycosidic bonds in NSPs due to the lack of endogenous β-glucanases and β-xylanases in their digestive tract and hence they cannot use dietary NSPs as an energy source (Kuz'mina, 1996; Sinha *et al.*, 2011; Dalsgaard *et al.*, 2012). Nevertheless, as previously indicated, aquafeeds contain a variety of plant-based ingredients from cereals and legumes and NSPs are always present in feeds in variable amounts.

10.2.2 NSPs and their interactions in fish digestion

Similar to terrestrial monogastric animals, two main mechanisms of action for NSPs have been described for fish and with the NSPs classified according to their water-binding capacity into non-viscous water-insoluble compounds and viscous or water-soluble compounds (NRC, 2011). Some

of the components of the plant cell wall (insoluble fractions) encapsulate nutrients such as the protein and minerals in the endosperm of grains used in animal feed, affecting their digestion and absorption by fish and hence being eliminated via the faeces. On the other hand, the adverse effects of soluble NSPs in the fish gastrointestinal tract are associated with their high water-retention capacity. The viscous nature of the soluble NSPs can delay gastric emptying and digestive transit, decreasing the time for interaction between digestive enzymes and macromolecules (Storebakken and Austreng, 1987; Storebakken *et al.*, 1999). In addition, soluble NSPs can lead to alterations in gut morphology, native gut microbiome and mucus layer. Different effects related to changes in physiological and morphological effects on the digestive tract and intestinal microbiome have been described in several fish species (Sinha *et al.*, 2011). In general, the presence of soluble NSPs in fish diets results in an increase in viscosity and dry matter decrease of the digesta. This negatively affects the digestibility, absorption and retention of dietary nutrients in several fish species such as salmonids (Storebakken, 1985; Refstie *et al.*, 1999), African catfish (*Clarias gariepinus*) (Leenhouwers *et al.*, 2006, 2007a), common carp (*Cyprinus carpio*) (Hossain *et al.*, 2001) and tilapia (*Oreochromis niloticus*) (Leenhouwers *et al.*, 2007b; Haidar *et al.*, 2016). Reduction of protein digestibility has been reported by several authors who evaluated the inclusion of NSPs from guar gum and soybeans in rainbow trout and Atlantic salmon (Storebakken, 1985; Mwachireya *et al.*, 1999; Refstie *et al.*, 1999), as well as in non-carnivorous fish species (Leenhouwers *et al.*, 2006). In addition, it has been postulated that NSPs negatively influence lipid breakdown in the intestine through binding to bile salts, lipids and cholesterol, thereby affecting nutrient assimilation.

An increase in digesta viscosity has been reported to reduce gastric emptying and digestive transit in fish, producing alterations in plasma cholesterol and glucose levels (Shimeno *et al.*, 1992; Kaushik *et al.*, 1995; Refstie *et al.*, 1999; Hossain *et al.*, 2001; Kraugerud *et al.*, 2007; Leenhouwers *et al.*, 2007a).

Equally, reports suggest that NSPs can interact with minerals through ionic interactions with the carboxyl groups of galacturonic acid, negatively affecting the absorption of ions in fish fed diets with a high content of NSPs (Kraugerud *et al.*, 2007; Leenhouwers *et al.*, 2007b; Øvrum and Storebakken, 2007).

All these described alterations directly or indirectly affect fish growth, as observed in rainbow trout fed a diet rich in galacto-mannan from guar gum (mannose and gal-actose: 58 and 42 g/kg, respectively), in-cluded at the level of 10% in the diet, which resulted in a 30% reduction of growth and a change in body fat content from 5.1 to 2.7% (Storebakken, 1985). Similarly, Hossain *et al.* (2001) found that dietary inclusion of galactomannan-rich endosperm separated from *Sesbania aculeata* seeds at 72, 108 and 144 g/kg levels resulted in higher whole-body moisture and lower corporal crude protein, lipid and energy content in com-mon carp compared with the control diet. Hossain *et al.* (2003) observed a reduction in growth rate and alterations in body com-position (higher whole-body moisture and lower corporal lipid and energy) of tilapia fed with dietary levels of sesbania endo-sperm above 58 g/kg diet. Other reports sug-gest that NSPs from detoxified *Jatropha cur-cas* seed meal (DJSM) can considerably affect nutrient utilization, fish growth, and produce alterations in fish body compos-ition when the fishmeal protein fraction of the diet is replaced by 75 and 62.5% DJSM in common carp and rainbow trout, respect-ively (Kumar *et al.*, 2008, 2010). In contrast, Leenhouwers *et al.* (2006, 2007a) reported no effect of NSPs on growth performance with an increase in intestinal viscosity. This background should justify more research on the digestive and physiological mechanisms involved when fish are fed plant-based diets containing moderate to high levels of NSPs.

10.2.3 Mechanisms of action of NSP-degrading enzymes

As mentioned previously, fish can hydro-lyse α-glycosidic bonds through their endogen-ous intestinal α-amylases, breaking down the starch into simpler sugars to obtain energy. However, they are incapable of hydrolysing the β-glycosidic bonds of NSPs (NRC, 2011) and sugars from cellulose, hemicellulose and other derivatives (Ray *et al.*, 2012). There-fore, exogenous supplementation with NSP-degrading enzymes is required to ameliorate the negative effects of the NSPs on fish di-gestive functions and/or promote the break-down of NSPs into smaller oligosaccharides with prebiotic-like functions, to be utilized by the microbiota. While the application of such enzymes as additives in feeds for poultry and pigs has been extensively investigated (Campbell and Bedford, 1992; Bedford, 2000; Kiarie *et al.*, 2013; Choct, 2015) and commercial products are used worldwide, the use of NSP-degrading enzymes in aqua-culture is not as widely implemented.

Three main positive effects resulting from enzymatic degradation of NSPs in the digestive tract of terrestrial monogastrics have been described: (i) the reduction in viscosity of the digesta; (ii) the hydrolysis of insoluble fibre fractions of the cell wall in grains; and (iii) the benefits associated with the modulation of the digestive microbiota (Simon, 1998; Masey O'Neill *et al.*, 2014; Aftab and Bedford, 2018; Bedford, 2018).

The first effect of NSP-degrading en-zymes is characterized by the content of sol-uble carbohydrates present in some cereal grains (wheat, triticale, oats, rye, barley) and an increase in the viscosity of the digesta. This results in slower digestive transit rates, accumulation of particulate matter for mi-crobial adhesion and proliferation of harm-ful bacteria (Vahjen *et al.*, 1998). In the case of fish, an increase in viscosity of the diges-ta reduces the access of digestive enzymes to dietary nutrients, slowing the digestion rate and affecting their digestibility (Bedford, 2000) and absorption (German and Bittong, 2009; Shi *et al.*, 2017).

The second effect resulting from the use of NSP-degrading enzymes is related to the release of nutrients trapped within the insoluble fibrous cell wall of cereals and legumes (the 'cage effect'). As in pigs and poultry, fish do not produce endogenous en-zymes able to digest fibre within the cell walls enabling access to these trapped nutrients.

Thus, the application of exogenous enzymes able to disrupt the cell walls allows water permeation and facilitates access of endogenous proteases and amylases to improve the hydrolysis of dietary protein and starch, improving their digestion and absorption.

The third mechanism of NSP-degrading enzymes is related to the modulation of the digestive microbiota through changes in the substrate used by the gut-associated bacterial population. NSP-degrading enzymes release oligosaccharides, promoting beneficial bacterial fermentation and changing the production of volatile fatty acids as well as the microbiota production and profile (Bedford, 2018). The oligosaccharides produced by NSP-degrading enzymes are not available to the endogenous digestive enzymes of the animals, thereby reaching the distal intestine to act as prebiotics. Craig *et al.* (2020) concluded that broiler chickens fed wheat-based diets supplemented with xylanase had similar effects on NSP concentration and volatile fatty acids in the caeca as broilers fed wheat-based diets supplemented with xylo-oligosaccharides. This observation suggests benefits of xylanase supplementation beyond digesta viscosity reduction and the release of extra nutrients. It is hypothesized that xylo-oligosaccharides with prebiotic proprieties can selectively stimulate beneficial bacteria (*Bifidobacterium*, *Lactobacillus*) while suppressing deleterious bacteria (*Salmonella*, *Clostridium*, *Campylobacter*, *Escherichia coli*) (Thammarutwasik *et al.*, 2009). Despite the complex mode of action, there are reports evidencing the desirable effect of xylo-oligosaccharides on the beneficial bacteria populations in both terrestrial monogastric animals (Adeola and Cowieson, 2011) and fish (Castillo and Gatlin, 2015).

10.2.4 NSP-degrading enzymes and responses in fish nutrition

The study of the effects of exogenous carbohydrase enzyme supplementation in pigs and poultry has been well described as a convenient nutritional strategy to get more energy and nutrients from feeds but also to maintain the normal function and health of the gastrointestinal tract (Choct and Cadogan, 2001; Partridge, 2001; Jackson, 2010; Svihus, 2010; Adeola and Cowieson, 2011; Bedford, 2018).

Sinha *et al.* (2011) reviewed the impact of NSPs on fish, and Castillo and Gatlin (2015) presented a comprehensive summary of the effects of NSP-degrading enzymes in fish nutrition. Most studies suggest that the supplementation of fish diets with NSP-degrading enzymes is beneficial for protein and energy utilization and fish growth performance (Carter *et al.*, 1994; Stone *et al.*, 2003; Kumar *et al.*, 2005, 2006a,b,c, 2009; Ai *et al.*, 2007; Farhangi and Carter, 2007; Lin *et al.*, 2007; Yildirim and Turan, 2010; Dalsgaard *et al.*, 2012; Ghomi *et al.*, 2012; Goda *et al.*, 2012; Zhou *et al.*, 2013; Jiang *et al.*, 2014; Zamini *et al.*, 2014). However other studies reported slight or no effect of NSP-degrading enzymes on nutrient utilization by fish (Ng and Chong, 2002; Ogunkoya *et al.*, 2006; Farhangi and Carter, 2007; Yigit and Olmez, 2011; Dalsgaard *et al.*, 2012; Adeoye *et al.*, 2016; Ramos *et al.*, 2017). The use of NSP-degrading enzymes in fish diets, alone or combined with other exogenous enzymes (e.g. amylases, phytases, proteases), as well as the species-specific differences in fish digestive systems might explain the variable responses observed in the literature.

For example, Jiang *et al.* (2014) studied the effects of xylanase supplementation on *C. carpio* fed a plant-based diet. The authors observed improved growth performance, higher activity of intestinal trypsin, chymotrypsin, lipase and amylase enzymes, and alterations in the microflora favouring *Lactobacillus* over *Aeromonas* and *E. coli* in the fish intestine. More recently, Ramos *et al.* (2017) observed that the use of an enzymatic complex (carbohydrases, phytase and proteases) in diets for *Mugil liza* juveniles did not improve animal performance or influence biometrical indices. However, enzyme supplementation increased bone Ca content and the lipid content in the peritoneal cavity, and reduced the intestinal damage caused by the soybean meal-based diet (even at low doses).

Adeoye *et al.* (2016) evaluated the effects of commercial NSP-degrading enzymes (xylanase, β-glucanase and cellulase) on growth and general health status in Nile tilapia. Dietary exogenous carbohydrases improved intestinal health and altered the community of intestinal bacteria, but no differences were found in growth rate and feed conversion efficiency compared with fish fed the diet without enzyme supplementation. The authors pointed out that further quantitative studies are necessary to confirm how exogenous carbohydrases modulate intestinal microbiota and if these modulations contribute towards the improved growth performance of the host.

Maas *et al.* (2018) studied the effect of phytase, xylanase and their combination on growth performance and nutrient utilization in Nile tilapia. When xylanase (4000 U/kg) was supplemented to a plant-based diet as the only exogenous enzyme source, the carbohydrase did not result in any improvement in fish growth but enhanced the digestibility of dry matter, crude protein, carbohydrates and energy. However, fish fed the diet supplemented with both phytase and xylanase showed a higher growth than fish fed only the phytase-supplemented diet. The authors suggested that better protein digestibility and retention efficiency by fish were the reasons for such a beneficial effect of both enzymes on growth. More recently, Maas *et al.* (2019) evaluated the combined effect of phytase 1000 FTU/kg and xylanase 4000 U/kg in different plant-based diets. The authors found that enzyme supplementation affected the absolute growth and feed conversion ratio, while the digestibility of NSP, total energy, ash, P and Ca improved with enzyme supplementation. They concluded that the effectiveness of the enzymes was dependent on the amount of NSP-rich ingredients in the diet. Nevertheless, in this case, the effects of the xylanase and phytase were not evaluated separately.

Different findings reported in the literature suggest that the three mechanisms postulated to explain the beneficial effects of NSP-degrading enzymes on nutrient digestibility and retention efficiency, that consequently can or cannot be translated into better growth rate in fish, are inconsistent. Therefore, prediction of the response to NSP-degrading enzymes as may occur with other groups of exogenous enzymes, such as the phytases, is not possible today. However, the described different responses to the supplementation can be partially explained because the studies have been conducted using a wide diversity of enzyme combinations, from single enzymes to multi-enzyme complexes (carbohydrases, proteases and phytase; Table 10.1). Moreover, these studies have been conducted on fish species showing a great diversity of feeding habits and gastrointestinal digestive features. These differences in the relative importance of the stomach and intestinal digestion phases, specific for each species, make it difficult to compare results between studies when NSP-degrading enzymes are used as a dietary supplement in fish species. More studies will be needed to understand the predominance of the postulated mechanisms whereby NSP-degrading enzymes reduce the antinutritional effects of soluble and insoluble NSPs in aquaculture.

10.3 Inositol Phosphate Isomers (InsPs) and InsPs-Degrading Enzymes

10.3.1 Phytic acid (InsP$_6$) and its interactions in fish digestion

Phytic acid (*myo*-inositol(1,2,3,4,5,6)hexakis(dihydrogen phosphate); InsP$_6$), and its salts are the main storage form of P in cereals and legumes. Phytate is accumulated in grains during their development and maturation, accompanied by other storage macromolecules such as proteins, starch and lipids. In mature seeds used as raw material for aquafeeds, the InsPs are mainly accumulated in the form of InsP$_6$ (90–95%), with small proportions of InsP$_5$ and InsP$_4$ esters (Pontoppidan *et al.*, 2007). P bound to the inositol molecule has a very low bioavailability in terrestrial monogastrics (Selle and Ravindran, 2007, 2008) as well as in fish, due to the lack of phytase in their gastrointestinal tract (Morales *et al.*, 2016).

Table 10.1. Summary of trials testing for the effects of enzymatic and multi-enzymatic blends in diets for fish.

Enzymatic blend	Enzymes included	Fish species	Reference
Single NSP carbohydrase	Cellulase	*Oreochromis niloticus*	Yigit and Olmez (2011)
	Cellulase	*Ctenopharyngodon idella*	Zhou *et al.* (2013)
	Xylanase	*Clarias gariepinus*	Babalola (2006)
	Xylanase	*Cyprinus carpio* var. Jian	Jiang *et al.* (2014)
	Xylanase	*O. niloticus*	Maas *et al.* (2018)
Two NSP carbohydrases	β-Glucanase, β-xylanase	*Bidyanus bidyanus*	Stone *et al.* (2003)
Multi-carbohydrases	Xylanase, β-glucanase, β-amylase, cellulase, pectinase	*C. gariepinus*	Yildirim and Turan (2010)
Carbohydrase + phytase	Xylanase, phytase	*O. niloticus* × *Oreochromis mossambicus*	Wallace *et al.* (2016)
	Xylanase, phytase	*O. niloticus*	Maas *et al.* (2019)
Multi-enzymatic blends	Trypsin, alkaline protease, acid protease, amyloglucosidase, amylase, cellulase	*Salmo salar*	Carter *et al.* (1994)
	Protease, cellulase, xylanase, α-galactosidase, amylase	*Oreochromis* sp.	Ng and Chong (2002); Ng *et al.* (2002)
	Protease, xylanase, amylase, cellulase, β-glucanase	*Oncorhynchus mykiss*	Ogunkoya *et al.* (2006)
	Protease, hemicellulases, α-galactosidase	*O. mykiss*	Farhangi and Carter (2007)
	Protease, β-glucanase, xylanase	*O. niloticus* × *Oreochromis aureus*	Lin *et al.* (2007)
	Phytase, glucanase, pentosanase, cellulase, xylanase	*Lateolabrax japonicus*	Ai *et al.* (2007)
	Protease, phytase, xylanase, cellulase, pectinase, β-glucanase, α-amylase, lipase	*Huso huso*	Ghomi *et al.* (2012)
	Protease, xylanase, β-glucanase	*O. mykiss*	Dalsgaard *et al.* (2012)
	Protease, xylanase, cellulase, pectinase, β-glucanase, α-amylase, lipase, phytase, phosphatase	*Salmo trutta*	Zamini *et al.* (2014)
	Xylanase, endo-β-mannanase, cellulase, α-galactosidase, amylase	*S. trutta*	Zamini *et al.* (2014)
	Protease, xylanase, phytase	*O. niloticus*	Adeoye *et al.* (2016)
	Xylanases, β-glucanases, pectinases, phytase, α-galactosidase, aspartate-protease, metalloprotease	*Mugil liza*	Ramos *et al.* (2017)

Despite grains having endogenous phytase, capable of dephosphorylating the InsPs during germination, this endogenous phytase is labile to high temperatures and is deactivated during the feed extrusion process. Therefore, the presence of unavailable P in the form of InsPs in the diet results in a potential deficiency of P that can produce decreases in growth performance and fish health (Sugiura *et al.*, 2004). To avoid P deficiencies, a bioavailable inorganic P source must be added to the diet (e.g. monocalcium, monosodium or monoammonium phosphate); however, if a phytase enzyme is not used, the undigested InsPs will reach the environment in the faeces (Morales *et al.*, 2018).

The chemical structure of $InsP_6$ is quite stable, and its large number of phosphate moieties confers to the molecule 12 replaceable reactive sites with negative charges in complete dissociation, where three to nine are dissociated under the pH of the gastrointestinal tract. For example, in Atlantic salmon (*Salmo salar*) fed continuously, the pH in the stomach contents ranges from 4.0 to 5.2, while that of the chyme in the distal intestine varies between 8.2 and 8.7. Other studies reported lower pH values, close to 2.0, in the stomach content of several fish species (Krogdahl *et al.*, 2015). Under such conditions, the dissociated $InsP_6$ has the potential ability to bind to different positively charged mineral ions, such as Zn^{2+}, Cu^{2+}, Ni^{2+}, Co^{2+}, Mn^{2+}, Ca^{2+} and Fe^{2+} (in that order of stability) (Cheryan, 1980), reducing their bioavailability. Different studies have reported the negative effect of $InsP_6$ on the digestibility and retention efficiency of Zn, Mg, Ca and Cu in fish (Storebakken *et al.*, 1998; Sugiura *et al.*, 2001).

Another type of interaction between $InsP_6$ and dietary nutrients is related to its ability to bind proteins and amino acids both in terrestrial monogastrics (Selle *et al.*, 2000; Cowieson *et al.*, 2006) and fish (Kumar *et al.*, 2012; Morales *et al.*, 2016). The presence of protein–$InsP_6$ complexes in feed ingredients, the formation of binary and ternary complexes with soluble protein released by digestion and the inhibition of proteolytic enzymes are the primary modes of action that can affect protein digestion within the gastrointestinal tract. Depending on the pH, InsPs form binary (protein–$InsP_6$) or ternary (protein–mineral–$InsP_6$) complexes (Kies *et al.*, 2006). Phytic acid–protein interactions by binary complexes occur through ionic bonds between $InsP_6$ and basic amino acid residues at pH values below the isoelectric point of proteins. Under these conditions, the anionic groups of $InsP_6$ interact with the cationic groups of the protein to form binary complexes. The basic amino acids arginine, lysine and histidine are the most susceptible to chelation. Once gastric digesta pass through the proximal intestine, most dietary proteins reach their isoelectric point, therefore the $InsP_6$ is gradually released from the $InsP_6$–protein complexes enabling ternary protein–cation–$InsP_6$ complexes.

These ternary complexes are formed by a cationic bridge, presumably Ca^{2+}, when the digesta pH rises above 5.0–6.0 and proteins acquire a net negative charge.

Moreover, protein–$InsP_6$ complexes may interact with functional proteins such as digestive proteases in pig, poultry and fish (Kies *et al.*, 2006; Selle *et al.*, 2006; Morales *et al.*, 2011, 2014). There is a general consensus that binary $InsP_6$–protein complexes are more relevant than the ternary ones, affecting the proteolytic efficacy of gastric pepsin in two ways: (i) through the inhibition of pepsin due to its precipitation as a pepsin–InsPs complex; and (ii) through the reduction in the bioaccessibility of pepsin substrates (dietary protein). Both modes of action can affect the release of pepsin products, which partially regulate pancreatic secretory activity (Santos-Hernández *et al.*, 2018).

Similarly, Khan and Ghosh (2013) reported that dietary $InsP_6$ reduced to a different extent the activity of digestive amylase in rohu carp (*Labeo rohita*), catla (*Catla catla*) and mrigal (*Cirrhinus mrigala*), depending on the concentration of $InsP_6$ in the digesta. Interactions between $InsP_6$ and lipids through lipophytin complexes formed between $InsP_6$, a cation and lipids have been previously reported in poultry (Leeson, 1993), suggesting that metallic soaps in the intestinal lumen may reduce energy utilization from lipids. Despite no reports being found in the literature about the identification of lipophytin complexes in fish species, some studies reported a higher apparent digestibility of lipid when $InsP_6$-degrading enzymes were supplemented in fish diets (Goda, 2007; Liu *et al.*, 2013a,b; Roy *et al.*, 2014). Studying the effect of $InsP_6$ on feed intake, feed utilization and feeding-related gene expression hormones, Liu *et al.* (2014) observed that diets with high content of $InsP_6$ decreased the expression of some genes responsible for appetite.

Many years of research on the varied deleterious effects of dietary $InsP_6$ supports the supplementation of plant-based aquafeeds with exogenous phytases as a more efficient way to improve nutrient assimilation, growth and health in fish, and also to alleviate environmental pollution due to nutrient discharges.

10.3.2 Considerations about the use of phytases as fish feed additives

The relevant factors that influence the benefits of phytases in plant-based diets for fish, and how the inclusion of this additive might improve their protein and P bioavailability, were discussed previously by Morales *et al.* (2016). A comprehensive review of mechanisms of action of phytases in fish can be found in Cao *et al.* (2007), Kumar *et al.* (2012), Dersjant-Li *et al.* (2015) and Lemos and Tacon (2017). This section addresses how phytase may improve feed utilization in cold- and warmwater fish species and discusses the main challenges facing the optimization of the enzyme activity in aquafeeds.

Phytase catalyses the sequential release of P to produce lower *myo*-inositol phosphate esters, from $InsP_5$ to $InsP_1$ (Debnath *et al.*, 2005). Phytases are acidic, neutral or alkaline phosphatases, depending on the functional pH profile of the enzyme. However, histidine acid phosphatases are the most widely used commercial phytate-degrading enzymes in animal farming. The most common fungal phytases used for decades in animal feeds were obtained from *Aspergillus niger* and *Peniophora lycii*, whereas bacterial phytases, mainly from *E. coli* expressed in *Pichia pastoris* and *Schizosaccharomyces pombe*, gained participation in recent years. Depending on their origin, these enzymes differ in functional pH range; stability to pH, temperature and digestive proteases; and substrate specificity. New phytases recently developed by commercial companies offer improved efficacy and resistance, such as the phytases from *E. coli* and *Buttiauxella* sp. expressed in *Trichoderma reesei* and from *Citrobacter braakii* expressed in *Aspergillus oryzae*.

Other types of phytases can be found as endogenous enzymes in cereal and legume seeds (e.g. β-propeller phytases, cysteine phosphatases, purple acid phosphatases), although their effect is not considered relevant mainly due to their low activity and low stability to the high temperatures (>100°C) used during the extrusion of aquafeeds. Phytase activity can also be found in the microbiota of ruminants and to a lesser extent in the colon/hindgut of pigs and caeca of poultry (Schlemmer *et al.*, 2001; Selle and Ravindran, 2007). However, exogenous phytate-degrading enzyme supplementation is required to enable relevant dephosphorylation in the gastrointestinal tract of non-ruminant animals. In fish, the efficiency of dephosphorylation by endogenous phytase present in the digestive tract is variable and related to the different feeding habits of the species, as well as to the anatomy and physiology of the digestive tract.

Ellestad *et al.* (2002) evaluated the phytate dephosphorylation efficacy by the endogenous phytase activity in the intestinal brush border of a carnivorous fish species (hybrid striped bass, *Morone chrysops* × *Morone saxatilis*) and two omnivorous fish species, tilapia and carp, observing that the dietary $InsP_6$ content was reduced by 50% in tilapia, whereas the hybrid bass and the carp reduced dietary $InsP_6$ by only 2%. Moreover, Denstadli *et al.* (2006) found that between 5 and 15% of the dietary $InsP_6$ can be reduced by rainbow trout. Similar results were observed in this species by Morales *et al.* (2015), who reported a 17–22% reduction in the content of $InsP_6$ in the digesta in absence of exogenous phytase supplementation.

When phytase is used as an aquafeed additive, the enzyme is exposed to different physical-chemical conditions that can alter its activity. Therefore, for efficient phytate hydrolysis within the fish stomach, the enzyme must be able to withstand stressing factors like high temperature during feed preparation, as well as low gastric pH and the presence of pepsin. The first stressing condition for the phytase is presented during the manufacture of the diet. There are three places where the phytase must resist high temperatures: the conditioner, the extruder and the dryer. In the conditioner, the raw feed ingredients (including phytase) are mixed with steam, water, and often oils or other liquid ingredients, and the temperature of the mash can rise up to (95°C) (Strahm,

2000; Beyer, 2007). The extruder barrel is where temperature and pressure are transferred to the mash before the pellet is formed through the die. Within the extruder, pressure and temperature increase rapidly and can be in the range of 20–40 bar and 100–150°C, respectively. Third, the wet pellets from the extruder are directed to the dryer to reduce the moisture of the pellets below 10% in order to ensure a satisfactory conservation, and the air temperature of the dryer can range from 100 to 150°C. Although a high extrusion temperature is thought to improve the nutritional quality of pellets (Barrows *et al.*, 2007; Morken *et al.*, 2012; Sørensen, 2012; Bowzer *et al.*, 2016), it can also impair thermolabile phytases. Most phytases are functional between 40 and 70°C (Greiner and Konietzny, 2010), and when the temperature surpasses 80°C the activity of the enzyme is negatively affected (Dersjant-Li *et al.*, 2015). Developing heat-stable phytases (Li, J. *et al.*, 2019) and the development of thermo-protective matrices/coatings for commercial phytases are imperative to reduce activity losses during aquafeed production.

To avoid the loss of phytase activity generated by high-temperature processes, the pretreatment of plant ingredients with phytase before the extrusion process may be an option (Cheng and Hardy, 2003; Denstadli *et al.*, 2007). However, pretreatment requires modifications to the industrial process that are not always technically feasible and may raise the costs of manufacture of aquafeeds. A practical solution currently used by the industry is the application of the enzyme in a liquid form during the oil coating after the pellets are extruded, dried and cooled (Vielma *et al.*, 2004; Denstadli *et al.*, 2007). In a recent study, Pontes *et al.* (2019) observed that the inclusion of phytase 1500 FTU/kg before extrusion resulted in an apparent P digestibility in Nile tilapia of 33%, whereas the same dose applied after extrusion (as liquid form) increased apparent P digestibility to 86%. It is clear that using granulated/powder phytase mixed in the dry mixture of ingredients before the pellet extrusion, on one hand, or as liquid form after pelleting, on the other, produces different results and that

feed manufacturing conditions must be considered to optimize the enzyme response in fish.

Once fish ingest the pellets, two main factors modulate the activity of the phytase: (i) the water temperature; and (ii) the pH of the digesta in the gastrointestinal tract. Regardless of whether the enzyme is used in warmwater fish species (20 to 30°C) or coldwater fish species (5 to 20°C), the environmental temperature is considerably lower than the temperature of homeothermic animals and consequently the optimum temperature for most commercial microbial phytases. Previous *in vitro* studies simulating the gastric digestion of the rainbow trout in winter (6°C) and summer (16°C) temperatures reported changes in the dephosphorylation rate of $InsP_6$, suggesting that enzymatic degradation of $InsP_6$ may be severely affected by low temperatures (Morales *et al.*, 2011). Comparing the phytase pretreatment of plant ingredients and phytase coating in pelleted diet for Atlantic salmon, Denstadli *et al.* (2007) concluded that the pre-incubation prior to extrusion might be a more rational method to increase mineral availability in fish reared in cold water (8°C).

One way to potentially compensate for the effect of low temperature in coldwater fish species is the inclusion of a higher dose of phytase in the diet. For example, the inclusion of 4000 FTU phytase/kg in a rainbow trout diet improved growth, feed conversion, and mineral (P, Ca, Mg) and protein utilization (Morales *et al.*, 2016). More recently, Lee *et al.* (2020) concluded that phytase supplementation could be a useful tool to reduce inorganic P inclusion in plant-based diets for trout reared at two different temperatures. The enhanced phytase from *E. coli* supplemented in trout fed low-P diets stimulated growth and nutrient utilization at 11 and 15°C. These recent findings suggest that the use of phytase as a fish feed additive has a very interesting potential in coldwater fish species such as trout and salmon.

Both $InsP_6$ and phytase are primarily affected by pH changes taking place during gastrointestinal digestion. The solubility of the InsPs is largely pH-dependent, being soluble at low pH but forming insoluble InsP$_6$–cation complexes when the pH rises above 4 (Grynspan and Cheryan, 1983). Taking this into account, InsP$_6$ must be hydrolysed as quickly as possible by phytase in the upper part of the digestive tract to counteract its antinutritional effects (Dersjant-Li *et al.*, 2015). An important factor influencing the effectiveness of the process is the buffering capacity (BC) of the diet. As a result of such BC, the pH of the stomach increases during feeding, prior to the secretion of hydrochloric acid and gastric pepsinogen. Several hours after feeding, the pH of the gastric content drops and the digesta is emptied to the proximal intestine, where the pH gradually rises due to the pancreatic secretions. The pH changes in the stomach content often show a wave pattern affected by the BC of the dietary ingredients, the use of organic acids or their salts as a feed additive, the feeding frequency and size of the feed ration, fish age and water temperature, among other fish intrinsic and environmental factors.

Phytic acid is more soluble at lower pH and therefore most commercial phytases work well under the acidic conditions present in fish stomach; hence, InsP$_6$ is more available to be enzymatically hydrolysed within this organ. Regardless of their fungal or bacterial origin, 80% of the optimal dephosphorylating activity of the enzymes ranges between pH 3.0 and 5.5 (Menezes-Blackburn *et al.*, 2015). *E. coli* phytase is active over a wide pH range, with an optimum close to 4.5, but this can vary slightly depending on the production technology and expression organism, whereas it seems that phytases from *C. braakii* and *Buttiauxella* sp. work better under more acidic conditions (pH 4.0 and 3.5, respectively). Therefore, it can be suggested that the activity of added phytases in carnivorous fish such as trout, salmon and catfish, as well as in other species able to drop the pH of the stomach content to values close to the optimum of the enzymes, will be different to that in herbivorous/omnivorous fish lacking acid digestion. This can partially explain the variable responses obtained when phytase is included in diets for fish species with

different feeding habits (Kumar *et al.*, 2012; Lemos and Tacon, 2017).

The resistance to both the acidic conditions of the stomach and the presence of gastric pepsin are highly desirable features for commercial phytases used as a feed additive. *In vitro* studies simulating the gastrointestinal tract of rainbow trout suggest that exposure to gastric digestion resulted in a significant decrease in the activity of the phytases from *A. niger* and *P. lycii* (Kumar *et al.*, 2003). In the same study, the authors observed that *E. coli* phytase was more resistant than the fungal phytases, not only when exposed to gastric pepsin, but also to intestinal trypsin and chymotrypsin. Menezes-Blackburn *et al.* (2015) also described that phytase from *E. coli* was more resistant to a simulated gastric digestion, including or not porcine pepsin, than those from *A. niger* or *P. lycii*. In fish, Morales *et al.* (2011) evaluated the effect of rainbow trout pepsin present in crude stomach extracts on the activity of two commercial phytases of bacterial and fungal origin. They concluded that phytase from *E. coli* could be more active and stable than that obtained from *P. lycii* under the gastric environment of these carnivorous fish.

10.3.3 Responses to phytate-degrading enzymes in fish species

The effects of dietary supplementation with phytase have been evaluated in a number of coldwater fish species (e.g. Atlantic salmon, rainbow trout), temperate-water species (e.g. European seabass *Dicentrarchus labrax*, striped bass) and warmwater fish species (Nile tilapia, rohu carp, red seabream *Pagrus major*, Australian catfish *Tandanus tandanus*, channel catfish *Ictalurus punctatus*, African catfish, pangas catfish *Pangasius pangasius*, pacu *Piaractus mesopotamicus*, milkfish *Chanos chanos*, carp *Carassius auratus* and grass carp *Ctenopharyngodon idellus*, among others). The comparative beneficial effects of using the enzyme on nutrient digestibility and fish performance were well described by Kumar *et al.* (2012) and Lemos and Tacon (2017).

In general, in coldwater fish species, the supplementation of the plant-based diets with phytase results in a better dietary P digestibility. For example, in rainbow trout, most studies testing phytase doses from 500 up to 6000 FTU/kg diet suggest a clear dose-dependent response and the optimum phytase doses for P digestibility are close to 1000 FTU/kg (Sugiura *et al.*, 2001; Cheng *et al.*, 2004; Vielma *et al.*, 2004; Wang *et al.*, 2009; Vandenberg *et al.*, 2012; Verlhac-Trichet *et al.*, 2014). For the same fish species, the improvement in P digestibility due to the phytase supplementation ranged between 17% (Lanari *et al.*, 1998) and 100% or more (Sugiura *et al.*, 2001; Cheng *et al.*, 2004; Dalsgaard *et al.*, 2009; Verlhac-Trichet *et al.*, 2014; Morales *et al.*, 2015). In these studies, the digestibilities of Zn, Mg, Mn, Ca and Fe were also higher with phytase supplementation. Similar responses were observed for Atlantic salmon, with a positive dose–response from 250 up to 4000 FTU/kg and 81% improvement in dietary P digestibility (Carter and Sajjadi, 2011).

However, a recent study suggests that the response to dietary supplementation with phytase may be different in rainbow trout and Atlantic salmon (Greiling *et al.*, 2019). While faecal disappearance of $InsP_6$ was similar in both fish species when no phytase was included in the diet (about 8%), a dose of 6-phytase from *A. oryzae* of 2800 FTU/kg resulted in faecal disappearance of $InsP_6$ of 32% in salmon and 82% in rainbow trout. Moreover, the hydrolysis of the different moieties of InsPs progressed to a greater extent in rainbow trout. As a consequence, the supplementation with phytase showed that total P digestibility increased from 17 to 24% in Atlantic salmon and from 33 to 70% in rainbow trout. The authors suggested that this surprisingly big difference between two coldwater fish species with similar digestive functions could be explained considering that freshwater fish usually present a lower stomach pH than marine fish (Márquez *et al.*, 2012). This acidic condition could have reduced the strength of the cation–phytate complexes making them more sensitive to the action of phytase, as pointed out by Maenz (2001).

However, it must be outlined that rearing water temperatures were 12.0°C for salmon and 15.4°C for trout and this could enhance (to a certain extent) phytase activity within the stomach of the latter species.

The high increment in P digestibility found in the described study agrees with previous results obtained in the same fish species by Morales *et al.* (2015), who reported an increment in apparent P digestibility from 38 to 73% when a plant-based diet with similar content of total P was supplemented with 6-phytase from *E. coli* of 4000 FTU/kg and fish were reared between 11 and 15°C. Another recent study, aimed to evaluate the effect of phytase on the performance and nutrient retention efficiency of rainbow trout fed low-P plant-based diets, reported P digestibilities of 25, 55 and 82% when the diet included 0, 500 and 2500 FTU/kg, respectively, of the same 6-phytase from *E. coli* (Lee *et al.*, 2020). Results obtained in these last studies suggest that 1000 FTU phytase/kg may not be enough to maximize $InsP_6$ dephosphorylation in coldwater fish species and more phytase would be required when water temperature is quite low, as occurs in the farming of salmonids. In this sense, it can be expected that warmwater fish species should offer a better response to phytase supplementation, considering that most species are reared at water temperatures at least 10°C higher. The recent reviews by Kumar *et al.* (2012) and Lemos and Tacon (2017) highlight that the beneficial effects of phytase on the digestibility of nutrients when feeding these species on plant-based diets were mainly observed for P (>30% gain) and other trace minerals, protein (2–18%), lipid (26–65%), energy (4–16%) and amino acids (5–12%). Given that carnivorous, omnivorous and herbivorous warmwater fish species have substantial anatomical and physiological differences in their digestive tracts, further studies will be necessary to maximize the effect of phytase for a given species.

Lastly, different studies reported that phytase added to plant-based diets improved phytate-P bioavailability from 20 to 60% and reduced the P loading to the environment by between 30 and 50% in several fish species such as rainbow trout (Rodehutscord and Pfeffer, 1995; Lanari *et al.*, 1998; Forster *et al.*, 1999; Sugiura *et al.*, 2001; Morales *et al.*, 2015), Atlantic salmon (Storebakken *et al.*, 1998), tilapia (Goda, 2007) and carp (Schaefer and Koppe, 1995). On account of these studies, it can be stated that the use of phytase in aquafeed is imperative to reduce the negative impact caused by the release of nutrients to the aquatic environment.

10.3.4   Phytase strategy for extra-phosphoric effects

An enzyme dose high enough to hydrolyse dietary InsPs quickly and thus eliminate its negative antinutritional effects in the early stages of the digestive process is often commercially known as 'superdosing'. It is assumed that higher doses of phytase can result not only in a higher phytate-P bioavailability but also in other extra-phosphoric benefits for the fish, as well as other monogastric animals. As suggested by Cowieson *et al.* (2011), the extra-phosphoric benefits of high doses of phytase in the diet are not only a higher digestibility of dietary amino acids and minerals, but also an increased bioavailability of metal cofactors for endogenous enzymes or a decrease of endogenous loss of protein. The mechanisms postulated for such extra-phosphoric benefits are mainly related to the formation of $InsP_6$–protein complexes and their interactions with digestive enzymes, being related to different factors like the solubility of proteins at a given pH in the presence of divalent cations and the functional properties of the phytase (pH range, substrate affinity, resistance to gastric pepsin).

Several studies reported better digestion of dietary protein when high phytase doses (3000–4000 FTU/kg) were used in fish diets (Vandenberg *et al.*, 2011, 2012; Morales *et al.*, 2015). As pointed out by Morales *et al.* (2016), in fish species with a functional stomach, the quick hydrolysis of the insoluble $InsP_6$–protein complexes present in the diet begins with the formation of lower InsPs esters ($InsP_5$, followed by $InsP_4$ and

$InsP_3$), thus avoiding the *de novo* formation of $InsP_6$–protein complexes. Superdosing of phytase may contribute to increasing the protein solubility concentration of the digesta during the early stages of gastric digestion, increasing dietary protein bioavailability and decreasing at the same time the negative effect of $InsP_6$ on the gastric pepsin activity. The net result would be a more effective protein hydrolysis. Moreover, the fast destruction of $InsP_6$ reduces the formation of $InsP_6$–Ca complexes able to bind to intestinal proteases (Selle *et al.*, 2000; Kies *et al.*, 2006; Morales *et al.*, 2011, 2013, 2014).

This quick dephosphorylation of $InsP_6$ in the upper part of the digestive tract can be a favourable strategy to improve dietary nutrient utilization and to reduce the excretion of undigested nutrients to the water when replacing expensive animal proteins by cheaper alternative plant-protein ingredients with relative high levels of native phytic acid (Morales *et al.*, 2016).

10.4   Other Enzymes

10.4.1   Exogenous proteases in fish nutrition

As the pressure on world protein supply increases and the industry becomes more competitive, aquafeed manufacturers are looking to develop nutritionally adequate but cost-effective diets using high levels of plant-protein ingredients. Within this context, exogenous protease supplementation is gaining attention in recent years as a possible nutritional strategy to reduce the crude protein content in the diets, with a presumably beneficial effect related to the reduction of undigested protein released to the water through fish faeces (Castillo and Gatlin, 2015).

Research on exogenous proteases as aquafeed additives is not as extensive as that of phytase and NSP-degrading enzymes, but there are a number of studies on this topic supporting an increase in the digestibility of protein and other nutrients in coldwater fish species such as rainbow trout (Drew *et al.*, 2005; Dalsgaard *et al.*, 2012, 2016) and warmwater fish species such as tilapia (*O. niloticus* × *Oreochromis aureus*) (Li *et al.*, 2016; Li, X.Q. *et al.*, 2019).

The hypothetical mechanism of action of exogenous proteases suggests a deficiency of fish endogenous proteases, therefore dietary protein can be more efficiently hydrolysed to lower-molecular-weight peptides and bioavailable amino acids, improving their utilization and promoting fish growth. However, in most cases, the effects of exogenous proteases were studied when forming part of a multi-enzyme complex with phytase, amylase and NSP-degrading enzymes, making it difficult to assess the precise effect of the enzyme on nutrient bioavailability, utilization and fish growth (Carter *et al.*, 1994; Farhangi and Carter, 2007; Lin *et al.*, 2007; Dalsgaard *et al.*, 2012; Ghomi *et al.*, 2012). Only a few studies evaluated the effect of single exogenous proteases in fish. For instance, Adeoye *et al.* (2016) studied the effects of an exogenous commercial serine protease from *Bacillus licheniformis* on growth and general health status of Nile tilapia. Supplementation of the diet with 15,000 U protease/kg diet did not result in better growth or feed conversion efficiency compared with the control diet, although fish survival rate was higher. The authors hypothesized that the potential beneficial effects of the enzyme could have been irrelevant since the study was carried out using a diet with a high content of crude protein (40%), exceeding the requirement for fish maintenance and growth. In a similar study performed using the same dose of 15,000 U protease/kg diet, but diets with lower protein content (26–28% crude protein), the authors observed clear benefits on apparent protein digestibility, protein retention efficiency, feed conversion efficiency and fish growth rate (Ragaa *et al.*, 2017).

As suggested by Leinonen and Williams (2015) when studying the effects of dietary proteases on N emissions from broiler production, further research would be useful to quantify the potential beneficial effect of their use combined to a strategy of reduction in the contents of dietary protein in order to decrease undigested faecal protein and excreted soluble ammonium to the water. This could be particularly relevant in aquafeeds designed for recirculation aquaculture systems. In addition, the interaction of endogenous proteases with exogenous proteases supplemented in fish feed and its regulation through the dynamic changes in digestive function must be better understood.

10.4.2 Exogenous amylases in fish nutrition

In general, a dietary level of up to 20% starch is considered adequate for marine and coldwater fish species, whereas higher levels can be digested by fresh- and warmwater fish due to differences in the activity of their intestinal amylase (Wilson, 1994). Once the raw plant ingredients used to produce aquafeed are conditioned and extruded then more starch is gelatinized, making it more susceptible to the action of digestive α-amylase; the net result being a more efficient digestion and nutritive utilization by fish (Romano and Kumar, 2018). Therefore, a high content of starch in the diet or a deficient gelatinization may affect carbohydrate digestion in the digestive tract of fish. This effect is likely to be more profound in carnivorous species, where the activity of α-amylase is usually lower than in omnivore and herbivore species.

Several studies, as reviewed by Romano and Kumar (2018), evaluated the effects of including α-amylase in fish diets with different degrees of starch gelatinization. The authors concluded that, as a general trend, starch digestibility increases with the degree of starch gelatinization but the effect on growth rate is highly variable. In fact, most reports suggest that the beneficial effect of the enzyme on fish growth occurs when the starch is not or poorly gelatinized. Stone *et al.* (2003) evaluated the effects of a commercial exogenous α-amylase on the digestibility of wheat starch in silver perch (*Bidyanus bidyanus*), observing a positive effect of the enzyme on the digestibility of raw starch, whereas the digestibility of gelatinized starch was unaffected. The authors suggested that the use of α-amylase is useful if diets contain uncooked raw starch, but unnecessary if gelatinization is achieved through heat processing. Similarly, Kumar *et al.* (2006a,b,c, 2009) in different studies with rohu carp evaluated the use of different doses of α-amylase in diets including both gelatinized and non-gelatinized maize and two different levels of dietary protein. Results suggest that fish performance was better when the non-gelatinized maize was used, regardless of protein level and α-amylase feed supplementation.

The number of studies about the effects of α-amylase in fish diets is very limited in comparison to those conducted in terrestrial monogastrics. Nevertheless, more research is needed on this topic, considering the positive responses observed on starch digestion in aquafeeds containing a significant fraction of non-gelatinized starch and particularly when supplied to carnivorous fish species, which have low inherent amylase activity. There is no doubt that aquaculture will grow over the next decades on the basis of aquafeeds with a high content of plant-protein ingredients that often present significant amounts of raw starch. In this regard, the use of α-amylase as a single-enzyme source, or combined with other carbohydrases, might have an interesting potential similar to that reported in pig and poultry diets.

10.5   Outlook

Aquaculture is currently, and will be in the future, part of the solution to cover the gap between the increasing global demand for fish products for human consumption and the decreasing offer coming from fisheries. With a global aquafeed production estimated at 41 MMT for 2019 (Alltech, 2020) that shows a clear trend to increase in the future, more alternative plant-protein ingredients to produce aquafeeds will be needed. However, the presence of different ANFs in such plant ingredients will require innovative solutions based on the use of enzymatic and functional feed additives to ensure that aquaculture continues to grow sustainably.

The use of enzymes like phytase, xylanase, β-glucanase, cellulase, amylase and protease, used as a single-enzyme additive or as a blend, will contribute to a more efficient use of plant and feed ingredients. Despite the wide variety of different environments and feeding habits presented by fish species, most studies reported that the use of exogenous enzymes improves nutrient digestibility, absorption and retention, resulting in better growth and feed conversion efficiency and, in some cases, positive stimulation of the immune system. As in terrestrial non-ruminants, phytase is the enzyme producing the most significant benefits associated with nutrient utilization by fish fed plant-based diets. Currently, the molecular mechanisms of action of phytase on InsPs and their direct and indirect benefits on the digestibility of P and other minerals, dietary protein, endogenous proteases, starch and lipids are relatively very well defined in fish (Cao *et al.*, 2007; Kumar *et al.*, 2012; Dersjant-Li *et al.*, 2015; Morales *et al.*, 2016; Lemos and Tacon, 2017).

In contrast, the mechanisms whereby NSP-degrading enzymes result in better nutrient utilization, growth performance and health in non-ruminant animals, including fish, are still debated (Bedford, 2018). The great diversity of fish species of relevance in aquaculture, their feeding habits, anatomy and digestive functions, added to the fact that fish are ectothermic organisms that live at temperatures below the optimum functional temperature of most commercial enzymes, justify further research when selecting the type, combination and dose of phytase and carbohydrases for aquafeeds. In addition to those focused on phytase and NSP-degrading enzymes, more studies are needed to assess the direct and indirect effects of using exogenous serine proteases to ensure more effective protein digestion in fish, allowing for reduced protein content in diets. Similarly, additional studies are required to evaluate the effects of using exogenous α-amylase to improve the digestibility of non-gelatinized starch from plant ingredients used in aquafeeds for carnivorous fish species.

In fish nutrition, it is still imperative to define updated nutritional models, considering not only the bioavailable nutrients supplied by dietary ingredients, but also the bioavailability of additional nutrients resulting from the use of exogenous enzymes. Quantitative matrices of bioavailable nutrients from enzymatic origin are already developed for terrestrial non-ruminant production animals, in particular, to predict how much bioavailable P from InsPs will be available due to phytase activity. However, further studies would be necessary to develop a specific matrix of nutrients for aquafeed considering the target fish species, the stage of life and the environmental conditions. These advances would not only contribute to the production of more efficient and low-cost aquafeeds but also be key to develop a new generation of eco-friendly aquafeeds.

References

Adeola, O. and Cowieson, A.J. (2011) Opportunities and challenges in using exogenous enzymes to improve nonruminant animal production. *Journal of Animal Science* 89, 3189–3218.

Adeoye, A.A., Jaramillo-Torres, A., Fox, S.W., Merrifield, D.L. and Davies, S.J. (2016) Supplementation of formulated diets for tilapia (*Oreochromis niloticus*) with selected exogenous enzymes: overall performance and effects on intestinal histology and microbiota. *Animal Feed Science and Technology* 215, 133–143.

Aftab, U. and Bedford, M.R. (2018) The use of NSP enzymes in poultry nutrition: myths and realities. *World's Poultry Science Journal* 74, 1–10.

Ai, Q., Mai, K., Zhang, W., Xu, W., Tan, B., *et al.* (2007) Effects of exogenous enzymes (phytase, non-starch polysaccharide enzyme) in diets on growth, feed utilization, nitrogen and phosphorus excretion of Japanese seabass, *Lateolabrax japonicus*. *Comparative Biochemistry and Physiology – Part A: Molecular & Integrative Physiology* 147, 502–508.

Alltech (2020) Alltech® 2020 Global Feed Survey. Available at: https://www.alltech.com/sites/default/files/GFS_Brochure_2020.pdf (accessed 7 October 2021).

Arbige, M.V., Shetty, J.K. and Chotani, G.K. (2019) Industrial enzymology: the next chapter. *Trends in Biotechnology* 37, 1355–1366.

Babalola, T.O.O. (2006) The effects of feeding Moina, microdiet and xylanase supplemented microdiet on growth and survival of *Clarias gariepinus* (Burchell) larvae. *Nigerian Journal of Fisheries* 2/3, 205–217.

Bach Knudsen, K.E. (1997) Carbohydrate and lignin contents of plant materials used in animal feeding. *Animal Feed Science and Technology* 67, 319–338.

Bailey, R.W. (1973) Structural carbohydrates. In: Butler, G.W. and Bailey, R.W. (eds) *Chemistry and Biochemistry of Herbage*. Academic Press, New York, pp. 157–211.

Barrows, F.T., Stone, D.A.J. and Hardy, R.W. (2007) The effects of extrusion conditions on the nutritional value of soybean meal for rainbow trout (*Oncorhynchus mykiss*). *Aquaculture* 265, 244–252.

Bedford, M.R. (2000) Exogenous enzymes in monogastric nutrition – their current value and future benefits. *Animal Feed Science and Technology* 86, 1–13.

Bedford, M.R. (2018) The evolution and application of enzymes in the animal feed industry: the role of data interpretation. *British Poultry Science* 59, 486–493.

Bengtsson, S., Åman, P. and Graham, H. (1990) Chemical studies on mixed-linked β-glucans in hull-less barley cultivars giving different hypocholesterolemic responses in chickens. *Journal of Agricultural and Food Chemistry* 52, 435–445.

Beyer, K. (2007) Preconditioning of pet foods, aquatic and livestock feeds. In: Riaz, M.N. (ed.) *Extruders and Expanders in Pet Food, Aquatic and Livestock Feeds*. Agrimedia GmbH, Clenze, Germany, pp. 175–190.

Bowzer, J., Page, M. and Trushenski, J.T. (2016) Extrusion temperature and pellet size interact to influence growth performance of hybrid striped bass fed industrially compounded aquafeeds. *North American Journal of Aquaculture* 78, 284–294.

Campbell, G.L. and Bedford, M.R. (1992) Enzyme applications for monogastric feeds: a review. *Canadian Journal of Animal Science* 72, 449–466.

Cao, L., Wang, W., Yang, C., Yang, Y., Diana, J., *et al.* (2007) Application of microbial phytase in fish feed. *Enzyme and Microbial Technology* 40, 497–507.

Carter, C.G. and Sajjadi, M. (2011) Low fishmeal diets for Atlantic salmon, *Salmo salar* L., using soy protein concentrate treated with graded levels of phytase. *Aquaculture International* 19, 434–444.

Carter, C.G., Houlihan, D.F., Buchanan, B. and Mitchell, A.I. (1994) Growth and feed utilization efficiencies of seawater Atlantic salmon, *Salmo salar* L., fed a diet containing supplementary enzymes. *Aquaculture Research* 25, 37–46.

Castillo, S. and Gatlin, D.M. (2015) Dietary supplementation of exogenous carbohydrase enzymes in fish nutrition: a review. *Aquaculture* 435, 286–292.

Cheng, Z.J. and Hardy, R.W. (2003) Effects of extrusion and expelling processing, and microbial phytase supplementation on apparent digestibility coefficients of nutrients in full-fat soybeans for rainbow trout (*Oncorhynchus mykiss*). *Aquaculture* 218, 501–514.

Cheng, Z.J., Hardy, R.W., Verlhac, V. and Gabaudan, J. (2004) Effects of microbial phytase supplementation and dosage on apparent digestibility coefficients of nutrients and dry matter in soybean product-based diets for rainbow trout *Oncorhynchus mykiss*. *Journal of the World Aquaculture Society* 35, 1–15.

Cheryan, M. (1980) Phytic acid interactions in food systems. *CRC Critical Reviews in Food Science and Nutrition* 13, 297–335.

Choct, M. (2015) Feed non-starch polysaccharides for monogastric animals: classification and function. *Animal Production Science* 55, 1360–1366.

Choct, M. and Cadogan, D.J. (2001) How effective are supplemental enzymes in pig diets? In: Cranwell, P.D. (ed.) *Manipulating Pig Production VIII: Proceedings of the 8th Biennial Conference of the Australasian Pig Science Association (APSA), Adelaide, South Australia*. APSA, Werribee, Australia, pp. 240–247.

Cowieson, A.J., Acamovic, T. and Bedford, M.R. (2006) Phytic acid and phytase: implications for protein utilization by poultry. *Poultry Science* 85, 878–885.

Cowieson, A.J., Wilcock, P. and Bedford, M.R. (2011) Super-dosing effects of phytase in poultry and other monogastrics. *World's Poultry Science Journal* 67, 225–235.

Craig, A.D., Khattak, F., Hastie, P., Bedford, M.R. and Olukosi, O.A. (2020) Xylanase and xylo-oligosaccharide prebiotic improve the growth performance and concentration of potentially prebiotic oligosaccharides in the ileum of broiler chickens. *British Poultry Science* 61, 70–78.

Dalsgaard, J., Ekmann, K.S., Pedersen, P.B. and Verlhac, V. (2009) Effect of supplemented fungal phytase on performance and phosphorus availability by phosphorus-depleted juvenile rainbow trout (*Oncorhynchus mykiss*), and on the magnitude and composition of phosphorus waste output. *Aquaculture* 286, 105–112.

Dalsgaard, J., Verlhac, V., Hjermitslev, N.H., Ekmann, K.S., Fischer, M., *et al.* (2012) Effects of exogenous enzymes on apparent nutrient digestibility in rainbow trout (*Oncorhynchus mykiss*) fed diets with high inclusion of plant-based protein. *Animal Feed Science and Technology* 171, 181–191.

Dalsgaard, J., Bach Knudsen, K.E., Verlhac, V., Ekmann, K.S. and Pedersen, P.B. (2016) Supplementing enzymes to extruded, soybean-based diet improves breakdown of non-starch polysaccharides in rainbow trout (*Oncorhynchus mykiss*). *Aquaculture Nutrition* 22, 419–426.

Debnath, D., Pal, A.K., Narottam, P.S., Jain, K.K., Yengkokpam, S. and Mukherjee, S.C. (2005) Effect of dietary microbial phytase supplementation on growth and nutrient digestibility of *Pangasius pangasius* (Hamilton) fingerlings. *Aquaculture Research* 36, 180–187.

Denstadli, V., Skrede, A., Krogdahl, Å., Sahlstrøm, S. and Storebakken, T. (2006) Feed intake, growth, feed in Atlantic salmon (*Salmo salar* L.) fed graded levels of phytic acid. *Aquaculture* 256, 365–376.

Denstadli, V., Storebakken, T., Svihus, B. and Skrede, A. (2007) A comparison of online phytase pre-treatment of vegetable feed ingredients and phytase coating in diets for Atlantic salmon *Salmo salar* L. reared in cold water. *Aquaculture* 269, 414–426.

Dersjant-Li, Y., Awati, A., Schulze, H. and Partridge, G. (2015) Phytase in non-ruminant animal nutrition: a critical review on phytase activities in the gastrointestinal tract and influencing factors. *Journal of the Science of Food and Agriculture* 95, 878–896.

Drew, M.D., Racza, V.J., Gauthierb, R. and Thiessen, D.L. (2005) Effect of adding protease to coextruded flax:pea or canola:pea products on nutrient digestibility and growth performance of rainbow trout (*Oncorhynchus mykiss*). *Animal Feed Science and Technology* 119, 117–128.

Ebringerová, A. (2006) Structural diversity and application potential of hemicelluloses. *Macromolecular Symposia* 232, 1–12.

Ellestad, L.E., Angel, R. and Soares, J.H. Jr (2002) Intestinal phytase II: a comparison of activity and *in vivo* phytate hydrolysis in three teleost species with differing digestive strategies. *Fish Physiology and Biochemistry* 26, 259–273.

FAO (2018) *The State of World Fisheries and Aquaculture 2018 – Meeting the Sustainable Development Goals*. Food and Agriculture Organization of the United Nations, Rome.

Farhangi, M. and Carter, C.G. (2007) Effect of enzyme supplementation to dehulled lupin-based diets on growth, feed efficiency, nutrient digestibility and carcass composition of rainbow trout, *Oncorhynchus mykiss* (Walbaum). *Aquaculture Research* 38, 1274–1282.

Forster, I., Higgs, D.A., Dosanjh, B.S., Rowshandeli, M. and Parr, J. (1999) Potential for dietary phytase to improve the nutritive value of canola protein concentrate and decrease phosphorus output in rainbow trout (*Oncorhynchus mykiss*) held in 11°C fresh water. *Aquaculture* 179, 109–125.

Francis, G., Makkar, H.P.S. and Becker, K. (2001) Antinutritional factors present in plant-derived alternate fish feed ingredients and their effects in fish. *Aquaculture* 199, 197–227.

Gatlin, D.M. III, Barrows, F.T., Bellis, D., Brown, P., Campen, J., *et al.* (2007) Expanding the utilization of sustainable plant products in aquafeeds – a review. *Aquaculture Research* 38, 551–579.

German, D.P. and Bittong, R.A. (2009) Digestive enzyme activities and gastrointestinal fermentation in wood-eating catfishes. *Journal of Comparative Physiology B: Biochemical, Systemic, and Environmental Physiology* 179, 1025–1042.

Ghomi, M.R., Shahriari, R., Langroudi, H.F., Nikoo, M. and von Elert, E. (2012) Effects of exogenous dietary enzyme on growth, body composition, and fatty acid profiles of cultured great sturgeon *Huso huso* fingerlings. *Aquaculture International* 20, 249–254.

Goda, A. (2007) Effect of dietary soybean meal and phytase levels on growth, feed utilization and phosphorus discharge for Nile tilapia (*Oreochromis niloticus* L.). *Journal of Fisheries and Aquatic Science* 2, 248–263.

Goda, A., Mabrouk, H., Wafa, M. and El-Afifi, T. (2012) Effect of using baker's yeast and exogenous digestive enzymes as growth promoters on growth, feed utilization and hematological indices of Nile tilapia, *Oreochromis niloticus* fingerlings. *Journal of Agricultural Science and Technology B* 2, 15–28.

Greiling, A.M., Tschesche, C., Baardsen, G., Kröckel, S., Koppe, W. and Rodehutscord, M. (2019) Effects of phosphate and phytase supplementation on phytate degradation in rainbow trout (*Oncorhynchus mykiss* W.) and Atlantic salmon (*Salmo salar* L.). *Aquaculture* 503, 467–474.

Greiner, R. and Konietzny, U. (2010) Phytases: biochemistry, enzymology and characteristics relevant to animal feed use. In: Bedford, M.R. and Partridge, G.G. (eds) *Enzymes in Farm Animal Nutrition*, 2nd edn. CAB International, Wallingford, UK, pp. 96–128.

Grynspan, F. and Cheryan, M. (1983) Calcium phytate: effect of pH and molar ratio on *in vitro* solubility. *Journal of the American Oil Chemists' Society* 60, 1761–1764.

Haidar, M.N., Petie, M., Heinsbroek, L.T.N., Verreth, J.A.J. and Schrama, J.W. (2016) The effect of type of carbohydrate (starch vs. nonstarch polysaccharides) on nutrients digestibility, energy retention and maintenance requirements in Nile tilapia. *Aquaculture* 463, 241–247.

Hardy, R.W. (2010) Utilization of plant proteins in fish diets: effects of global demand and supplies of fish meal. *Aquaculture Research* 41, 770–776.

Hossain, M.A., Focken, U. and Becker, K. (2001) Galactomannan-rich endosperm of sesbania (*Sesbania aculeate*) seeds responsible for retardation of growth and feed utilisation in common carp, *Cyprinus carpio* L. *Aquaculture* 203, 121–132.

Hossain, M.A., Focken, U. and Becker, K. (2003) Antinutritive effects of galactomannan-rich endosperm of sesbania (*Sesbania aculeata*) seeds on growth and feed utilisation in tilapia, *Oreochromis niloticus*. *Aquaculture Research* 34, 1171–1179.

Jackson, M.E. (2010) Mannanase, alpha-galactosidase and pectinase. In: Bedford, M.R. and Partridge, G.G. (eds) *Enzymes in Farm Animal Nutrition*, 2nd edn. CAB International, Wallingford, UK, pp. 54–84.

Jiang, T.T., Feng, L., Liu, Y., Jiang, W.D., Jiang, J., *et al.* (2014) Effects of exogenous xylanase supplementation in plant protein-enriched diets on growth performance, intestinal enzyme activities and microflora of juvenile Jian carp (*Cyprinus carpio* var. Jian). *Aquaculture Nutrition* 20, 632–645.

Kaushik, S.J., Cravedi, J.P., Lalles, J.P., Sumpter, J., Fauconneau, B. and Laroche, M. (1995) Partial or total replacement of fish meal by soybean protein on the growth, protein utilisation, potential estrogenic or antigenic effects, cholesterolemia and flesh quality in rainbow trout, *Oncorhynchus mykiss*. *Aquaculture* 133, 257–274.

Khan, A. and Ghosh, K. (2013) Phytic acid-induced inhibition of digestive protease and α-amylase in three Indian major carps: an *in vitro* study. *Journal of the World Aquaculture Society* 44, 853–859.

Kiarie, E., Romero, L.F. and Nyachoti, C.M. (2013) The role of added feed enzymes in promoting gut health in swine and poultry. *Nutrition Research Reviews* 26, 71–88.

Kies, A.K., De Jonge, L.H., Kemme, P.A. and Jongbloed, A.W. (2006) Interaction between protein, phytate, and microbial phytase *in vitro* studies. *Journal of Agricultural and Food Chemistry* 54, 1753–1758.

Kraugerud, O.F., Penn, M., Storebakken, T., Refstie, S., Krogdahl, Å. and Svihus, B. (2007) Nutrient digestibilities and gut function in Atlantic salmon (*Salmo salar*) fed diets with cellulose or non-starch polysaccharides from soy. *Aquaculture* 273, 96–107.

Krogdahl, A., Hemre, G.I. and Mommsen, T.P. (2005) Carbohydrates in fish nutrition: digestion and absorption in postlarval stages. *Aquaculture Nutrition* 11, 103–122.

Krogdahl, A., Penn, M., Thorsen, J., Refstie, S. and Bakke, A.M. (2010) Important antinutrients in plant feedstuffs for aquaculture: an update on recent findings regarding responses in salmonids. *Aquaculture Research* 41, 333–344.

Krogdahl, A., Sundby, A. and Holm, H. (2015) Characteristics of digestive processes in Atlantic salmon (*Salmo salar*). Enzyme pH optima, chyme pH, and enzyme activities. *Aquaculture* 449, 27–36.

Kumar, S., Sahu, N., Pal, A., Choudhury, D., Yengkokpam, S. and Mukherjee, S. (2005) Effect of dietary carbohydrate on haematology, respiratory burst activity and histological changes in *L. rohita* juveniles. *Fish & Shellfish Immunology* 19, 331–344.

Kumar, S., Sahu, N. and Pal, A. (2006a) Non-gelatinized corn supplemented with microbial α-amylase at sub-optimal protein in the diet of *Labeo rohita* (Hamilton) fingerlings increases cell size of muscle. *Journal of Fisheries and Aquatic Science* 1, 102–111.

Kumar, S., Sahu, N., Pal, A., Choudhury, D. and Mukherjee, S. (2006b) Non-gelatinized corn supplemented with α-amylase at sub-optimum protein level enhances the growth of *Labeo rohita* (Hamilton) fingerlings. *Aquaculture Research* 37, 284–292.

Kumar, S., Sahu, N., Pal, A., Choudhury, D. and Mukherjee, S. (2006c) Studies on digestibility and digestive enzyme activities in *Labeo rohita* (Hamilton) juveniles: effect of microbial α-amylase supplementation in non-gelatinized or gelatinized corn-based diet at two protein levels. *Fish Physiology and Biochemistry* 32, 209–220.

Kumar, S., Sahu, N., Pal, A., Sagar, V., Sinha, A.K. and Baruah, K. (2009) Modulation of key metabolic enzyme of *Labeo rohita* (Hamilton) juvenile: effect of dietary starch type, protein level and exogenous α-amylase in the diet. *Fish Physiology and Biochemistry* 35, 301–315.

Kumar, V., Miasnikov, A., Sands, J.S. and Simmins, P.H. (2003) *In vitro* activities of three phytases under different pH and protease challenges. In: Paterson, J.E. (ed.) *Manipulating Pig Production IX: Proceedings of the 9th Biennial Conference of the Australasian Pig Science Association (APSA), Fremantle, Western Australia.* APSA, Werribee, Australia, p. 164.

Kumar, V., Makkar, H.P.S. and Becker, K. (2008) Detoxification of *Jatropha curcas* seed meal and its utilisation as a protein source in fish diet. *Comparative Biochemistry and Physiology – Part A: Molecular & Integrative Physiology* 151, 13–14.

Kumar, V., Makkar, H.P.S. and Becker, K. (2010) Nutritional, physiological and haematological responses in rainbow trout (*Oncorhynchus mykiss*) juveniles fed detoxified *Jatropha curcas* kernel meal. *Aquaculture Nutrition* 17, 451–467.

Kumar, V., Sinha, A.K., Makkar, H.P.S., De Boeck, G. and Becker, K. (2012) Phytate and phytase in fish nutrition. *Journal of Animal Physiology and Animal Nutrition* 96, 335–364.

Kuz'mina, V.V. (1996) Influence of age on digestive enzyme activity in some freshwater teleosts. *Aquaculture* 148, 25–37.

Lanari, D., D'Agaro, E. and Turri, C. (1998) Use of nonlinear regression to evaluate the effects of phytase enzyme treatment of plant protein diets for rainbow trout, *Oncorhynchus mykiss*. *Aquaculture* 161, 345–356.

Lee, S.A., Lupatsch, I., Gomes, G.A. and Bedford, M.R. (2020) An advanced *Escherichia coli* phytase improves performance and retention of phosphorus and nitrogen in rainbow trout (*Oncorhynchus mykiss*) fed low phosphorus plant-based diets, at 11°C and 15°C. *Aquaculture* 516, 734549.

Leenhouwers, J.I., Adjei, B.D., Verreth, J.A.J. and Schrama, J.W. (2006) Digesta viscosity, nutrient digestibility and organ weights in African catfish (*Clarias gariepinus*) fed diets supplemented with different levels of a soluble non-starch polysaccharide. *Aquaculture Nutrition* 12, 111–116.

Leenhouwers, J.I., Ter, V.M., Verreth, J.A.J. and Schrama, J.W. (2007a) Digesta characteristics and performance of African catfish (*Clarias gariepinus*) fed cereal grains that differ in viscosity. *Aquaculture* 264, 330–341.

Leenhouwers, J.I., Ortega, R.C., Verreth, J.A.J. and Schrama, J.W. (2007b) Digesta characteristics in relation to nutrient digestibility and mineral absorption in Nile tilapia (*Oreochromis niloticus* L.) fed cereal grains of increasing viscosity. *Aquaculture* 273, 556–565.

Leeson, S. (1993) Recent advances in fat utilisation by poultry. In: Farrell, D.J. (ed.) *Recent Advances in Animal Nutrition in Australia.* The University of New England, Armidale, Australia, pp. 170–181.

Leinonen, I. and Williams, A.G. (2015) Effects of dietary protease on nitrogen emissions from broiler production: a holistic comparison using life cycle assessment. *Journal of the Science of Food and Agriculture* 95, 3041–3046.

Lemos, D. and Tacon, A.G.J. (2017) Use of phytases in fish and shrimp feeds: a review. *Reviews in Aquaculture* 9, 266–282.

Li, J., Li, X., Gai, Y., Sun, Y. and Zhang, D. (2019) Evolution of *E. coli* phytase for increased thermostability guided by rational parameters. *Journal of Microbiology and Biotechnology* 29, 419–428.

Li, X.Q., Chai, X.Q., Liu, D.Y., Chowdhury, M.A.K. and Leng, X.J. (2016) Effects of temperature and feed processing on protease activity and dietary protease on growths of white shrimp, *Litopenaeus vannamei*, and tilapia, *Oreochromis niloticus* × *O. aureus*. *Aquaculture Nutrition* 22, 1283–1292.

Li, X.Q., Zhang, X.Q., Kabir Chowdhury, M.A., Zhang, Y. and Leng, X.J. (2019) Dietary phytase and protease improved growth and nutrient utilization in tilapia (*Oreochromis niloticus* × *Oreochromis aureus*) fed low phosphorus and fishmeal-free diets. *Aquaculture Nutrition* 25, 46–55.

Lin, S., Mai, K. and Tan, B. (2007) Effects of exogenous enzyme supplementation in diets on growth and feed utilization in tilapia, *Oreochromis niloticus* × *O. aureus*. *Aquaculture Research* 38, 1645–1653.

Liu, L.W., Luo, Y.W., Hou, H.L., Pan, J. and Zhang, W. (2013a) Partial replacement of monocalcium phosphate with neutral phytase in diets for grass carp, *Ctenopharyngodon idellus*. *Journal of Applied Ichthyology* 29, 520–525.

Liu, L.W., Su, J.M., Zhang, T., Liang, X.F. and Luo, Y.L. (2013b) Apparent digestibility of nutrients in grass carp (*Ctenopharyngodon idellus*) diet supplemented with graded levels of neutral phytase using pretreatment and spraying methods. *Aquaculture Nutrition* 19, 91–99.

Liu, L., Zhou, Y., Wu, J., Zhang, W., Abbas, K., *et al.* (2014) Supplemental graded levels of neutral phytase using pretreatment and spraying methods in the diet of grass carp, *Ctenopharyngodon idellus*. *Aquaculture Research* 45, 1932–1941.

Maas, R.M., Verdegem, M.C.J., Dersjant-Li, Y. and Schrama, J.W. (2018) The effect of phytase, xylanase and their combination on growth performance and nutrient utilization in Nile tilapia. *Aquaculture* 487, 7–14.

Maas, R.M., Verdegem, M.C.J. and Schrama, J.W. (2019) Effect of non-starch polysaccharide composition and enzyme supplementation on growth performance and nutrient digestibility in Nile tilapia (*Oreochromis niloticus*). *Aquaculture Nutrition* 25, 622–632.

Maenz, D.D. (2001) Enzymatic characteristics of phytases as they relate to their use in animal feeds. In: Bedford, M.R. and Partridge, G.G. (eds) *Enzymes in Farm Animal Nutrition*, 1st edn. CAB International, Wallingford, UK, pp. 61–84.

Mares, D.J. and Stone, B.A. (1973) Studies on wheat endosperm. II. Properties of the wall components and studies on their organisation in the wall. *Australian Journal of Biological Sciences* 26, 813–830.

Márquez, L., Robles, R., Morales, G.A. and Moyano, F.J. (2012) Gut pH as a limiting factor for digestive proteolysis in cultured juveniles of the gilthead sea bream (*Sparus aurata*). *Fish Physiology and Biochemistry* 38, 859–869.

Masey O'Neill, H.V., Smith, J.A. and Bedford, M.R. (2014) Multicarbohydrase enzymes for non-ruminants. *Asian-Australasian Journal of Animal Sciences* 27, 290–301.

Menezes-Blackburn, D., Gabler, S. and Greiner, R. (2015) Performance of seven commercial phytases in an *in vitro* simulation of poultry digestive tract. *Journal of Agricultural and Food Chemistry* 63, 6142–6149.

Montagne, L., Pluske, J.R. and Hampson, D.J. (2003) A review of interactions between dietary fibre and the intestinal mucosa, and their consequences on digestive health in young non-ruminant animals. *Animal Feed Science and Technology* 108, 95–117.

Morales, G.A., Moyano, F.J. and Marquez, L. (2011) *In vitro* assessment of the effects of phytate and phytase on nitrogen and phosphorus bioaccessibility within fish digestive tract. *Animal Feed Science and Technology* 170, 209–221.

Morales, G.A., Saenz de Rodrigañez, M.A., Márquez, L., Díaz, M. and Moyano, F.J. (2013) Solubilisation of protein fractions induced by *Escherichia coli* phytase and its effects on *in vitro* fish digestion of plant proteins. *Animal Feed Science and Technology* 181, 54–64.

Morales, G.A., Márquez, L., Saenz de Rodrigañez, M.A., Bermúdez, L., Robles, R. and Moyano, F.J. (2014) Effect of phytase supplementation of a plant-based diet on phosphorus and nitrogen bioavailability in sea bream *Sparus aurata*. *Aquaculture Nutrition* 20, 172–182.

Morales, G.A., Denstadli, V., Collins, S.A., Mydland, L.T., Moyano, F.J. and Øverland, M. (2015) Phytase and sodium diformate supplementation in a plant-based diet improves protein and minerals utilization in rainbow trout (*Oncorhynchus mykiss*). *Aquaculture Nutrition* 22, 1301–1311.

Morales, G.A., Márquez, L., Hernández, A.J. and Moyano, F.J. (2016) Phytase effects on protein and phosphorus bioavailability in fish diets. In: Walk, C.L., Kühn, I., Stein, H.H., Kidd, M.T. and Rodehutscord, M. (eds) *Phytate Destruction – Consequences for Precision Animal Nutrition*, Wageningen Academic Publishers, Wageningen, the Netherlands, pp. 129–165.

Morales, G.A., Azcuy, R.L., Casaretto, M.E., Márquez, L., Hernández, A.J., *et al.* (2018) Effect of different inorganic phosphorus sources on growth performance, digestibility, retention efficiency and discharge of nutrients in rainbow trout. *Aquaculture* 495, 568–574.

Morken, T., Moyano, F.J., Márquez, L., Sørensen, M., Mydland, L.T. and Øverland, M. (2012) Effects of heat treatment and sodium diformate on amino acid composition, *in vivo* digestibility in mink and *in vitro* bioavailability using digestive enzymes from Atlantic salmon. *Animal Feed Science and Technology* 178, 84–94.

Mwachireya, S.A., Beames, R.M., Higgs, D.A. and Dosanjh, B.S. (1999) Digestibility of canola protein products derived from the physical, enzymatic and chemical processing of commercial canola meal in rainbow trout *Oncorhynchus mykiss* (Walbaum) held in fresh water. *Aquaculture Nutrition* 5, 73–82.

Ng, W.K. and Chong, K.K. (2002) The nutritive value of palm kernel and the effect of enzyme supplementation in practical diets for red hybrid tilapia (*Oreochromis* sp). *Asian Fisheries Science* 15, 167–176.

Ng, W.K., Lim, H.A., Lim, S.L. and Ibrahim, C.O. (2002) Nutritive value of palm kernel meal pretreated with enzyme or fermented with *Trichoderma koningii* (Oudemans) as a dietary ingredient for red hybrid tilapia (*Oreochromis* sp.). *Aquaculture Research* 33, 1199–1207.

NRC (2011) *Nutrient Requirements of Fish and Shrimp*. National Academies Press, Washington, DC.

Ogunkoya, A.E., Page, G.I., Adewolu, M.A. and Bureau, D.P. (2006) Dietary incorporation of soybean meal and exogenous enzyme cocktail can affect physical characteristics of faecal material egested by rainbow trout (*Oncorhynchus mykiss*). *Aquaculture* 254, 466–475.

Øvrum, H.J. and Storebakken, T. (2007) Effects of cellulose inclusions on pellet quality and digestibility of main nutrients and minerals in rainbow trout (*Oncorhynchus mykiss*). *Aquaculture* 272, 458–465.

Partridge, G.G. (2001) The role and efficacy of carbohydrase enzymes in pig nutrition. In: Bedford, M.R. and Partridge, G.G. (eds) *Enzymes in Farm Animal Nutrition*, 1st edn. CAB International, Wallingford, UK, pp. 161–198.

Perlin, A.S. (1951) Isolation and composition of the soluble pentosans of wheat flours. *Cereal Chemistry* 28, 370–391.

Pontes, T.C., França, W.G., Dutra, F.M., Portz, L. and Ballester, E.L.C. (2019) Evaluation of the phytase enzyme in granulated and liquid forms for Nile tilapia (*Oreochromis niloticus*). *Archivos de Zootecnia* 68, 158–163.

Pontoppidan, K., Pettersson, D. and Sandberg, A.S. (2007) *Peniophora lycii* phytase is stable and degrades phytate and solubilises minerals *in vitro* during simulation of gastrointestinal digestion in the pig. *Journal of the Science of Food and Agriculture* 87, 2700–2708.

Ragaa, N.M., Elala, N.M.A., Kamal, A.M. and Kamel, N.F. (2017) Effect of a serine-protease on performance parameters and protein digestibility of cultured *Oreochromis niloticus* fed diets with different protein levels. *Pakistan Journal of Nutrition* 6, 148–154.

Ramos, L.R.V., Pedrosa, V.F., Mori, A., De Andrade, C.F.F., Romano, L.A., *et al.* (2017) Exogenous enzyme complex prevents intestinal soybean meal induced enteritis in *Mugil liza* (Valenciennes, 1836) juvenile. *Annals of the Brazilian Academy of Sciences* 89, 341–353.

Ray, A.K., Ghosh, K. and Ringo, E. (2012) Enzyme-producing bacteria isolated from fish gut: a review. *Aquaculture Nutrition* 18, 465–492.

Refstie, S., Svihus, B., Shearer, K.D. and Storebakken, T. (1999) Nutrient digestibility in Atlantic salmon and broiler chickens related to viscosity and non-starch polysaccharide content in different soybean products. *Aquaculture* 79, 331–345.

Rodehutscord, M. and Pfeffer, E. (1995) Effects of supplemental microbial phytase on phosphorus digestibility and utilization in rainbow trout, *Oncorhynchus mykiss*. *Water Science and Technology* 31, 143–147.

Romano, N. and Kumar, V. (2018) Starch gelatinization on the physical characteristics of aquafeeds and subsequent implications to the productivity in farmed aquatic animals. *Reviews in Aquaculture* 11, 1271–1284.

Roy, T., Banerjee, G., Dan, S.K., Ghosh, P. and Ray, A.K. (2014) Improvement of nutritive value of sesame oil-seed meal in formulated diets for rohu, *Labeo rohita* (Hamilton), fingerlings after fermentation with two phytase producing bacterial strains isolated from fish gut. *Aquaculture International* 22, 633–652.

Santos-Hernández, C., Miralles, B., Amigo, L. and Recio, I. (2018) Intestinal signaling of proteins and digestion derived products relevant to satiety. *Journal of Agricultural and Food Chemistry* 66, 10123–10131.

Schaefer, A. and Koppe, W.M. (1995) Effect of a microbial phytase on utilization of native phosphorus by carp in a diet based on soybean meal. *Water Science and Technology* 31, 149–155.

Schlemmer, U., Jany, K.D., Berk, A., Schulz, E. and Rechkemmer, G. (2001) Degradation of phytate in the gut of pigs – pathway of gastro-intestinal inositol phosphate hydrolysis and enzymes involved. *Archives of Animal Nutrition* 55, 255–280.

Selle, P.H. and Ravindran, V. (2007) Microbial phytase in poultry nutrition. *Animal Feed Science and Technology* 135, 1–41.

Selle, P.H. and Ravindran, V. (2008) Phytate-degrading enzymes in pig nutrition. *Livestock Science* 113, 99–122.

Selle, P.H., Ravindran, V., Caldwell, R.A. and Bryden, W.L. (2000) Phytate and phytase: consequences for protein utilization. *Nutrition Research Reviews* 13, 255–278.

Selle, P.H., Ravindran, V., Bryden, W.L. and Scott, T. (2006) Influence of dietary phytate and exogenous phytase on amino acid digestibility in poultry: a review. *Journal of Poultry Science* 43, 89–103.

Shi, X., Luo, Z., Chen, F., Huang, C., Zhu, X.-M. and Liu, X. (2017) Effects of dietary cellulase addition on growth performance, nutrient digestibility and digestive enzyme activities of juvenile crucian carp *Carassius auratus*. *Aquaculture Nutrition* 23, 618–628.

Shimeno, S., Hosokawa, H., Yamane, R., Masumoto, T. and Uneno, S.I. (1992) Change in nutritive value of de-fatted soybean meal with duration of heating time for yellowtail. *Nippon Suisan Gakkaishi* 58, 1351–1359.

Simon, O. (1998) The mode of action of NSP hydrolysing enzymes in the gastrointestinal tract. *Journal of Animal and Feed Sciences* 7, 115–123.

Sinha, A.K., Kumar, V., Makkar, H.P.S., De Boeck, G. and Becker, K. (2011) Non-starch polysaccharides and their role in fish nutrition – a review. *Food Chemistry* 127, 1409–1426.

Sørensen, M. (2012) A review of the effects of ingredient composition and processing conditions on the physical qualities of extruded high-energy fish feed as measured by prevailing methods. *Aquaculture Nutrition* 18, 233–248.

Stone, D.A.J., Allan, G.I. and Anderson, A.J. (2003) Carbohydrate utilization by juvenile silver perch, *Bidyanus bidyanus* (Mitchell). IV. Can dietary enzymes increase digestible energy from wheat starch, wheat and dehulled lupin? *Aquaculture Research* 34, 135–147.

Storebakken, T. (1985) Binders in fish feeds: I. Effect of alginate and guar gum on growth, digestibility, feed intake and passage through the gastrointestinal tract of rainbow trout. *Aquaculture* 47, 11–26.

Storebakken, T. and Austreng, E. (1987) Binders in fish feeds: II. Effect of different alginates on digestibility of macronutrients in rainbow trout. *Aquaculture* 60, 121–131.

Storebakken, T., Shearer, K.D. and Roem, A.J. (1998) Availability of protein, phosphorus and other elements in fish meal, soy-protein concentrate and phytase-treated soy-protein-concentrate-based diets to Atlantic salmon, *Salmo salar*. *Aquaculture* 161, 365–379.

Storebakken, T., Kvien, I.S., Shearer, K.D., Grisdale-Helland, B. and Helland, S.J. (1999) Estimation of gastro-intestinal evacuation rate in Atlantic salmon (*Salmo salar*) using inert markers and collection of faeces by sieving: evacuation of diets with fish meal, soybean meal or bacterial meal. *Aquaculture* 172, 291–299.

Strahm, B.S. (2000) Preconditioning. In: Riaz, M.N. (ed.) *Extruders in Food Applications*. Technomic Publishing Company, Inc., Lancaster, Pennsylvania, pp. 115–126.

Sugiura, S.H., Gabaudan, J., Dong, F.M. and Hardy, R.W. (2001) Dietary microbial phytase supplementation and the utilization of phosphorus, trace minerals and protein by rainbow trout *Oncorhynchus mykiss* (Walbaum) fed soybean meal-based diets. *Aquaculture Research* 32, 583–592.

Sugiura, S.H., Hardy, R.W. and Roberts, R.J. (2004) The pathology of phosphorus deficiency in fish – a review. *Journal of Fish Diseases* 27, 255–265.

Svihus, B. (2010) Effect of digestive tract conditions, feed processing and ingredients on response to NSP enzymes. In: Bedford, M.R. and Partridge, G.G. (eds) *Enzymes in Farm Animal Nutrition*, 2nd edn. CAB International, Wallingford, UK, pp. 129–159.

Thakur, B.R., Singh, R.K. and Handa, A.K. (1997) Chemistry and uses of pectin – a review. *Critical Reviews in Food Science and Nutrition* 37, 47–73.

Thammarutwasik, P., Hongpattarakere, T., Chantachum, S., Kijroongrojana, K., Itharat, A., *et al.* (2009) Prebiotics – a review. *Songklanakarin Journal of Science and Technology* 31, 401–408.

Vahjen, W., Glaser, K., Schafer, K. and Simon, O. (1998) Influence of xylanase-supplemented feed on the development of selected bacterial groups in the intestinal tract of broiler chicks. *Journal of Agricultural Science* 130, 489–500.

van Barneveld, R.J. (1999) Understanding the nutritional chemistry of lupin (*Lupinus* spp.) seed to improve livestock production efficiency. *Nutrition Research Reviews* 12, 203–230.

Vandenberg, G.W., Scott, S.L., Sarker, P.K., Dallaire, V. and Noüe, J. (2011) Encapsulation of microbial phytase: effects on phosphorus bioavailability in rainbow trout (*Oncorhynchus mykiss*). *Animal Feed Science and Technology* 169, 230–243.

Vandenberg, G.W., Scott, S.L. and Noüe, J. (2012) Factors affecting nutrient digestibility in rainbow trout (*Oncorhynchus mykiss*) fed a plant protein-based diet supplemented with microbial phytase. *Aquaculture Nutrition* 18, 369–379.

Verlhac-Trichet, V., Vielma, J., Dias, J., Rema, P., Santigosa, E., *et al.* (2014) The efficacy of a novel microbial 6-phytase expressed in *Aspergillus oryzae* on the performance and phosphorus utilization of cold- and warm-water fish: rainbow trout, *Oncorhynchus mykiss*, and Nile tilapia, *Oreochromis niloticus*. *Journal of the World Aquaculture Society* 45, 367–379.

Vielma, J., Ruohonen, K., Gabaudan, J. and Vogel, K. (2004) Top-spraying soybean meal-based diets with phytase improves protein and mineral digestibilities but not lysine utilization in rainbow trout, *Oncorhynchus mykiss* (Walbaum). *Aquaculture Research* 35, 955–964.

Wallace, B.J.L., Murray, F.J. and Little, D.C. (2016) Effects of β-xylanase and 6-phytase on digestibility, trace mineral utilisation and growth in juvenile red tilapia, *Oreochromis niloticus* (Linnaeus, 1758) × *O. mossambicus* (Peters, 1852), fed declining fishmeal diets. *Journal of Applied Ichthyology* 32, 471–479.

Wang, F., Yang, Y.H., Han, Z.Z., Dong, H.W., Yang, C.H. and Zou, Z.Y. (2009) Effects of phytase pretreatment of soybean meal and phytase-sprayed in diets on growth, apparent digestibility coefficient and nutrient excretion of rainbow trout (*Oncorhynchus mykiss* Walbaum). *Aquaculture International* 17, 143–157.

Wilson, R.P. (1994) Utilization of dietary carbohydrate by fish. *Aquaculture* 124, 67–80.

Yigit, N.O. and Olmez, M. (2011) Effects of cellulase addition to canola meal in tilapia (*Oreochromis niloticus* L.) diets. *Aquaculture Nutrition* 17, 494–500.

Yildirim, Y.B. and Turan, F. (2010) Effects of exogenous enzyme supplementation in diets on growth and feed utilization in African catfish, *Clarias gariepinus*. *Journal of Animal and Veterinary Advances* 9, 327–331.

Zamini, A., Kanani, H., Esmaeili, A., Ramezani, S. and Zoriezahra, S. (2014) Effects of two dietary exogenous multi-enzyme supplementation, Natuzyme® and beta-mannanase (Hemicell®), on growth and blood parameters of Caspian salmon (*Salmo trutta caspius*). *Comparative Clinical Pathology* 23, 187–192.

Zhou, Y., Yuan, X., Liang, X., Fang, L., Li, J., *et al.* (2013) Enhancement of growth and intestinal flora in grass carp: the effect of exogenous cellulase. *Aquaculture* 416–417, 1–7.

11 Analysis of Enzymes, Principles and Challenges: Developments in Feed Enzyme Analysis

Noel Sheehan*

AB Vista, Ystrad Mynach, UK

11.1 Introduction

Traditional methods for analysing enzyme activity by 'wet chemistry' methods, as described in the previous edition of this book (Sheehan, 2010), whether in products, premixes or feeds, have posed challenges in the modern laboratory. These challenges include the repetitiveness of the work that was difficult to automate and utilized substrates and methodologies that did not always fully define the enzyme activity and required laboratory facilities with the equipment and management systems to handle hazardous chemicals. Over the past decade, however, there have been significant developments in both methods and equipment that have helped alleviate such constraints. This has enabled the larger service laboratories downstream of the production process, where there is a commercial imperative to provide analysis results in a relevant time frame, to increase throughput and decrease turnaround time. It has also increased the agility of the smaller laboratories involved in analysis of finished feed. Developments over the past decade include:

1. New types of laboratory equipment have allowed laboratories to partially automate the assay workflow in traditional enzyme 'wet chemistry' methods, such as outlined in Section 11.2.

2. Immunoassay methods such as ELISAs and lateral flow devices (LFDs) have been used routinely in the last 10 years to detect their specific target enzyme products in-feed. Immunoassay in general offers greater specificity for the analyte than wet chemistry analysis. Plate-based ELISA is suited to high throughput, including full automation of the assay workflow in a laboratory environment, while LFDs provide quick tests that can provide results within minutes with elementary laboratory technology and skills.

3. A new method for measuring phytase activity, based on measuring the reduction in turbidity of a phytic acid ($InsP_6$)–lysozyme complex, that offers a faster, safer alternative to the traditional wet chemistry analysis for phytases and that additionally is adaptable to high-throughput screening.

4. A new method for analysing xylanases has also become available. Traditional substrates manufactured by extracting the xylan from wheat and beech are not well-defined chemically and may vary from batch to batch or with different manufacturers. The new assay, called the XylX6 assay, uses a chemically defined colorimetric

**Email: noelsheehan@abvista.com

©CAB International 2022. *Enzymes in Farm Animal Nutrition, 3rd Edition* (M. Bedford *et al.* eds)
DOI: 10.1079/9781789241563.0011

synthetic substrate based on a xylo-oligosaccharide (XOS) tagged with a *p*-nitrophenol molecule at one end and with a blocker at the other end to prevent degradation by β-xylosidase. The ultimate release of the *p*-nitrophenol by endoxylanase results in yellow colour that is easily measured. Unlike the traditional reducing sugar methods, no boiling step or harsh chemicals are required, thus facilitating automation.

5. A new method for analysing proteases has become available as well. Traditional substrates include casein and haemoglobin, and the assay utilizes precipitation that requires centrifugation or filtration. The new assay, relatively new to the feed industry, uses a chemically defined colorimetric synthetic substrate, Suc-Ala-Ala-Pro-Phe-pNA. Protease cleaves the substrate, releasing the chromogen *p*-nitroaniline (pNA). The amount of released yellow pNA colour is proportional to the protease activity of the enzyme and results in a yellow colour that is easily measured. Like the new xylanase method, no boiling step or harsh chemicals are required, thus facilitating automation and ease of use.

6. In the past, analysis of enzyme activity from vitamin/mineral premixes was particularly fraught with problems due to the high content of interfering mineral ions in the extraction step. Now, a simple workaround, of mixing the premix into blank feed, allows premixes to be analysed by an existing method developed for feed analysis.

11.2   Partial Automation of Wet Chemistry-Type Assays is Possible

Analysis of feed enzymes, whether in feed samples or in premixes and products, by traditional wet chemistry methods can be time-consuming. This is because it can be difficult to achieve full workflow automation when steps such as centrifugation or boiling are involved. However, in recent years, it has become possible to achieve some partial workflow automation, with examples below including the use of plate readers, multichannel pipettors with variable tip spacing and automated diluter systems.

In the International Organization for Standardization (ISO) phytase method (Gizzi *et al.*, 2008; ISO, 2009), it is stipulated to have three reaction tubes and two blank tubes = five test-tubes per feed extract that is assayed. As each sample will have duplicate or triplicate extractions, on a busy day, analysing approximately 16 samples, with duplicate extractions, plus at least one positive and negative control extraction and calibration curve tubes, generates approximately 200 test-tubes that will require reading on a spectrophotometer. The typical options for this are to pour the solutions into a cuvette, place into the spectrophotometer cell and take the reading: either manually in a lab notebook or on a printout from the spectrophotometer to be transcribed later into an electronic format; or typed directly into an electronic sheet (some laboratories will not allow this last option for data traceability reasons). In addition, for transferring the solutions to the spectrophotometer, some laboratories use a sipper accessory. The sipper is a pump system that supplies the solution from a test-tube or beaker directly into the sample compartment and so offers health and safety benefits over the manual method. However, when using this, the cycle to complete a reading on the sipper can be even longer than the manual method (due to the need for washing between samples) and thus can further increase the time for this process.

At our laboratories we have adopted two strategies to semi-automate this process. First, instead of taking a reading in a spectrophotometer, we have switched to taking the readings on 96-well plates. This follows the same Beer–Lambert rule as a spectrophotometer, with just the caveat that in a spectrophotometer the distance is fixed usually to 10 mm by the width of the cuvette. In a plate reader, this is variable depending on the depth of the liquid. In our work, we have found that in a typical 96-well flat-bottom plate, 0.3 ml gives a very similar absorbance to the cuvette. Even with this efficiency, it is still relatively time-consuming to pipette an aliquot from each tube on to the plate, one at a time.

A further efficiency is to use a multichannel pipettor with variable tip-spacing. Standard multichannel pipettors have the distance between channels fixed so it is not possible to use these to transfer liquids from a test-tube rack to a 96-well plate. However, using multichannel pipettor with variable tip-spacing means the channels can be moved further apart to aspirate the liquid from the tubes and then moved closer together for dispensing to the plate. Using these two strategies can result in savings of many hours of repetitive work and can semi-automate what are quite 'old-fashioned' methods and prevent queues to use laboratory equipment.

Similarly, in running the assays on the feed enzyme additive, the dilution process needed to bring the sample into the range that can be detected in the assay can often be quite a time-consuming step; due to the high activity of the samples to be analysed, multiple serial dilutions are required, often involving pipetting small volumes of liquid where small errors of 1–2 µl could result in a 2–4% error in the analysis. With potentially three serial dilution steps for the highest-activity samples, this could result in a compounded error of 6–12% just on the dilution steps alone, therefore it is very important to carry out these steps with a great deal of accuracy. Manual pipetting by a human will always be subject to some error and therefore a preferred method would be to use a diluter system. From our experience where an analyst had 24 extractions on which to perform dilutions, where the dilutions were also being recorded on an analytical balance, diluting the samples could take >60 min whereas using an automated dilution system can cut this process down to <20 min.

Using these strategies can result in savings of many hours of repetitive work and can semi-automate what are quite 'old-fashioned' methods, with the speed of the new strategies preventing queues to use laboratory equipment as well.

11.3   Use of Immunoassay Techniques

Immunoassays use antibodies as the detecting ('capture') reagents. Antibodies are glycoproteins produced by specific cells of the immune systems of animals in response to stimulation by a foreign substance. The foreign substance that elicits the production of a specific antibody is referred to as an antigen. The attribute of an antibody that makes it useful as a reagent in a diagnostic kit is its capacity to bind with high specificity and affinity to the antigen that elicited its production. Immunoassay methods involve two different techniques: ELISA (enzyme-linked immunosorbent assay) or LFD (immunochromatography lateral flow device). Immunoassays are already a widely used tool in agriculture, for example for analysis of mycotoxins (Chu, 1984) and more recently for the analysis of genetically modified proteins (Grothaus et al., 2006). Additionally, ELISA has also been developed to detect heparinase enzyme activity and the assay preferentially detects the 8+50 kDa active heparinase heterodimer versus the latent 65 kDa pro-enzyme (Shafat et al., 2006).

While the wet chemistry methods remain the typical industry methods for enzyme analysis, AB Vista are using an alternative technology, based on immunoassay techniques, to analyse enzyme activity in feeds. To detect the AB Vista enzyme activities in feed, antibodies were produced that are specific to the folded, active xylanase or phytase protein. These are highly specific and do not react with similar commercial enzymes such as other Escherichia coli phytases. These antibodies are then incorporated, in what is typically referred to as a 'sandwich ELISA', into a diagnostic kit (Graham and Sheehan, 2013). For the actual analysis, the feed sample is milled and extracted in much the same way as it would be for a traditional wet chemistry method, an aliquot of the extract centrifuged, the supernatant diluted (if necessary, according to the activity of the sample and the range of the kit) and then analysed using the diagnostic ELISA kit. This kit contains an antibody-coated (antibodies immobilized to the plate) 96-well microplate, an enzyme-conjugated secondary antibody, standards, controls, an enzyme substrate for colour development, washing buffer and sample extraction buffer. As shown in Fig. 11.1, on addition of the diluted extract to the ELISA well, the antibodies coated on to the plate wells capture the target enzyme protein

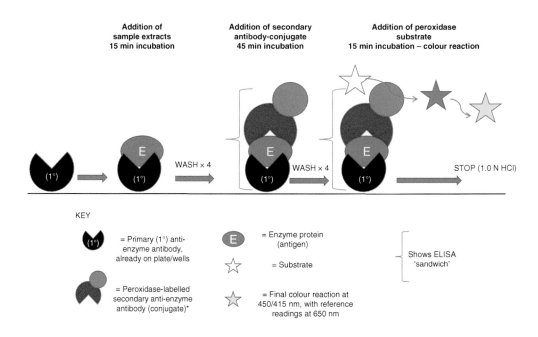

Fig. 11.1. ELISA sandwich assay. (Author's own figure.)

and after a set time, the plate is washed to remove the feed extract and any unbound antigen. Another antibody, conjugated to a horseradish peroxidase enzyme, is then added, which also binds to the enzyme protein, forming the ELISA 'sandwich'. After another wash step, a substrate for the peroxidase is added, which produces a colour reaction. The enzyme activity in the test sample is quantified by reference to a series of calibrator solutions also containing the active enzyme, alongside a positive and negative control sample that are always included in every assay run to monitor the performance of the assay carried out that day.

The advantages of ELISA are the high specificity and high signal-to-noise ratio; plus, at least after the initial step, it is unlikely that anything from the sample will interfere with the subsequent detection of bound antigen, whereas in other wet chemistry methods there is always the possibility of feed sample components being carried through the extraction and dilution. ELISA is a well-established and worldwide technology, using essentially harmless reagents,

and there is a whole range of equipment available that can thus be used to turn feed analysis into a high-throughput endeavour. Even when using the manual assay it is possible for an analyst, using multi-channel pipettors, to analyse 40 tests relatively easily in a half a day, while by comparison with the older wet chemistry methods, an analyst could probably only analyse half that number of samples and with significantly greater effort as well. Automated systems are also available to run ELISA analysis. While the effort to mill samples, do the extractions and dilute samples is still required in both ELISA and wet chemistry, once at this stage, the automated systems offer the analyst the walk-away option of loading samples into the analyser and returning approximately two hours later for the results.

LFDs for the detection of AB Vista enzymes use the same 'sandwich' principle as ELISA, except with a different detection mechanism. In ELISA, the detection mechanism is based on producing hydrogen peroxide which then reacts with a chromophore to produce a colour. LFDs use typically an

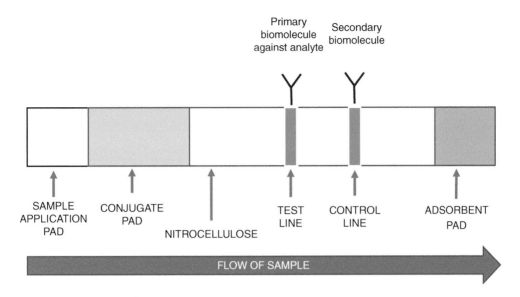

Fig. 11.2. The layout of an LFD. (Author's own figure, based on example in Grothaus *et al.*, 2006.)

antibody in the system labelled with a coloured particle that can be seen visually, the most common being colloidal gold.

A typical LFD, as shown in Fig. 11.2 (and, for example, in Grothaus *et al.*, 2006), consists of a sample application pad, a conjugate pad, a nitrocellulose membrane and a wicking (adsorbent) pad assembled on a thin plastic backing. The principle behind the LFD is that a liquid sample (or its extract) containing the analyte of interest moves through simple capillary flow through the LFD. There are different zones in the LFD strips which contain molecules that can interact with the analyte if present in the sample.

To use the LFD for detection of phytase in-feed, for instance, a portion of feed (e.g. 10 g) is first extracted by adding 100–150 ml of tap water and with vigorous shaking by hand for 30 s. The solid particles are then allowed to settle, and an aliquot of the liquid (extract) is added to a small vial.

The end of the test strip with the sample pad is then dipped into the vial and allowed to remain there for 5 min for the test to take place. Once the LFD test strip is added to the extract, the liquid then begins moving by simple capillary flow laterally through the strip with the sample pad

providing some additional filtration to prevent large particles blocking the flow of liquid. (In some LFDs, the sample pad may also be treated to adjust the sample properties, such as the pH.)

At the first stage of the test the liquid sample flows through the conjugate pad, which contains at least one mobile capture antibody that is specific to the phytase protein (analyte/antigen) and also contains another mobile antibody that does not capture the phytase protein, with both of these antibodies being gold labelled. As the sample flows through this, the mobile capture antibody will form a complex by binding the phytase (MBC–Phy).

At the next stage of the test, the liquid will now contain mobile capture antibody (i.e. that which has not bound the phytase due to being in excess), MBC–Phy and the second antibody specific to the check-zone antigen. The first zone is designed to capture the phytase protein and so then forms the antibody sandwich. For a sample with phytase protein present, this accumulates at this zone until this becomes visible to the naked eye as a line across the LFD. Liquid continues to flow along the strip to the second zone and at this second zone the non-capture antibody will bind to the check-zone antigen, also producing a visible line to show that the test has worked (liquid flowed properly). This provides a very simple visual technology with three options:

1. One test line visible = test has worked but the sample is negative for phytase.
2. Two test lines visible = test has worked and the sample is positive for phytase.
3. No line visible = test has not worked, repeat.

More advanced versions of the technology can be used that enable the results to be more quantitative when combined with a scanner (Davis and Roberts, 2013; Koczula and Gallotta, 2016). At AB Vista laboratories, in combination with our technology partner, Envirologix, we have validated this technology for use in global markets for the analysis of phytase and xylanase in-feed (see Fig. 11.3).

The advantages of this LFD technology, whether just for the yes/no qualitative answer or for the more quantitative approach, is of course the simplicity. A drop of sample extract is added to the test strip, or the strip is dipped into the extract in a small vial, wait five minutes and results are available. The latter quantitative option offers significant benefits to small laboratories such as found

within a feed mill, with just a means to grind the sample homogeneously (preferably a laboratory-grade mill), the scanner and some glassware. Although no specialist skills are required, some analytical thoroughness is required from the person running the analysis to ensure the best, most accurate and precise results.

11.4   A Novel Method to Analyse Phytase

Current wet chemistry phytase methods are relatively time-consuming and the dangerous chemicals used represent significant barriers for many laboratories, especially the smaller, less well-equipped laboratories, where investment in local exhaust ventilation devices such as fume cabinets is required to prepare reagents and perform the assay, and for the administrative burden that using these chemicals generates. While the immunoassay techniques as described in Section 11.3 offer a high-throughput method that resolves many of these problems, the initial development of the antibodies is relatively expensive and provides assay methods that are specific to a particular phytase molecule.

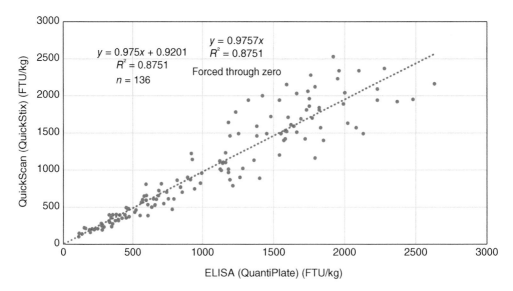

Fig. 11.3. Analysis of samples for Quantum® Blue phytase by two different methods, internal data. The *x*-axis refers to feed samples analysed for Quantum Blue by the established ELISA plate method, while the *y*-axis refers to the same samples analysed using the LFD with scanner method. (Author's own figure.)

A new method for measuring phytase activity, based on measuring the reduction in turbidity of an $InsP_6$–lysozyme complex, that offers a faster, safer alternative to the traditional wet chemistry analysis of phytases and that additionally is adaptable to high-throughput screening has recently been developed (Tran et al., 2011). In that study, five phytases (of which four were commercial products used in the feed industry) were tested including two from E. coli, one from Bacillus sp., one from Aspergillus niger and another from Peniophora lycii. The isoelectric point (pI) of a protein is the pH at which the protein has no net charge. The authors noted that $InsP_6$–protein complexes are usually turbid at a pH lower than the pI of the protein. Lysozyme has a pI between 10.5 and 11.0 (Alderton et al., 1945). Therefore, lysozyme offered opportunities to produce a substrate that would have, at time zero of any enzyme assay, a high level of turbidity, measured as optical density in a plate reader or spectrophotometer at 600 nm (OD_{600}), across a range of different pH values relevant to the animal feed industry. In initial studies to determine the optimum combination of $InsP_6$ and lysozyme, Tran and co-workers determined a ratio of 1.5:1, or more specifically 0.3:0.23 mM of $InsP_6$:lysozyme. Using this combination of $InsP_6$:lysozyme produced optimal substrate complexes for analysing phytase in the pH range of 2.5–5.5 due to:

- excellent stability of these complexes (no loss of turbidity when stored refrigerated, at 5–8°C, for several months); and
- similar turbidity across the pH range – this would be important so that small fluctuations in pH due to instrument uncertainty would not cause variability in assays.

This substrate then was used to analyse the five different phytases and the decrease in turbidity was shown to have a linear correlation with the increase in the release of inorganic phosphate (Pi). The release of one international unit, one micromole of Pi per minute, was correlated to a 3.03-unit OD decrease per minute at OD_{600}.

As with the new xylanase method discussed in Section 11.5 below, it is unlikely

that this method will immediately gain a widespread acceptance and replace the older methods that use more toxic chemicals, especially in the quality control/service environment, where end-point assays are usually favoured over kinetic assays and where the current methods are heavily embedded in the industry. This method is/will also be dependent on the quality of and the steady supply of the phytic acid and lysozyme substrate and having the exact molarity of each well defined. If past history just in the supply of phytic acid is an indicator, specific products may be discontinued with little notice by large chemical suppliers from their catalogues.

In the work as presented by Tran et al. (2011), this method was used primarily on relatively high-activity products. As the phytase produced at the enzyme manufacturing plant moves through the supply chain, into such sample matrices as premixes, blends, complementary feeds and finished feeds for different target species, the activity per kilogram of sample becomes lower and the possible interferences become more prevalent. The sensitivity of this new method is lower than existing methods: 'feed samples containing maize and soy flour and E. coli phytase variant 1 at 400–2300 FTU/kg could be assayed by the kinetic method, whereas with a phytase level at 200 FTU/kg or lower in the feed the kinetic method was not suitable because the incubation needed to be overnight' (Tran et al., 2011). So, this method is probably not suitable, without further development, for phytase analysis in feed. For comparison, the ISO 30024:2009(E) phytase method quotes 20 and 60 U/kg as the limit of detection and limit of quantification, respectively (ISO, 2009). Generally, to increase the sensitivity in assays the options are to increase the time or temperature of the assay or to move the pH closer to the optimum. The suggestion would be that if feeds <200 U/kg require an overnight assay, then even feeds of 200–500 FTU/kg would probably need an extended assay of several hours. 'Real-world' feeds are also likely to contain minerals and other ingredients, and with this lack of sensitivity in the assay for commercial feeds comes the imperative to avoid diluting the sample. This means, however, that a key strategy to avoid matrix effects interfering in analysis, namely that of diluting out these matrix effects, would not be available when analysing feeds by this method. One possibility for further improvement to the Tran *et al.* (2011) method is to use a pretreatment of the samples to reduce background interference, one example being to desalt the feed extract using PD-10 desalting columns with molecular weight cut-off of 2500. Nevertheless, such a pretreatment would still further dilute the sample. Alternatively, as described by Kim and Lei (2005), samples can be concentrated and cleaned using a combination of a 0.45 µm filtration followed by the use of spin columns with a molecular weight cut-off of 30,000. While these might add extra complexity by adding two extra steps, this could clean up the feed sample, providing assurance that components in the sample matrix, such as other proteins or fats, low-molecular-weight mineral ions and phytic acid originating from the feed sample, are no longer able to interfere with the assay. The result would be reduced variability in the analysis with the added benefit that the spin columns can also concentrate the sample, which might help to adapt this method to lower-activity feed samples.

In other potential future developments, it has been shown already that an enzymatic method can be used for measuring Pi. This technology also avoids using the traditional toxic and/or corrosive chemicals associated with measuring phosphate. Instead, the Pi analysis can be carried out enzymatically with a phosphate detection method relying on the use of purine nucleoside phosphorylase (PN-Pase) and 2-amino-6-mercapto-7-methylpurine ribonucleoside (MESG) (Webb, 1992). The reaction between Pi and MESG can be measured on a spectrophotometer at 360 nm. News from within the industry suggests this technology is close to being commercialized into an easy-to-use kit form in 2021.

11.5   A New Way to Analyse Xylanase

As discussed in the second edition of this book (Sheehan, 2010), the most popular

method of analysing carbohydrase enzymes such as cellulase (EC 3.2.1.4), β-glucanase (EC 3.21.6), mannanase (EC 3.2.1.78) and xylanase (EC 3.2.1.8) activity, especially in high-activity samples such as products, premixes and blends, is via the DNS method (McCleary and McGeough, 2015). In this method, 3,5-dinitrosalicylic acid (DNS) is used in a reagent to detect production of reducing sugars by carbohydrases. Despite the widespread use of this methodology, there are limitations. Although the method is typically used to measure the more relevant endo-acting enzymes, it does not distinguish between the reducing sugar that is produced when, for example, a xylanase catalyses the breakdown of a xylan substrate into XOS versus the xylose reducing sugar that is produced by the action of β-xylosidase (EC 3.2.1.37). In animal feeding, it is the former enzyme that is considered to be beneficial and breaking down the xylan substrate completely to xylose would be considered detrimental (Schutte, 1990; Schutte *et al.*, 1992). So, if comparing two enzyme products, this method might overestimate the activity differences or potentially their effect in the animal if a significant β-xylosidase activity was present in the one and not the other. The DNS method is also dependent on a boiling step which makes full automation impossible. The boiling step may also produce additional reducing sugars that overestimate activity (McCleary and McGeough, 2015) and this can also make it difficult to standardize the assay across different laboratories with different boiling apparatus. The DNS method utilizes native polysaccharide substrates that are liable to batch-to-batch differences in composition and purity (Bailey *et al.*, 1992), as well as interruptions in supply, without consultation of the feed industry (previously many laboratories were using the birch xylan from Sigma-Aldrich to measure xylanase activity, but Sigma-Aldrich discontinued this during the last decade, meaning many laboratories had to switch to and validate the use of beechwood xylan instead).

To address these concerns, a new substrate has been developed to measure xylanase that:

- is more chemically defined and can therefore address some of the industry and research issues such as detecting only endoxylanase activity and not accidentally also detecting β-xylosidase; and
- provides a substrate that offers the potential for greater automation and a more standardized way of measuring activity (Mangan *et al.*, 2017).

This new substrate utilizes three 'tricks':

1. To begin with, it uses tried-and-tested technology that is already used to measure disaccharidases, which is the chemical *p*-nitrophenol. In the feed industry, for example, this is already used to measure α-galactosidase (EC 3.2.1.22). For measuring α-galactosidase, a galactose is tagged at the reducing end with *p*-nitrophenol, which resembles a glucose molecule, to produce the substrate *p*-nitrophenyl-α-galactopyranoside. In the bound state *p*-nitrophenol is colourless but in the unbound state, and especially in alkaline solution, it forms a yellow colour that is easily detectable in spectrophotometers and plate readers; thus the substrate is colourless, but the breakdown of the substrate releases the yellow colour to detect the enzyme activity. Similar disaccharide substrates exist for the measurement of β-galactosidase, β-xylosidase and many others. In the case of this novel xylanase substrate, the first step in the development was therefore to add a *p*-nitrophenol molecule to the reducing end of an XOS (X5) molecule.

2. This substrate would also be susceptible to β-xylosidase, so the next step was to block the other non-reducing end of the XOS in a two-stage process. The first stage was to add a glucose to the non-reducing end and the second was to create an acetal group on that glucose. This process results in the substrate 4,6-*O*-(3-ketobutylidene)-4-nitrophenyl-β-45-*O*-glucosylxylopentaoside, which to a xylanase enzyme 'looks' like an X7 oligosaccharide.

3. Finally, in order to be able to quantify the xylanase enzyme post-hydrolysis of the substrate, an analytical kit has been developed around this substrate so that the xylanase reaction is also coupled with sat-

urating levels of β-xylosidase. This means that the smaller *p*-nitrophenyl-XOS fragment released by the xylanase is now broken down to xylose and free *p*-nitrophenol and the yellow colour formed relates stoichiometrically to the xylanase catalytic event (Mangan *et al.*, 2017).

The exact sequence is as shown in Fig. 11.4. This provides a very elegant solution to some of the problems faced in xylanase analysis, especially for research laboratories studying xylanases in digesta samples, for example. Historically though, the older methods are associated with product registrations so there will be a reluctance of laboratories to change to a new method which would create an extra workload for laboratories to validate this new method and for the regulatory teams to then update product registration dossiers.

In addition to this method, a similar new way of analysing β-glucanase, dubbed the 'MBG4 method', could also benefit the animal feed industry (Mangan *et al.*, 2016). Like the xylanase substrate, the new substrate contains the chromophore at one end and a blocking reagent at the other end. Conveniently though, in this MBG4 method, the enzyme will release the 4-nitrophenol chromophore without the need for the ancillary β-glucosidase.

11.6   A New Way to Analyse Protease

Traditional methods of analysing commercial proteases, especially in high-activity samples such as products, premixes and blends, use substrates such as casein or haemoglobin. The substrates, which are manufactured by extracting casein or haemoglobin from animal sources, may vary in purity or solubility from batch to batch or with different manufacturers and while relatively useful for quality control of products, are not well suited to in-feed analysis in terms of the detection mechanism and limit of detection and quantification. In these traditional methods the protease releases small peptides and amino acids from the casein or haemoglobin. The assay is stopped using trichloroacetic acid, which also precipitates

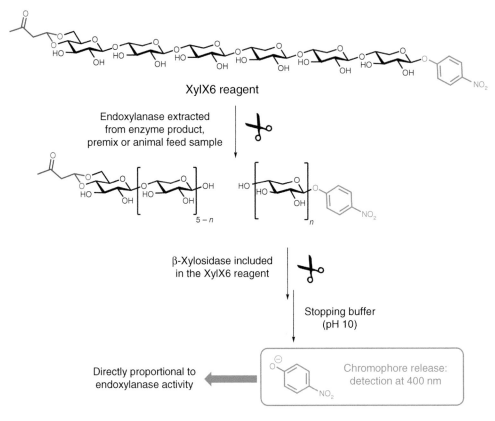

Fig. 11.4. How the XylX6 assay works. (From Mangan *et al.*, 2017. Figure used with permission from Megazyme.)

remaining larger peptides and protein material. The solubilized peptides are separated from the undigested proteins by centrifugation or filtration. The released peptides can then be quantified by using Folin's reagent (Anson, 1938).

An alternative assay, relatively new to the feed industry, uses a chemically defined colorimetric synthetic substrate Suc-Ala-Ala-Pro-Phe-pNA (National Center for Biotechnology Information, 2021). Protease cleaves the substrate, releasing the chromogen pNA. The amount of released yellow pNA is proportional to the protease activity of the enzyme and is measured photometrically at a wavelength of 405 nm. Unlike the traditional reducing sugar methods, no boiling step or harsh chemicals are required, thus facilitating automation. In addition, the detection method is highly specific and

as a result reduces the likelihood of interference from feed ingredients. This allows reliable determination of protease in feed samples (Cowieson *et al.*, 2020) in terms of both accuracy and resilience to the presence of interfering peptides and amino acids in the feed which act as 'false' or 'noise' activity when using the traditional assay on feeds without added protease.

11.7   A Workaround Way to Analyse Premixes Has Gained Widespread Acceptance

Historically, premixes have been analysed using the same methodology as used for products. This can present challenges during especially the extraction part of the workflow, where the components of the premix are at a relatively high concentration, and thus some strategies have included pH control using a buffer rather than just extracting in water and the addition of bovine serum albumin (BSA) and/or EDTA (ethylenediaminetetraacetic acid) or another similar chelating agent. These were discussed in the previous edition of this book (Sheehan, 2010). Anecdotally, it has been noticed that often enzyme activity is as expected in the final feed but in the intermediate premix stage it can be lower than expected, even with intervention strategies employed as described above. Many companies have essentially moved the premix analysis further downstream, so instead of trying to analyse the enzyme by the same method as the pure product, they have adopted the feed analysis methodology where the premix is mixed/diluted with what is essentially a blank (no enzyme) feed. This 'feed' is analysed and the results are related back to the original premix. The exact blank feed material varies slightly from laboratory to laboratory, with some using heat-treated wheat flour (VDLUFA, 2012) and others heat-treated maize meal. In our laboratories, we use a mixture of micronized wheat and micronized soya and have nicknamed this as the 'premix-feed method'.

Using this dry dilution technique enables accurate quantification of enzyme contents in vitamin/mineral premixes and has become widespread through the feed industry. Examples below are from some different EU registration documents for at least four different phytase products:

- 'Based on the performance characteristics presented, the EURL recommends for official control the ring-trial validated colorimetric method (EN ISO 30024) for the determination of 6-phytase in premixtures (after dilution with heat-treated whole grain flour)' (EFSA Panel on Additives and Products or Substances used in Animal Feed (FEEDAP), 2012).
- 'The Applicant quantified the phytase activity in premixture samples ... by first diluting the samples with heat treated whole grain wheat flour or maize and then analysing them as feedingstuffs' (European Commission Directorate General Joint Research Centre, 2016).
- 'Furthermore, the Applicant applied ... the ring-trial validated colorimetric method (VDLUFA 27.1.3) for the quantification of the phytase activity in premixtures' (EFSA Panel on Additives and Products or Substances used in Animal Feed (FEEDAP), 2017).
- 'The ring-trial validated VDLUFA 27.1.3 and VDLUFA 27.1.4 methods describing the preparation of feed additives and premixtures for quantification of the phytase activity' (European Commission Directorate General Joint Research Centre, 2018).
- 'VDLUFA 27.1.3 method, based on a solid dilution using maize meal, describing ... preparation of premixtures for quantification of the phytase activity .... This combination of methods has been ring-trial validated for premixtures with phytase activities .... These performance characteristics are in good agreement with those reported in the VDLUFA 27.1.4 /EN ISO 30024 combination thus confirming the applicability to the analysis of the products ... well as the extension of scope to premixtures' (European Commission Directorate General Joint Research Centre, 2019).

Benefits of the premix-feed method include:

1. Validation showed higher measured phytase activity in premixes compared with direct methods for measuring phytase activity in premixes, as shown in Fig. 11.5.
2. Use of cheap, easy-to-source ingredients (micronized wheat and/or micronized soya) versus many different, some quite expensive, chemicals (BSA, EDTA, sodium acetate, phytic acid, ammonium metavanadate, acetic acid, nitric acid).

The premix-feed method, when combined with ELISA, gives:

1. Specificity for specific phytase and xylanase in premixes and will not work for

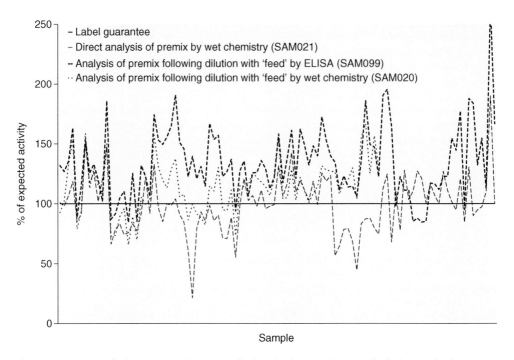

Fig. 11.5. Recovery of phytase activity by premix-feed method versus direct method, showing higher recoveries by the premix-feed method compared with direct methods. SAM refers to the laboratory method. (Author's own figure.)

premixes containing other phytases or xylanases, or feed-derived enzymes whether from the cereals themselves or fungal contaminants.

2. Improvements in workflow. ELISA uses essentially non-hazardous reagents that are easier to prepare, so the hazards for laboratory staff are significantly reduced compared with wet chemistry methods which use strong acids and ammonium metavanandate. Health and safety (e.g. COSHH (Control of Substances Hazardous to Health) in the UK; OSHA (Occupational Safety and Health Administration) in the USA) administrative work is thus also significantly reduced.

3. Non-hazardous waste.

4. Opportunities for high throughput using automated ELISA systems.

5. Benefits for new laboratories, including only having to set up two methods, avoiding having to set up four methods, and the capability to do premixes and feeds using the same methodology and equipment.

Limitations of the premix-feed method are:

1. The dry dilution step has a quantitative effect on results, unlike other preparation steps. As this is done separately from the actual assay, often by a different person performing the analysis, this has to be managed carefully, to avoid errors.

2. There is an extra milling step.

3. Since this concept was introduced (VD-LUFA, 2012), changes have been introduced to the wet chemistry methods, as described in Section 11.2, that have made them quicker and more automated. Maybe the wet chemistry methods have 'caught up' in ease of use?

11.8   Note on Extraction of Enzyme Activities from Any Matrix

All the methods mentioned above rely on the enzyme being quantitatively recovered from the matrix of interest, whether it is the enzyme product itself, a mineral/vitamin premix containing the enzyme or finished feed. While workarounds for controlling and removing the variation and interference of compounds in the premix or finished feeds are described in this chapter, one issue that needs to be addressed is the variation between enzyme products with regard to their 'extractability'. Some enzymes are coated, which may demand specific extraction buffers. Others may require specific pH extraction buffers in order to ensure that all the enzyme is removed from the matrix (Basu *et al.*, 2007). Regardless, it is important to note that there is not a 'one size fits all' approach in every case due to the idiosyncrasies of the products currently on the marketplace and thus it is prudent to consult with the manufacturer regarding any specific extraction or assay conditions required.

References

Alderton, G., Ward, W.H. and Fevold, H.L. (1945) Isolation of lysozyme from egg white. *Journal of Biological Chemistry* 157, 43–58.

Anson, M.L. (1938) The estimation of pepsin, trypsin, papain and cathepsin with hemoglobin. *Journal of General Physiology* 22, 79–89.

Bailey, M.J., Biely, P. and Poutanen, K. (1992) Interlaboratory testing of methods for assay of xylanase activity. *Journal of Biotechnology* 23, 257–270.

Basu, S.S., Winslow, S., Nelson, A., Ono, M. and Betts, S. (2007) Extraction methods and assays for feed enzymes. *WO/2007/002192*. World Intellectual Property Organization, Geneva, Switzerland.

Chu, F.S. (1984) Immunoassays for analysis of mycotoxins. *Journal of Food Protection* 47, 562–569.

Cowieson, A.J., Bhuiyan, M.M., Sorbara, J.O.B., Pappenberger, G., Pedersen, M.B. and Choct, M. (2020) Contribution of individual broilers to variation in amino acid digestibility in soybean meal and the efficacy of an exogenous monocomponent protease. *Poultry Science* 99, 1075–1083.

Davis, A.H. and Roberts, R.W. (2013) QuickTox™ Kit for QuickScan Ochratoxin-A. *Journal of AOAC International* 96, 1019–1025.

EFSA Panel on Additives and Products or Substances used in Animal Feed (FEEDAP) (2012) Scientific opinion on the safety and efficacy of Phyzyme XP (6-phytase) as a feed additive for minor poultry species. *EFSA Journal* 10, 2619. Available at: https://efsa.onlinelibrary.wiley.com/doi/pdf/10.2903/j.efsa.2012.2619 (accessed 3 March 2021).

EFSA Panel on Additives and Products or Substances used in Animal Feed (FEEDAP) (2017) Safety and efficacy of Natuphos® E (6-phytase) as a feed additive for avian and porcine species. *EFSA Journal* 15, 5024. Available at: https://efsa.onlinelibrary.wiley.com/doi/pdf/10.2903/j.efsa.2017.5024 (accessed 7 October 2021).

European Commission Directorate General Joint Research Centre (2016) Evaluation Report on the Analytical Methods submitted in connection with the Application for Authorisation of a Feed Additive according to Regulation (EC) No 1831/2003. Axtra® PHY 20000 TPT2 (FAD-2015-0048; CRL/150029). Available at: https://ec.europa.eu/jrc/sites/jrcsh/files/finirep-fad-2015-0048-axtra-phy-20000tpt2.pdf (accessed 3 March 2021).

European Commission Directorate General Joint Research Centre (2018) Evaluation Report on the Analytical Methods submitted in connection with the Application for Authorisation of a Feed Additive according to Regulation (EC) No 1831/2003. Ronozyme® HiPhos (FAD-2017-0021; CRL/160038). Available at: https://ec.europa.eu/jrc/sites/jrcsh/files/finrep-fad-2017-0021-ronozyme_hiphos.pdf (accessed 3 March 2021).

European Commission Directorate General Joint Research Centre (2019) Evaluation Report on the Analytical Methods submitted in connection with the Application for Authorisation of a Feed Additive according to Regulation (EC) No 1831/2003. Preparation of 6-phytase (EC 3.1.3.26) (FAD-2019-0042; CRL/190023). Available at: https://ec.europa.eu/jrc/sites/jrcsh/files/finrep_fad-2019-0042_optiphos_plus_porcine.pdf (accessed 3 March 2021).

Gizzi, G., Thyregod, P., von Holst, C., Bertin, G., Vogel, K., *et al.* (2008) Determination of phytase activity in feed: interlaboratory study. *Journal of AOAC International* 91, 259–267.

Graham, H. and Sheehan, N. (2013) Cost-effective and convenient xylanase enzyme analysis. Available at: https://www.allaboutfeed.net/Feed-Additives/Articles/2013/11/Cost-effective-and-convenient-xylanase-enzyme-analysis-1395820W/ (accessed 13 August 2020).

Grothaus, G.D., Bandla, M., Currier, T., Giroux, R., Jenkins, R.G., *et al.* (2006) Immunoassay as an analytical tool in agricultural biotechnology. *Journal of AOAC International* 89, 913–928.

ISO (International Organization for Standardization) (2009) *ISO 30024:2009. Animal Feeding Stuffs – Determination of Phytase Activity*. ISO, Geneva, Switzerland.

Kim, T.W. and Lei, X.G. (2005) An improved method for a rapid determination of phytase activity in animal feed. *Journal of Animal Science* 83, 1062–1067.

Koczula, K.M. and Gallotta, A. (2016) Lateral flow assays. *Essays in Biochemistry* 60, 111–120.

Mangan, D., Liadova, A., Ivory, R. and McCleary, B.V. (2016) Novel approaches to the automated assay of β-glucanase and lichenase activity. *Carbohydrate Research* 435, 162–172.

Mangan, D., Cornaggia, C., Liadova, A., McCormack, N., Ivory, R., *et al.* (2017) Novel substrates for the automated and manual assay of endo-1,4-β-xylanase. *Carbohydrate Research* 445, 14–22.

McCleary, B.V. and McGeough, P. (2015) A comparison of polysaccharide substrates and reducing sugar methods for the measurement of endo-1,4-β-xylanase. *Applied Biochemistry and Biotechnology* 177, 1152–1163.

National Center for Biotechnology Information (2021) PubChem Compound Summary for CID 5496888, N-Succinyl-ala-ala-pro-phe-p-nitroanilide. Available at: https://pubchem.ncbi.nlm.nih.gov/compound/N-Succinyl-ala-ala-pro-phe-p-nitroanilide (accessed 3 March 2021).

Schutte, J.B. (1990) Nutritional implications and metabolizable energy value of D-xylose and L-arabinose in chicks. *Poultry Science* 69, 1724–1730.

Schutte, J.B., de Jong, J., van Weerden, E.J. and van Baak, M.J. (1992) Nutritional value of D-xylose and L-arabinose for broiler chicks. *British Poultry Science* 33, 89–100.

Shafat, I., Zcharia, E., Nisman, B., Nadir, Y., Nakhoul, F., *et al.* (2006) An ELISA method for the detection and quantification of human heparanase. *Biochemical and Biophysical Research Communications* 341, 958–963.

Sheehan, N. (2010) Analysis of enzymes, principles and problems: developments in enzyme analysis. In: Bedford, M.R. and Partridge, G.G. (2001) *Enzymes in Farm Animal Nutrition*, 2nd edn. CAB International, Wallingford, UK, pp. 260–272.

Tran, T.T., Hatti-Kaul, R., Dalsgaard, S. and Yu, S. (2011) A simple and fast kinetic assay for phytases using phytic acid–protein complex as substrate. *Analytical Biochemistry* 410, 177–184.

VDLUFA (Association of German Agricultural Analytic and Research Institutes eV) (ed.) (2012) Method 27.1.3: Preparation of mineral feeds and mineral premixtures for the determination of the phytase activity. In: *Methods Book III: The Chemical Analysis of Feedingstuffs*, 3rd edn, 8th supplementary volume. VDLUFA-Publishing House, Darmstadt, Germany.

Webb, M.R. (1992) A continuous spectrophotometric assay for inorganic phosphate and for measuring phosphate release kinetics in biological systems. *Proceedings of the National Academy of Sciences USA* 89, 4884–4887.

12 Delivery and Stabilization of Enzymes in Animal Feed

Douglas Dale*, Todd Becker, Michael Reichman and Sam Maurer
IFF, Palo Alto, California, USA

12.1 Introduction

Exogenous enzymes provide a vital function in various animal feed applications. Amylases, cellulases, xylanases and proteases increase the digestibility and availability of nutrients to the animal by breaking down the feed to more bioavailable forms and reducing specific antinutrients naturally present in certain feed raw materials. Phytases, the single largest supplementary enzyme activity in feed, break down the phytic acid, releasing phosphate. This allows the feed producer to decrease the amount of inorganic phosphate added to the feed, resulting in less phosphate release to the environment. In addition, the breakdown of phytic acid disrupts its chelating properties, which releases more nutrients to be available to the animal. In all, without added enzymes, the quality of the feed would be reduced significantly. However, delivering the enzymes to the animal requires that the activity is fully present after both production and storage of the feed. During the feed production process, enzymes can be exposed to extreme temperatures, moisture and physical forces leading to loss of activity and resultant animal performance. In order to ensure that the enzymes will maintain their essential function, enzyme producers have employed multiple approaches to protect them from the extreme conditions experienced during feed production.

12.1.1 The market for pelleting-stable feed enzymes

Sales of animal feed enzymes exceeded US$1.1 billion in 2016 and are projected to exceed US$2.0 billion by 2024. The dominant application globally for feed enzymes is to enhance the nutrient availability and digestibility of maize- and soy-based diets for poultry and swine. Phytases are responsible for about 40% of global sales, with the balance comprised of proteases and non-starch polysaccharide-degrading enzymes – such as xylanases, cellulases, β-glucanases and pectinases (Ploegmakers, 2017).

The major global suppliers of feed enzymes are IFF, Novozymes/DSM, BASF, Adisseo and AB Vista; smaller players include Enmex, Elanco, BioResource International, Beldem, Advanced Enzymes, Cargill, ADM, CHR Hansen, Biovet and numerous Chinese suppliers.

*Email: doug.dale@iff.com

©CAB International 2022. *Enzymes in Farm Animal Nutrition, 3rd Edition* (M. Bedford *et al.* eds)
DOI: 10.1079/9781789241563.0012

12.1.2 Application of enzymes in feed

While dry admixtures of maize, soy, vitamins and other feed additives – referred to as 'mash' feed – can be provided directly to poultry and swine, pelleted feed is generally the preferred format. Pellets provide the benefits of uniform consistency, ease of provision and flow in feed troughs, and less feed wastage by the animals. While liquid enzymes can be sprayed on to the exterior of preformed feed pellets by post-pelleting liquid application (PPLA) systems, this route requires a considerable investment in specialized spraying equipment and is considered a more niche application globally.

The stability of exogenous enzyme products is of great importance throughout the supply chain, from production of the enzyme in fermenters to the addition of enzymes to animal feed. Enzyme products need to maintain activity by retaining their biological structure after long durations at elevated temperatures and humidity, and withstand undesired reactions with background sugars, oxidants and other added enzymes such as proteases, amylases and cellulases. The stability of an enzyme will be impacted by its various structural levels from amino acid sequence, post-translational modifications (such as glycosylation), local folded secondary structure and the three-dimensional folded tertiary structure (Puder *et al.*, 2009; Manning *et al.*, 2010). The stability of an enzyme can be improved through careful selection of the enzyme backbone and further engineering by the modification of the amino acid sequence of the enzyme.

12.1.3 Feed production process and impact on enzyme activity

Enzymes for animal feed can be delivered in multiple formats, both liquid and solid. Enzymes can be added to the feed production process at various points and, depending on this, they will be exposed to different stresses that can result in loss of activity and thereby risk inadequate performance when fed to the animals. When liquid enzyme products are added post-pelleting, this is the least stressful from a manufacturing perspective, but on the other hand will have a higher challenge than solid feed products for long-term shelf life. The production of solid feed products introduces stress points of varying types at multiple unit operations that can negatively impact the activity of the enzymes. Figure 12.1 is a schematic of the feed pelleting production process that indicates time and temperature exposure. Further information on the types of stresses is provided below.

12.1.3.1 Shear

Different degrees of shear are introduced at multiple locations. The first will occur in the blending operation. The blending equipment utilized is usually a ribbon or paddle mixer. Although generally viewed as low-stress operations, these mixers can impart high enough forces that will fracture or disrupt granulated enzyme products, making them more susceptible to other stresses (Van der Veen *et al.*, 2004). Similar levels of shear forces can be introduced in the conditioning process. The highest level of shear comes during pellet production. The degree of force will be dependent on the physical parameters of the die. Smaller diameter and longer length dies will have the highest degree of shear. In addition, the rate of processing as well as the components of the feed will influence the overall shear that the enzyme particles will encounter.

12.1.3.2 Moisture

Moisture is introduced naturally within the feed components. In addition, some manufacturers will intentionally add 2 to 4% water to the blending operation to help with downstream processing (Lundblad *et al.*, 2009). The majority of the moisture is introduced as high-pressure steam in the conditioning step. This moisture in combination with temperature is the highest degree of stress the enzyme product will encounter during the production process. Moisture on its own will have only a small impact on enzyme stability.

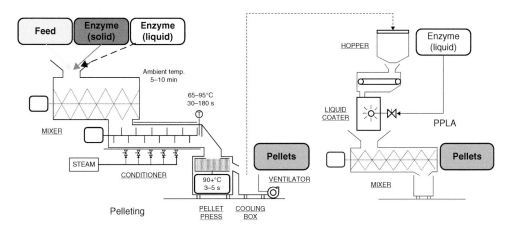

Fig. 12.1. Schematic of an animal feed production mill indicating unit operations and relative temperatures and times for each. (From Sorensen, 2019. Figure used with permission.)

12.1.3.3 Temperature

The main source of temperature exposure is generated during the conditioning step(s). Elevated temperatures, up to and exceeding 95°C, are established in the conditioner to pasteurize the feed as well as increase digestibility of some of the feed components. The exposure duration to these elevated temperatures in general is 30–90 s, but it could be up to 180 s in extreme cases. There is also a short, small spike in temperature of a few degrees Celsius as the feed passes through the pellet mill. Heat in this case is generated due to both friction and pressure. The elevated temperature in combination with moisture is the primary cause for enzyme activity loss during feed production (Rasmussen, 2010).

12.1.3.4 Pressure

There is also a transient pressure spike as the feed passes through the pellet mill. As mentioned above, this can result in a small temperature increase (3–5°C) (Truelock *et al.*, 2019). In addition, the pressure may have a detrimental impact on solid enzyme products resulting in exposure of the enzyme to other stresses due to fracturing or crushing of the enzyme granules.

12.1.4 Other sources of stress in animal feed production

12.1.4.1 Premixes

In many cases, enzymes are combined with other minor ingredients within the feed formulation to enable a more convenient addition process for the feed manufacturer. Other minor ingredients can include essential vitamins, minerals, amino acids and other miscellaneous feed additives. In some cases these components are incompatible with enzymes, as they may be hygroscopic in nature or negatively modify the enzyme (Sulabo *et al.*, 2011). This incompatibility can cause loss of enzyme activity during the life cycle of the premix due to moisture uptake or modification of the enzyme via oxidation.

12.1.4.2 Shelf life

Once the animal feed is produced, the enzyme must maintain its activity until it is consumed by the animal. The feed will be stored under ambient conditions which can include elevated temperatures and/or high humidity depending on the location of production. Both of these, like the stresses of the pelleting process, can lead to loss of enzyme performance. Although the extremes in stress are lower than in the pelleting process, the time element can be extended many months in certain circumstances. The shelf stability of the enzyme product itself is also of importance as label claims for expiry of the product can be up to 18 months. The product must be able to deliver the required activity at least up to this date, if not beyond. This is discussed further in Section 12.3.3.

As illustrated here, there are many conditions that enzymes must survive in order to provide their benefit to the animal. Hence, feed enzyme suppliers need to provide products that can be readily combined with the pre-pelleted feed and that are sufficiently stabilized to survive the feed pelleting process with high active enzyme recovery. This can be achieved either with an inherently thermostable enzyme delivered as a liquid formulation, or by use of a pelleting-stable granular formulation that can be blended into the pre-pelleted feed. This chapter highlights the approaches manufacturers have taken to address the challenge of delivering enzymes in feed application, with a focus on advances since the previous edition of this book (Bedford and Partridge, 2010).

12.2 Protein Stabilization Through Molecule Selection and Modification

Protein engineering to modify properties of enzymes is a well-established approach to address weaknesses or enhance desired characteristics in the molecule (Cervin *et al.*, 2014). The tools for this have advanced over the years to allow for thousands of variants to be generated in a short time period (Liu *et al.*, 2019). This allows researchers to explore many combinations of amino acid substitutions in rapid fashion. Beneficial properties can be combined to build on synergies of properties. In addition, shuffling of multiple enzyme backbones can be done to take advantage of combining beneficial properties into a single molecule (Lutz and Iamurri, 2017). Outlined below are several examples of engineering approaches that have been successfully applied to address the stresses in animal feed production mentioned previously.

12.2.1 Preventing thermal degradation

Of all the failure modes mentioned previously, thermal degradation is the most common and most harsh during the pelleting process due to the extreme temperatures in the presence of moisture for periods of up to several minutes. There are several approaches that can be taken to generate a more thermostable product. These include molecule selection, protein engineering and post-translational modifications.

12.2.1.1 Molecule selection

There are many natural sources of enzyme activities important for animal nutrition. Sources include bacterial, fungal and plant activities that can be applied. The natural enzyme backbone provides the starting point for any further engineering to improve properties (Cervin *et al.*, 2014). Starting with a molecule that already has some moderate thermal stability properties is best for further engineering. One approach is to source enzymes from extremophile organisms that would naturally have good thermal stability (Morgan *et al.*, 1995).

12.2.1.2 Protein engineering

Once an enzyme backbone has been identified, a common approach to further improve the thermal properties is to engineer the protein to maintain the tertiary and secondary structures as much as possible to prevent unfolding and possibly aggregation. Modifications that may improve the thermal stability include the introduction of disulfide bonds, additional salt bridges and increased structural packing to tighten the core of the protein. The thermal property of the enzyme molecule is usually expressed by the T_m, the temperature where half of the molecules have unfolded as measured by differential scanning calorimetry (DSC), for example. The increase in T_m can be correlated to improved survivability through the conditioning and pelleting process. This is described as pelleting recovery or yield: measured activity after pelleting divided by the measured activity prior to pelleting.

There are many examples where the T_m of an enzyme has been increased significantly (Lehmann, 2004; Miasnikov *et al.*, 2006; Nguyen and Winter, 2013; Trefzer *et al.*, 2013). Engineering the protein structure is one primary approach that enzyme suppliers use to improve their product offerings.

12.2.1.3 Post-translational modifications

During the pelleting process, the enzyme may unfold to some degree, but if aggregation can be prevented, the impact of unfolding can be minimal. It has been shown that by introducing glycosylation sites in the sequence, unfolding can be reduced and refolding enhanced. These sites will provide steric hindrance, preventing neighbouring unfolded molecules from aggregating (Hoiberg-Nielsen *et al.*, 2006). Upon cooling, the molecules can refold, thus maintaining their original activity. The concentration of glycosylation sites as well as the size of the glycan are dependent on the production organism. Not all microbes will decorate the enzymes to the same extent. Therefore, the choice of production host will also have an influence on the degree of refolding that can occur as a result of the level of glycosylation. It has also been found that some organisms express enzyme activities that remove glycans once they have been generated. In these cases, manufacturers can modify the organism so that they no longer produce the activity that removes the glycosylation. IFF demonstrated introduction of sites and removal of detrimental activity resulting in increased performance in pelleting (Gebert *et al.*, 2018). Novozymes has also demonstrated the benefit of glycosylation on stability during pelleting (Hoiberg-Nielsen *et al.*, 2006).

12.2.2 Preventing other failure modes through engineering

There are other modifications that can occur during processing and storage that can also impact the long-term stability and performance of enzymes. In some cases, these modifications can be silent as they do not impact the stability or the activity of the protein. However, when the modifications occur near the active site, they can be detrimental to enzyme performance. Two common modifications that have been encountered in feed production and storage are glycation and oxidation.

12.2.2.1 Glycation

Like oxidation, glycation can also influence the performance and stability of enzymes in feed. Although glycation can show up during pelleting, it is encountered more frequently during storage. Glycation occurs when sugars react with lysine side chains resulting in undesirable modifications. For some animal nutrition enzymes, the lysine side chain is located at a crucial position in the enzyme structure which when glycated could cause a loss in activity during the storage of the enzyme product. In addition, the glycation of proteins causes an undesirable increase in the brown colour of both granule and liquid products. The source of the sugars can be from fermentation carryover with the enzyme or introduced during the feed production process from feed components. The residual sugars that are contained in the filtered broth are reducing sugars such as glucose and mannose which can react with the lysine amino acids of the enzymes and cause glycation of the enzyme (Lund and Ray, 2017). Glycation is typically a more significant issue with solid products than liquids due to the low water content of the enzyme granules (Schmidt, 2004). There are several methods for reducing the likelihood of glycation including engineering the enzyme to replace lysine with an alternative amino acid or using processes such as diafiltration to reduce the amount of reducing sugars in the enzyme product (Gebert *et al.*, 2019).

12.2.2.2 Oxidation

Oxidation can also occur, but this event usually occurs post-production during storage. The oxidation event can be initiated by molecular oxygen or through radical-initiated reactions (Patel *et al.*, 2011). Regardless of the source, the result can negatively influence the performance of the enzyme, especially if the oxidized amino acid is near the active site of the enzyme. The activity of the enzyme can be reduced either by sterically preventing the substrate from entering the active site, or if the oxidized amino acid is involved with the chemistry of the enzyme reaction and is no longer able to carry out its function. Substituting the oxidizable amino acid with a non-reactive one through protein engineering is a common solution, as long as it does not impact function.

12.3   Stability During Formulation and Processing

In addition to stabilization approaches directly with the molecule, enzyme producers can protect the activity through physical means. Combinations of excipients in liquid formats can help maintain the enzyme structure. Encapsulation of the enzyme through multiple approaches can physically separate the enzyme from the process stresses and maintain the activity. These approaches in combination with molecule improvements can offer combined protection.

12.3.1   Impact of enzyme production

Enzymes used in industrial applications such as animal nutrition may not be completely purified and the background environment that the enzyme is exposed to throughout its storage life can affect various properties of the product (Blanch and Clark, 1995). These include activity loss, colour change and precipitate formation. The background environment is dependent on the production process used to make the enzyme. The most common production for animal nutrition enzymes is by submerged liquid fermentations using bacteria, yeast or fungi as the production organism. These organisms have been engineered to produce high quantities of the desired animal nutrition enzyme and the organisms require sugars, salts and metals to grow and produce

this specific enzyme. In addition, the organisms also produce side products including other native enzyme activities such as proteases which can degrade other enzymes during storage. The first step after the fermentation is the separation of the cells from the liquid. Because most animal nutrition enzymes are excreted enzymes, the cellular material contains very little of the enzyme product. However, the filtered fermentation broth can contain residual sugars, salt and other enzyme by-products which can cause undesired reactions with the production enzyme of interest and then cause a loss in activity over time during storage of the product.

12.3.2   Liquid enzyme formulation

Enzyme products used in animal nutrition applications require excipients to stabilize and prevent loss of activity during storage. The key excipients used in liquid formulations are polyols, sugars, salts, amino acids, preservatives and buffers. The most common polyols are sorbitol and glycerol, used as osmolytes to modify the interaction of the enzyme with the surrounding water molecules. Sorbitol and glycerol interact with the enzyme by either preferential exclusion or accumulation of the polyol from the 'hydration sphere' (Bagger *et al.*, 2003). The modification of the enzyme–water interaction by the polyol affects the rate of denaturation and aggregation, which can help to reduce the loss of structure that causes a loss of activity (Manning *et al.*, 2010). The polyol and its concentration affect the viscosity of the liquid formulation, which is important for post-pelleting application and addition of liquids to mash (Zhu *et al.*, 2010). The addition of sodium chloride or similar salts is used to lower the water activity of the liquid formulation preferably below 0.87 in order to decrease the risk of bacteria and yeast growth in the formulation (Scott, 1957; Leistner, 2000). Sodium chloride is the most common salt used to modify the water activity of the liquid formulation to help prevent growth of contaminant microorganisms during storage. In addition, preservatives such as potassium sorbate and sodium benzoate are added to prevent microbial contamination of the product. Liquid feed enzyme products are typically formulated at a pH range between 4.0 and 5.5 because most of them have maximal activity in this pH region (Menezes-Blackburn *et al.*, 2015). In addition, increasing the pH above this desired range increases the possibility for contamination from microorganisms and decreasing the pH below this desired range increases the activity of acidic proteases that can cause degradation of the enzyme. Citrate or phosphate buffers can be used to help maintain the liquid formulation in the desired pH range (EFSA, 2008a).

12.3.3   Solid enzyme formulation

In animal nutrition applications, enzymes are most commonly delivered in a solid format to improve pelleting and storage stability. In addition, the solid format will increase the safety of the product by reducing the potential for workers to be exposed to high levels of enzyme dust. Most solid enzyme products are added to the mash (mixture of all feed components) prior to pelleting and are required to stay active through the pelleting process with conditioner temperatures of 90 to 100°C and conditioner residence times typically ranging from 30 to 180 s. There are very few thermally stable enzymes that can stay active in such harsh environments. Enzyme manufacturers are constantly working on ways to increase the thermal stability of the enzymes while still maintaining the *in vivo* performance of the enzymes by modifying their amino acid sequences. In addition, enzyme manufacturers are continually developing new techniques and new formulations to increase the thermal stability of the solid format.

Solid products typically have longer storage stability than liquid products and are required to maintain activity over long durations at elevated temperatures and humidity. Most countries require regulatory filings to include data showing that the enzyme product will meet its declared specifications after storage under certain temperature conditions, typically 25, 35 and 40°C. In addition, the enzyme product is required to maintain activity in both premix and mash mixtures (EFSA, 2012). Homogeneity measurements are also required for solid products to ensure that there is good distribution of the enzyme product when added to feed. Typically, a coefficient of variation of less than or equal to 15% is required for European regulatory agencies (EFSA, 2008b).

12.3.3.1   Solid product forms

Current solid products can be classified into two main categories: coated or uncoated. A further classification of the current solid product offerings can be delineated by the processing technology used to make these products. Currently only IFF and Novozymes/ DSM have coated solids and these products are differentiated from competitor uncoated products because they can survive elevated temperature and long conditioner times while still maintaining significant amounts of activity (EFSA, 2012, 2016a,b). These coatings provide a moisture barrier to prevent steam introduced during the pelleting process from contacting the enzyme which will cause a loss of activity. The first attempts at a moisture barrier used a fat coating; while this provided a good moisture barrier, the dissolution rate of the fat *in vitro* and *in vivo* was slow, which prevented the enzyme from being released quickly and thereby reduced the effectiveness of the product. The more current coatings are made using a salt that is spray-coated on to the granule. The salt has a very high deliquescence point and does not absorb significant amounts of moisture or form hydrates; therefore, in high humidity or liquid environments the salt will dissolve but in lower humidity environments the salt will not absorb moisture. The dissolution rate of these salt coatings is of the order of 30 to 60 s, and they consequently release the enzyme into the animal gut without any significant delay. The main difference between the IFF and Novozymes products is the method of producing the solid granule. IFF uses spray coating while Novozymes uses high-shear granulation.

Uncoated solid products are also common; however, they have disadvantages with lower pelleting performance at elevated temperatures and long conditioner times. In addition, uncoated solid products have more exposure to moisture and other substances when stored in premix or feed, which may cause a decrease in storage stability compared with coated products (Sulabo *et al.*, 2011). The most common methods for producing uncoated solid products are low-shear granulation, spray drying and spray agglomeration. Low-shear granulation produces low payload and large particles due to the large amount of inert carrier material and binder needed to keep the granule from breaking apart. Enzyme manufacturers are moving away from spray drying and spray agglomeration due to dust exposure issues and the increased risk of enzyme sensitization (Basketter *et al.*, 2010). Spray-dried products have high payloads due to very low required binder concentrations which can be used to reduce the amount of product required for dosing. Illustrations of common solid enzyme formats and descriptions of their properties are given in Fig. 12.2.

One example of a solid application uses a dissolution system to dissolve spray-dried product in water and then spraying the dissolved enzyme either on to mash or in a post-pelleting application (Nollet, 2015). However, the exposure risk due to the spray-dried enzyme is extremely high and requires expensive and complicated containment equipment to adequately reduce that risk (Vanhanen *et al.*, 2001). Solid products have a higher risk of exposure than liquid products due to the generation of fine dust particles that can be suspended in air. This is an issue because enzymes are classified as respiratory sensitizers and have very strict exposure limits for workers (Vanhanen *et al.*, 2001). Coated solids provide the most protection against the formation of dust whereas spray-dried or spray-agglomerated solid products produce the most dust due to very small particle sizes, low densities and fragile particles that are prone to cracking and breaking (Basketter *et al.*, 2010). There is currently an occupational exposure limit for only one enzyme class, subtilisin, with a limit of 60 ng/m^3 based on at least one-hour sampling. There are no regulatory requirements for other enzymes, but solid enzyme products should be handled with great care to reduce dust exposure (Basketter *et al.*, 2010; AISE, 2014; De Vos *et al.*, 2018).

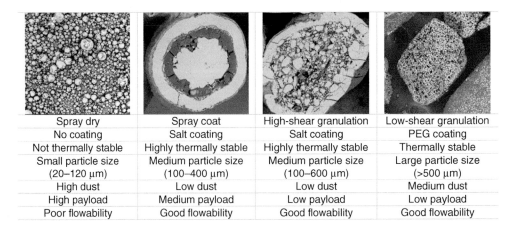

Spray dry	Spray coat	High-shear granulation	Low-shear granulation
No coating	Salt coating	Salt coating	PEG coating
Not thermally stable	Highly thermally stable	Highly thermally stable	Thermally stable
Small particle size (20–120 µm)	Medium particle size (100–400 µm)	Medium particle size (100–600 µm)	Large particle size (>500 µm)
High dust	Low dust	Low dust	Medium dust
High payload	Medium payload	Low payload	Low payload
Poor flowability	Good flowability	Good flowability	Good flowability

Fig. 12.2. Enzyme solid product form comparisons. PEG, polyethylene glycol. (Data from Becker *et al.*, 2010; Rasmussen, 2010; EFSA, 2012; Fru-Nji, 2012; Greiner and Konietzny, 2012; Marcussen *et al.*, 2016; De Jong *et al.*, 2017. Authors' own figure.)

12.4   Stability During Storage

Another challenge in the utilization of feed enzymes in animal nutrition is maintaining the stability of enzymes from their production at the plant through all steps of the distribution and feed application and their final consumption by the animal. Different steps in the distribution process present different challenges for maintaining the stability of the enzymes. Enzyme products typically have an advertised shelf life for delivery of enzyme activity over a period of time at specified storage conditions. A typical standard for both solid and liquid storage stability of feed enzymes is 70–95% retention of activity after 1 year of storage at 25°C at a relative humidity around 50%, with some products losing 50% or more activity when stored at temperatures in the range of 35–40°C and elevated relative humidity (EFSA, 2013, 2016b). Stability of enzyme activity is often higher when products are stored at 4°C (Sulabo et al., 2011); however, refrigeration of solid and liquid products is typically neither recommended in documentation supplied by feed enzyme manufacturers nor feasible in practical feed production.

12.4.1   Stability in diluted forms

Solid enzyme products will often be stored in the presence of other solid materials for an extended period of time. Such a material is added as a diluent at the site of manufacture, for example, in order to adjust the flowability of a solid powder or to dilute a highly concentrated solid granular product to deliver the target dose of enzyme activity. The water activity or hygroscopicity of such a diluent material may cause water uptake or desiccation of the enzyme powder, which could have either a stabilizing or destabilizing effect on the enzyme, depending on the properties of the enzyme and its stability in the solid product. If the enzyme in the solid product is moisture-sensitive, a filler material with a low water activity or high hygroscopicity could be selected to reduce the amount of moisture reaching the granular enzyme product. Types of materials commonly utilized as diluents in enzyme preparations include clays, starches and brans. These materials can also be present in the feed itself, introducing the potential for interaction with feed enzymes later in the feed pellet production process. For example, sepiolite is used as a lubricant for the pelleting process in some pelleting mixtures, and rice bran can be used as a source of nutrients (Samli et al., 2006; Jacob and Pescatore, 2012).

12.4.2   Stability in premix

After production, feed enzymes are often combined with other minor feed additives in a premix. Materials added to premixes can include small molecules and nutrients such as vitamins and minerals as well as agricultural products such as brans, starches, oils and probiotics. Limestone is also used as a typical carrier in premixes and is often present as a flow enhancer for other granular additives (Leeson and Summers, 2005). Typical recommendations for storage of premixes suggest that enzyme stability should be shown for at least 3 months, with 6 months stability or greater strongly preferred (ICCF, 2019). As is the case with diluents, the physical properties of the other additives in the premix, such as their physical strength, water uptake and potential for oxidation or other chemical interactions, can affect the stability of the enzyme. Just as enzymes can be engineered for stability in pelleting, the stability of the enzyme can be increased either through engineering of the molecule to resist the particular stresses imposed by the premix material or by isolating it within a protective matrix or layer. As in pelleting, coated enzymes typically show greater stability in premixes than non-coated enzymes. It has been reported that non-coated phytase enzymes showed poor stability after as little as 30 days stored in a premix (Sulabo et al., 2011). Abrasive materials used in premixes, including limestone, can also reduce the integrity of a feed enzyme, for example by disrupting the adhesion of the enzyme to its carrier, degrading its protective coating, or otherwise causing the enzyme-containing matrix to deteriorate in a way that is deleterious to the stability of the enzyme. It is not common for liquid feed enzymes to be dosed together with other activities in premixes.

12.4.3 Stability in feed pellets

Once pelleted, the feed enzymes must retain stability in the animal feed until consumption by the animal. Often, feed pellets are consumed by animals within days to weeks of production, although current industrial guidance suggests demonstrating enzyme stability in feed for 3 months after pelleting (ICCF, 2019). Depending on the delivery method for the feed enzyme, different types of interactions between the enzyme and the feed are possible. If delivered as a liquid, the enzyme might physically adsorb on to structures in the feed such as starches, lipids, proteins, or high-porosity substances such as clays. The enzyme might interact over a period of time with metals or other compounds added to the feed, particularly if residual moisture allows partial re-solubilization of the enzyme within its matrix. The feed may have different moisture uptake properties depending on the climate, weather and time of year, causing further moisture stress. Embedding the enzyme in a solid matrix or encasing it in a granular protective layer can help reduce the extent of direct interactions between the feed and the enzyme, but the integrity of such a matrix or layer may also be compromised during the pelleting process, allowing these interactions to occur. Patent claims for granular products mention improved friability or breaking strength of the solid materials (Markussen and Jensen, 2018). Even in PPLAs, failure modes introduced by physical and chemical interactions of enzymes with the feed must be explored over these timescales.

Many of the strategies used in stabilization of enzymes to survive pelleting will also have a positive impact on improving storage stability, such as reducing oxidation potential, protective glycosylation, or isolating the enzyme from environmental stresses using a protective matrix or layer (see Sections 12.2.1, 12.2.2 and 12.3.3). Protection of enzyme activity during pelleting often considers a relatively severe stress of elevated temperature, high moisture, high mechanical agitation and compression – delivered over a short period of time. In contrast, providing a stable shelf life for the enzyme often involves lower potential stresses with kinetics of the order of days, months or years (Sulabo *et al.*, 2011). Some of these processes highlighted earlier include glycation, deamidation and action by proteases in the case of liquid feed. The protein engineering and formulation stabilization strategies highlighted above will undoubtedly have a benefit, although applications testing under relevant conditions is always necessary to understand the response of any particular enzyme system to stress.

12.5 Conclusion

The utilization of enzymes is essential for the production of high-performing animal feed. However, the process from enzyme production to application in animal feed introduces several extreme conditions, such as pelleting, necessary to produce high-quality feed. Several of these forces can have a detrimental impact on enzyme activity in the final product. Manufacturers of enzymes have taken multiple approaches to ensure that the correct level of activity is delivered to the animal. The approaches can generally be categorized in two classes: (i) protein engineering; and (ii) formulation. In both cases, stability can be dramatically improved for processing and storage. In addition, combining the advantageous properties of both approaches can provide additive benefits for the enzyme product and potentially exceed the requirements of the industry.

References

AISE (2014) *Guiding Principles for the Safe Handling of Enzymes in Detergent Manufacture, Version 2*. International Association for Soaps, Detergents and Maintenance Products, Brussels. Available at: https://www.aise.eu/documents/document/20150603154309-20141202_summary_safe_handling_of_enzymes_in_detergent_finale.pdf (accessed 19 October 2021).

Bagger, H.L., Fuglsang, C.C. and Westh, P. (2003) Preferential binding of two compatible solutes to the glycan moieties of *Peniophora lycii* phytase. *Biochemistry* 42, 10295–10300. https://doi.org/10.1021/bi034693i

Basketter, D.A., Broekhuizen, C., Fieldsend, M., Kirkwood, S., Mascarenhas, R., *et al.* (2010) Defining occupational and consumer exposure limits for enzyme protein respiratory allergens under REACH. *Toxicology* 268, 165–170. https://doi.org/10.1016/j.tox.2009.12.014

Becker, N.T., Clarkson, K.A., Dale, D.A., Fryksdale, B., Gebert, M.S., *et al.* (2010) Stable, durable granules with active agents. *Patent US 20100124586 A1*.

Bedford, M.R. and Partridge, G.G. (eds) (2010) *Enzymes in Farm Animal Nutrition*, 2nd edn. CAB International, Wallingford, UK.

Blanch, H.W. and Clark, D.S. (1995) *Biochemical Engineering*. Marcel Dekker, New York.

Cervin, M., Kensch, O., Kettling, U., Kim, S., Leuthner, B., *et al.* (2014) Variant *Buttiauxella* sp. phytases having altered properties. *Patent EP 2,733,209 A2*.

De Jong, J.A., Woodworth, J., DeRouchey, J.M., Goodband, R.D., Tokach, M., *et al.* (2017) Stability of four commercial phytase products under increasing thermal conditioning temperatures. *Translational Animal Science* 1, 255–260. https://doi.org/10.2527/tas2017.0030

De Vos, C., Simonsen, M., van Oort, M., Autton, S., Alanen, A. and Van Caelenberg, T. (2018) *Industry Guidelines on the Safe Handling of Enzymes in the Bakery Supply Chain*. Association of Manufacturers and Formulators of Enzyme Products (AMFEP) and Federation of European Union Manufacturers and Suppliers of Ingredients to the Bakery, Confectionery and Patisserie Industries (Fedima), Brussels. Available at: https://amfep.org/publications/guidelines-on-the-safe-handling-of-enzymes-in-the-bakery-supply-chain/ (accessed 24 September 2021).

EFSA (2008a) Safety and efficacy of the product Quantum™ Phytase 5000 L and Quantum™ Phytase 2500 D (6-phytase) as a feed additive for chickens for fattening, laying hens, turkeys for fattening, ducks for fattening and piglets (weaned) – Scientific Opinion of the Panel on Additives and Products or Substances used in Animal Feed and the Panel on Genetically Modified Organisms. *EFSA Journal* 6, 627.

EFSA (2008b) Safety and efficacy of Phyzyme XP 10000 (TPT/L), 6-phytase, as feed additive for chickens for fattening, laying hens, ducks for fattening, turkeys for fattening, piglets (weaned), pigs for fattening and sows – Scientific Opinion of the Panel on Additives and Products or Substances used in Animal Feed. *EFSA Journal* 6, 915.

EFSA (2012) Scientific Opinion on the safety and efficacy of Ronozyme HiPhos GT (6-phytase) as feed additive for poultry and pigs. *EFSA Journal* 10, 2730.

EFSA (2013) Scientific Opinion on the safety and efficacy of Quantum® Blue (6-phytase) as a feed additive for laying hens and minor laying poultry species. *EFSA Journal* 11, 3433.

EFSA (2016a) Safety and efficacy of Axtra® PHY 20000 TPT2 (6-phytase) as a feed additive for poultry and porcine species. *EFSA Journal* 14, e04625.

EFSA (2016b) Scientific Opinion on the safety and efficacy of RONOZYME® HiPhos (6-phytase) as a feed additive for sows and fish. *EFSA Journal* 14, 4393.

Fru-Nji, F. (2012) Choosing the right phytase product for your application. In: *Proceedings of the Poultry Feed Quality Conference, Bangkok, Thailand, 9–10 July 2012*. Asian Agribiz, Bangkok, p. 25.

Gebert, M., Lee, S.K., Johnson, M. and Ward, M. (2018) Glycosylation as a stabilizer for phytase. *Patent US 9,894,917 B2*.

Gebert, M., Dalsgaard, S., Ortiz-Johnson, M., Garske, A. and Dale, D. (2019) Stable enzymes by glycation reduction. *Patent EP 3,068,879 B1*.

Greiner, R. and Konietzny, U. (2012) Update on characteristics of commercial phytases. In: AB Vista (ed.) *Proceedings of the International Phytase Summit*. AB Agri Ltd, Rome, pp. 96–107.

Hoiberg-Nielsen, R., Fuglsang, C., Arleth, L. and Westh, P. (2006) Interrelationships of glycosylation and aggregation kinetics for *Peniophora lycii* phytase. *Biochemistry* 45, 5057–5066. https://doi.org/10.1021/bi0522955

ICCF (2019) *Stability Testing of Feed Ingredients*. International Cooperation for Convergence of Technical Requirements for the Assessment of Feed Ingredients, Wiehl, Germany. Available at: https://iccffeed.org/wp-content/uploads/ICCF_GL_01-Stability-Testing-Step7.pdf (accessed 24 September 2021).

Jacob, J.P. and Pescatore, A.J. (2012) Using barley in poultry diets – a review. *Journal of Applied Poultry Research* 21, 915–940. https://doi.org/10.3382/japr.2012-00557

Leeson, S. and Summers, J.D. (2005) Ingredient evaluation and diet formulation. In: *Commercial Poultry Nutrition*, 3rd edn. Nottingham University Press, Nottingham, UK, pp. 9–121.

Lehmann, M. (2004) Phytases. *Patent US 6,720,174 B1*.

Leistner, L. (2000) Basic aspects of food preservation by hurdle technology. *International Journal of Food Microbiology* 55, 181–186. https://doi.org/10.1016/S0168-1605(00)00161-6

Liu, Q., Xun, G. and Feng, Y. (2019) The state-of-the-art strategies of protein engineering for enzyme stabilization. *Biotechnology Advances* 37, 530–537. https://doi.org/10.1016/j.biotechadv.2018.10.011

Lund, M.N. and Ray, C.A. (2017) Control of Maillard reactions in foods: strategies and chemical mechanisms. *Journal of Agricultural and Food Chemistry* 65, 4537–4552. https://doi.org/10.1021/acs.jafc.7b00882

Lundblad, K.K., Hancock, J.D., Behnke, K.C., Prestlokken, E., McKinney, L.J. and Sorrensen, M. (2009) Adding water into the mixer improves pellet quality and pelleting efficiency in diets for finishing pigs with and without use of expander. *Animal Feed Science and Technology* 150, 295–302. https://doi.org/10.1016/j.anifeedsci.2008.10.006

Lutz, S. and Iamurri, S. (2017) Protein engineering: past, present, and future. In: Bornscheuer, U. and Höhne, M. (eds) *Protein Engineering. Methods in Molecular Biology*, vol. 1685. Humana Press, New York, pp. 1–12.

Manning, M.C., Chou, D.K., Murphy, B.M., Payne, R.W. and Katayama, D.S. (2010) Stability of protein pharmaceuticals: an update. *Pharmaceutical Research* 27, 544–575. https://doi.org/10.1007/s11095-009-0045-6

Marcussen, E., Borup, F., Simonsen, O. and Kjaer Markussen, E. (2016) Enzyme granules. *Patent US 20160227817*.

Markussen, E. and Jensen, P.E. (2018) Enzyme granules for animal feed. *Patent EP 3072399 B1*.

Menezes-Blackburn, D., Gabler, S. and Greiner, R. (2015) Performance of seven commercial phytases in an *in vitro* simulation of poultry digestive tract. *Journal of Agricultural and Food Chemistry* 63, 6142–6149. https://doi.org/10.1021/acs.jafc.5b01996

Miasnikov, A., Kumar, V., Kensch, O., Pellengahr, K., Leuthner, B., *et al.* (2006) Enzymes. *Patent WO 2006/043178 A2*.

Morgan, A., Clarkson, K., Bodie, E. and Cuevas, W. (1995) Use of a thermostable enzyme as a feed additive. *Patent WO 9,529,997*.

Nguyen, K. and Winter, B. (2013) Polypeptide having phytase activity and increased temperature resistance of the enzyme activity, and nucleotide sequence coding said polypeptide. *Patent US 8,420,369 B2*.

Nollet, L. (2015) On site production of liquid feed enzymes: a unique globally applied tool. *International Poultry Production* 23(8), 35.

Patel, J., Kothari, R., Rashbehari, T., Ritter, N. and Tunga, B. (2011) Stability considerations for biopharmaceuticals: overview of protein and peptide degradation pathways. *BioProcess International* 9, 20.

Ploegmakers, M. (2017) Feed enzyme market to exceed US$2b by 2024. *All About Feed*. Available at: https://www.allaboutfeed.net/animal-feed/feed-additives/feed-enzyme-market-to-exceed-us2b-by-2024/ (accessed 19 October 2021).

Puder, K., Simonsen, O., Jørgensen, C. and Jensen, A. (2009) Phytase inactivation in the animal feed pelleting process. *New Biotechnology* 25, S234–S235.

Rasmussen, D.K. (2010) *Difference in Heat Stability of Phytase and Xylanase Products in Pig Feed*. Trial Report No. 875. Pig Research Centre, Danish Agriculture and Food Council, Copenhagen.

Samli, H.E., Senkoylu, N., Akyurek, H. and Agma, A. (2006) Using rice bran in laying hen diets. *Journal of Central European Agriculture* 7, 135–140.

Schmidt, S.J. (2004) Water and solids mobility in foods. *Advances in Food and Nutrition Research* 48, 1–101. https://doi.org/10.1016/S1043-4526(04)48001-2

Scott, W.J. (1957) Water relations of food spoilage microorganisms. *Advances in Food Research* 7, 83–127. https://doi.org/10.1016/S0065-2628(08)60247-5

Sorensen, P.L. (2019) *Standard Operating Procedure – Pelleting of Feed*. Teknologisk Institut, Kolding, Denmark, pp. 3–7.

Sulabo, R.C., Jones, C.K., Tokach, M.D., Goodband, R.D., Dritz, S.S., *et al.* (2011) Factors affecting storage stability of various commercial phytase sources. *Journal of Animal Science* 89, 4262–4271. https://doi.org/10.2527/jas.2011-3948

Trefzer, A., Alvardo, A., Kline, K., Steer, B., Solbak, A., *et al.* (2013) Phytases, nucleic acids encoding them and methods for making and using them. *Patent AU 2013204086 B2.*

Truelock, C.N., Ward, N.E., Wilson, J.W., Stark, C.R. and Paulk, C.B. (2019) Effect of pellet die thickness and conditioning temperature during the pelleting process on phytase stability. *Kansas Agricultural Experiment Station Research Reports* 5(8).

Van der Veen, M.E., van Iersel, D.G., van der Goot, A.J. and Boom, R.M. (2004) Shear-induced inactivation of α-amylase in a plain shear field. *Biotechnology Progress* 20, 1140–1145. https://doi.org/10.1021/bp049976w

Vanhanen, M., Tuomi, T., Tiikkainen, U., Tupasela, O., Tuomainen, A., *et al.* (2001) Sensitisation to enzymes in the animal feed industry. *Occupational & Environmental Medicine* 58, 119–123. https://doi.org/10.1136/oem.58.2.119

Zhu, C., Ma, Y. and Zhou, C. (2010) Densities and viscosities of sugar alcohol aqueous solutions. *Journal of Chemical & Engineering Data* 55, 3882–3885. https://doi.org/10.1021/je9010486

13 Poultry and Swine Gastrointestinal Systems Functionally Differ to Influence Feedstuff Digestion and Responses to Supplemental Enzymes

Edwin T. Moran Jr*

Auburn University, Auburn, Alabama, USA

13.1 Introduction

Although the gastrointestinal tracts of poultry and swine employ parallel tactics to effect digestion, substantial differences in anatomy and manipulation of digesta exist. In comparing the gastrointestinal tracts of birds with mammals, McWorter *et al.* (2009) noted that the avian species generally eat more food as a function of their metabolic size while having a relatively smaller intestine and shorter period to effect digestion. Complete feeds offered to fowl and swine are dominated by grain, grain by-products and plant protein concentrates, with animal by-products and added fat being secondary. While nutrient availabilities with most common feedstuffs are similar for both animals, many differences exist. Rostagno *et al.* (2005) provided nutrient availability data on several feedstuffs commonly used with poultry and swine. Although animals used in experimentation and terms of conduct differed by necessity, methodology employed in most measurements was the same. Specifically, values for per cent crude protein (CP) digestibility and apparent metabolizable energy (AME) were both based on amount of feedstuff consumed relative to complete collections of excreta. In most cases per cent CP digestibility between fowl and swine was similar; however, AME with swine frequently exhibited a meaningful advantage. Certain of the grains, grain by-products and other plant by-products usually provided these exceptions, particularly when diverse particulate sizes and/or meaningful amounts of non-starch carbohydrates were present (Table 13.1).

Enzyme supplementation of complete feeds has become a dominant practice with poultry and swine. Given the frequent AME advantage of swine with a variety of feedstuffs, then differences in response to supplemental enzymes may also exist. In agreement, matrix values assembled for supplemental enzymes intended for these animals vary to such an extent that confidence in their application is lacking (Shelton *et al.*, 2004; Cowieson, 2010; Bedford *et al.*, 2016). Implication of AME being affected apart from CP digestibility is supported by the absence of distinguishing alterations with amino acid availability between animals when using xylanase (Cowieson and Bedford, 2009), whereas differences in AME are indicated from studies using wheat. A series of wheats

---

*Email: moranet@auburn.edu

©CAB International 2022. *Enzymes in Farm Animal Nutrition, 3rd Edition* (M. Bedford *et al.* eds)
DOI: 10.1079/9781789241563.0013

Table 13.1. Digestible protein and energy values of feedstuffs used for poultry versus swine. (Selected values from Rostagno et al., 2005.)

		Maize		Wheat		Soybean oil meal (49%)	Poultry fat	Purified	
		Ground	Gluten meal	Ground	Shorts			Starch	Casein
% CP digestibility	Poultry	85.5	93.0	85.5	84.0	92.1	0	0	82.5
	Swine	87.0	93.0	86.8	78.0	91.0	0	0	82.5
AME (kcal/kg)	Poultry	3340	3696	3046	2321	2302	8687	3520	3520
	Swine	3381	3929	3260	2740	3253	8228	3625	3600

having a progressive increase in AME with poultry was observed to lose advantage from xylanase as their energy increased; however, differences with swine among wheats and when enzyme was supplemented could not be established (Ravindran, 2013).

Generally, enzyme supplements exert their primary effects during ingesta's transient residence in the gastric system with resulting advantages being realized in the small and/or large intestine. Small intestinal advantages can be attributed to improvements in lumen conditions, pancreatic enzyme effectiveness and net absorption of nutrients. Improvements involving the large intestine relate to alterations that had occurred to the non-starch polysaccharides (NSPs), enabling microflora to generate additional AME. The following is a cursory comparison of food progress through the gastrointestinal systems of fowl and swine together with the potential influences of supplemental enzymes.

13.2   Gastric System

13.2.1   Oral cavity responsibilities

Oral cavity responsibilities are preceded by food sourcing followed by prehension and sensory evaluation. Finding food depends on sight and smell, with hearing being a lesser-known quantity. In these respects, fowl and swine are opposites. Fowl have a poor sense of smell to find food compared with the extensive olfactory apparatus of swine. Conversely, the pig's eyes are far from acute while fowl are very adept at the use of vision. The oral cavity presents another extreme between these two simple-stomached animals. The fowl's beak is immobile and fixed in size, which feed particulates must accommodate. In turn, fowl saliva is restricted to being the viscous type that involves immediate lubrication and direct swallowing of prehended particles. Fowl preferably seize particulates commensurate with the size of the oral cavity thereby minimizing the surface area needed for lubrication during swallowing (Schiffman, 1966).

Fine particulates and/or mash feeds generally lead to wastage as well as extended work at consumption which invariably increases feed conversion (Yo et al., 1997; Favero et al., 2009). Separately, grains exhibiting viscosity from soluble hemicelluloses are known to combine with saliva and 'paste' mandibles when fine ground, to impede prehension. Grinding of grain can generate a wide array of particulates. Coarse particulates are dominated by the fibrous pericarp and aleurone, followed with medium sizes which are typically the flinty portion of the endosperm, while fines result from the floury endosperm. When these particulate sizes are fed separately, the coarse and medium ones with maize have favourable ileal digestibilities for dry matter, starch and gross energy, while being less than expected when fine (Mtei et al., 2019). Few taste buds exist within the beak, then their location at the back of the tongue and absence of oral fluidity minimize perception.

Swine have a mouth highly adaptable to feedstuffs of varying size and character. Both viscous and serous type saliva are released to enhance oral manipulation of food. Amylase is included with the serous saliva to complement that present with accompanying feed, while the viscous component lubricates mastication. Swine salivary amylase parallels its pancreatic component in the digestion of starch (Furuichi and Takahashi, 1989); however, a low activity exists compared with other mammals (Chauncey et al., 1963). Teeth are implicit to mastication with the extent of dentition being a function of age (Tucker and Widowski, 2009). A minimum complement exists at birth that is restricted to canines and incisors during milk intake, whereas the demands of solid food are accommodated by the progressive appearance of premolars and molars. The physical character of feed should be in synchrony with existing dentition for effective mastication and subsequent digestion. While supplemental enzymes are expected to have a minor influence on operation of the oral cavity per se, characteristics of ingesta entering the oesophagus can predispose their subsequent response to digestion once in the gastric system.

13.2.2 Storage of consumed food

This is the first responsibility of the gastric system and represented by the crop within fowl and the oesophageal and cardiac regions within the pig's stomach. The crop is completely separated from subsequent proventricular addition of gastric juice, as is maceration of lumen contents by the gizzard (Fig. 13.1). Oesophageal transfer of ingesta into the crop represents all size particulates originally prehended. Co-consumed water saturates fine particulates while disintegrating feed pellets; however, large particulates such as whole grains, their 'flinty' parts as well as fibrous areas largely maintain their original structure throughout crop storage.

The crop's mucosal lining harbours a microflora dominated by lactobacilli that 'seed' luminal contents to complement microbes accompanying ingesta (Champ *et al.*, 1983). Mucosal microbes are dense at the oesophageal entrance and sparse at distal aspects (Bayer *et al.*, 1975). Body temperature aids expansion of associated microbes that is further facilitated by being in an aqueous system under anaerobic conditions. Amylase is released by this microbial population to generate maltose and maltotriose from starch for use as their primary energy source. Resulting lactic acid with minor amounts of volatile fatty acids (VFAs) accrue to reduce pH (Öztürkcan, 1985). Resistant starches arising from heat treatments of grain and feed can impair amylase's ability at degrading starch and reduce pH (Szylit *et al.*, 1974; Moran, 2019a). Although amylase is normally present with a wide array of feedstuffs, natural activity varies from a high being encountered with grain to a minimum for soybean meal (Steiner *et al.*, 2007). Supplemental amylase when superimposed on all other sources leads to a collective effort at decreasing pH of the digesta. This decrease in pH could potentially approach the pK of 3.8 for lactic acid but the minimum usually approximates 5–6.

Amylase's ability at facilitating a reduction in pH can be impaired when confronted with large particulates that reduce granule

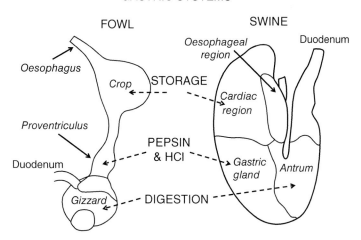

Fig. 13.1. Comparison of the gastric systems of fowl and swine. Fowl separate ingesta storage from subsequent addition of HCl and pepsin as well as formal digestion. Swine have each region immediately following one an other in the stomach. Each region entails common activities between animals. The overall purpose of gastric digestion is to improve aqueous compatibility of ingesta and enzymic release of nutrients for mucosal absorption. Most supplemental enzymes, particularly the carbohydrases, have their greatest impact during storage with subsequent advantages being realized in the small intestine and/or large intestine. Phytase enjoys a reduced pH created by microbes for action during storage as well as subsequent gastric digestion. (From Moran, 1982.)

exposure such as with the flinty parts of grain (Al-Rabadi *et al.*, 2009). Starch occlusion within the flinty endosperm largely involves adhering protein bodies dominated by the prolamines (Slack *et al.*, 1979). Dissolution of prolamines and granule release can be accomplished by supplemental proteases. Associated digestion not only exposes the granule surface but further hastens starch digestion by providing internal access with lateral exposure to the amylose helix (Tester *et al.*, 2007). Starch granules themselves have pores containing residual protein originating from their synthesis that impede entry of amylase (Huber and BeMiller, 1997). Many different supplemental proteases are possible; however, few favourably improve bird performance (Lee *et al.*, 2018a; Walk *et al.*, 2019). Effective proteases predominantly exhibit chymotrypsin type activity (Cowieson *et al.*, 2019) which is specific for internal cleavages at peptide bonds having amino acids expressing hydrophobic ends. Hydrophobic amino acids collectively represent the greatest proportion of most proteins; thus, increases in dietary protein usually result in greater proportions of chymotrypsin being released from the pancreas rather than either trypsin or the carboxypeptidases. In this respect, chymotrypsin would be adept at digesting the prolamines, which have an exceptional content of leucine and basis for their restricted solubility to dilute alcohol.

Strength at nutrient encapsulation is more extensive with cells of the aleurone layer and germ than endosperm. These cells harbour nascent enzymes employed during germination together with the bulk of kernel phytin (O'Dell and Boland, 1976; Rhodes and Stone, 2002). Extent of wall strength involves collaboration of an array of NSPs in conjunction with cellulose that varies among grains and cell location in the kernel (Knudsen, 2014). Aleurone protein is valued because of its desirable amino acid profile while phytin provides nutritionally important phosphorus and microminerals (Regvar *et al.*, 2011). Endosperm cell walls are weak and readily disassemble under aqueous conditions into soluble and/ or non-soluble hemicelluloses once in the crop (Hesselman and Åman, 1985; Bamforth and Kanauchi, 2001). Soluble forms may create varying viscosities and are prominent with wheat, barley and rye while the insoluble ones are more likely to occur with maize, sorghum and millet without altering aqueous character (Henry, 1985; Bengtsson, 1991; Kanauchi and Bamforth, 2001). Commercial sources of glucanase favour cleaving of the soluble forms to relieve the extent of viscosity while xylanases extend cleavage to the non-soluble forms and sturdy walls of the aleurone layer (Balance and Manners, 1978; Meng *et al.*, 2005). Combinations of both carbohydrases are of advantage when addressing the soluble viscous forms of fibre as well as structural ones (Cowieson *et al.*, 2010). Adding carbohydrases to maize diets when fine ground did not improve broiler performance and AME as much as when coarse (Kaczmarek *et al.*, 2014). Given that small amounts of structural proteins paralleling collagen cooperate with cell wall hemicelluloses to enhance strength, then supplemental protease (chymotrypsin) likely complements carbohydrase action (Robertson *et al.*, 1997).

Phytase would be minimally effective at the disassembly of phytin if not for the reduced pH enabled by microbially generated organic acids. Phytin has a very low solubility near neutrality which increases in concentration as pH decreases to improve phytase's ability at removing associated phosphorus (Kaufman and Kleinberg, 1971; Crea *et al.*, 2004). The addition of xylanase is envisaged to extend phytin destruction by phytase via its release from encapsulation. Understandably, total advantage when employing the full array of supplemental enzymes may not be additive compared with the summing of each one if used singly (Cowieson and Adeola, 2005; Cowieson *et al.*, 2019). Duration of ingesta in the crop influences the extent of microbial fermentation and potential action by supplemental enzymes. Such a delay is quite variable and largely relates to rapidity of intestinal nutrient recovery that is driven by needs of the body at-large (Rodrigues and Choct, 2018).

The pig's oesophagus conveys oral contents to the stomach. Unlike ingesta with fowl, mastication has minimized particulate size to increase surface exposure while the associated salivary amylase can foster an immediate but limited digestion of starch. Oesophageal mucosa upon entering the stomach harbours a microflora which seeds passing digesta to complement those accompanying consumed food in a manner paralleling the fowl's crop (Tannock and Smith, 1970; Barrow et al., 1971). Area of the stomach associated with ingesta storage is not separated from acid and pepsin addition or from formal gastric digestion as in fowl (Fig. 13.1). Essentially, the pig's stomach is a funnel collecting digesta in progressive layers that motility conveys from the cardiac area through the HCl- and pepsin-producing fundic zone to antral mixing. The pig's stomach seldom empties with motility but continually advances contents. Movement is initially weak in the cardiac region then gathers strength with a strong action being conducted in the antrum. Each successive layer in the cardiac region represents a progressive extent of anaerobic microbial activity and decreasing pH. The cardiac mucosa together with remaining aspects of the stomach have a mucous lining protective from lumen conditions (Pearson et al., 1980; Yakubov et al., 2007). However, the oesophageal surface is not protected and subject to 'conflicts' generated by adjacent microbial activity and pH. Prior mastication together with inclusion of salivary amylase predisposes an accentuated microbial population at the upper layers which can foster ulceration when using high-performance feeds, particularly when fine ground (Wolf et al., 2010). Such ulceration can be sufficiently serious to create mortality. Complications to the oesophageal mucosa from supplemental enzymes other than phytase likely depend on the nature of feedstuffs employed and intensity of animal production.

13.2.3 Formal gastric digestion

This is initiated with the addition of HCl followed by activation of accompanying pepsinogen once the pH approximates 2–3.

Gastric juice formation with fowl involves the proventriculus using oxnyticopeptic cells which form both HCl and pepsinogen, while the gastric gland area of swine relies on separate oxnytic and chief cells to produce HCl and pepsinogen, respectively. Motility retrieves 'seasoned' contents from the crop and cardiac area for inclusion of gastric juice before entry into the gizzard and stomach antrum, respectively. Supplemental enzymes may result in subtle alterations in operational pH without impairing gastric digestion. Supplementation with xylanase has been shown to increase gizzard pH while phytase may lead to a decrease, neither of which impacts broiler performance (Lee et al., 2018b).

Conditions existing during gastric digestion are deserving of comment. A substantial reduction in pH occurs that can further weaken plant cell wall associations among hemicelluloses to facilitate their rupture during intense motility. Viscosity resulting from solubilization of glucans and pentosans does not seem to impair gastric digestion with fowl as occurs during the subsequent recovery of nutrients from the small intestine (Haberer et al., 1998). Phytin protected by sturdy cell walls is of limited access to supplemental phytase while in the crop (Liao et al., 2005) until released through the forces of gizzard contractions (Truong et al., 2016). Phytases differing in pH optima continue to function during transition from storage through active gastric digestion although each may do so to differing extents (Yi and Kornegay, 1996; Onyango et al., 2005); however, other enzymes now encounter unfavourable conditions to be effective.

Destabilizing cellular structures enables dietary lipids whether added free and/or encapsulated to coalesce into a composite. Combining diverse lipids improves the likelihood of liquidity at body temperature, thereby improving subsequent emulsification and digestion. Organic acids and VFAs that are free remain largely nondissociated at low pH to be directly absorbed by either the gizzard musculature or antrum mucosa. These underlying tissues have substantial haemoglobin to accommodate oxygen and ability to rapidly consume these sources of energy. Entry of H^+ into microbes accompanying digesta may reduce the cytosolic pH of susceptible members to become lethal. Lysis of microbes not only decreases infectious threat and competition for nutrients but provides nutrition for the host. Pepsin focuses its attention on marginally soluble proteins that largely provide structural integrity of associated tissues. Pepsin's specificity is similar to chymotrypsin with cleavage at hydrophobic amino acids within the chain; however, gastric cleavage by pepsin is far more demanding for the preferred site to have a 'cluster' of hydrophobic amino acids that form hydrophobic bonds connecting adjacent chains. Such chain bonding is prominent with insoluble proteins such as found with animal connective tissue and associated with plant fibre.

Pepsin effectiveness at proteolysis appears to be compromised by the formation of protein complexes from phytic acid (Camus and Laporte, 1976). Such complexes likely depend on the presentation of cationic end groups of lysine, histidine and arginine that exist at low pH for complexation with corresponding anionic phosphates of phytic acid. Formation of these complexes directly with pepsin seems unlikely. Pepsin itself, along with structural proteins which represent its proteolytic objective, normally have minimal basic amino acids; however, pepsin's activation peptide is well endowed in this respect. Loss in pepsinogen may represent the primary complication to digestion. As a counter action, superdosing of phytase extends destruction of phytate thereby relieving potential threat to pepsin (Walk *et al.*, 2014). Hydrophobic bonding is nearly absent in the soluble albuminoid and globular proteins as typically represented by enzymes; thus, their demise by pepsin is generally spared (Moran, 2016a). Although this array of proteins usually has abundant basic amino acids that can potentially complex with phytic acid, such complexes are expected to disassemble once confronted with the neutral conditions of the small intestine and be digested by pancreatic enzymes once released.

The inclusion of HCl and pepsin into digesta is physically rigorous to complement earlier enzymic actions in the crop

and further weakened structural integrity. The gizzard is remarkably effective in this respect with the lumen being protected by a flexible koilin layer that parallels the unstirred water layer of intestine (Liman *et al.*, 2010; Moran, 2016b). As gizzard motility and the demands of particulate grinding increase, muscle mass adapts to accommodate need (Amerah and Ravindran, 2008). Eventually, a composite of fine particulates, colloids and soluble nutrients is formed for release into the small intestine. Retention of coarse material occurs by koilin ridging at the duodenal entrance of fowl as do similar structures appear prior to the pyloric valve of swine. Overburdening nutrient absorption in the duodenum of fowl has been shown to limit evacuations from the gizzard (Duke and Evanson, 1972; Duke *et al.*, 1975a), as is also expected with the pig's stomach.

13.3   Small Intestine

13.3.1   Anatomy and operation of the small intestine

The small intestine is different between fowl and swine (Moran, 1982). The fowl's duodenum progresses a considerable distance from gizzard through to the end of an intestinal loop formed by its association with the pancreas to where bile and pancreatic fluid enter. Jejunum subsequently continues to yolk sac remnant with ileum following to the caeco-colonic juncture. The duodenum is defined with swine as approximating the first 5% of intestine past the stomach's pyloric sphincter. Bile and pancreatic ducts enter the duodenum immediate to exit of gastric digesta. This beginning part of the intestine also expresses an accentuated thickness because of Brunner's glands in the mucosa that provide alkaline fluid to further aid neutralization. The last 5% of small intestine represents the ileum where an accentuated muscle layer is needed to peristaltically send a comparatively dense indigesta into the large intestine.

The intestinal wall in both animals comprises four major layers. The mucosa is initiated at the lumen followed by sub-mucosa, muscle layers and serosa, respectively. Minor layers of longitudinal and circular muscle fibres are also located within the mucosa and referred to as the *muscularis mucosae*. The major circular muscle dominates the intestinal wall with fowl while the *muscularis mucosae* fibres are prominent in swine (Moran, 1982). Such differences are important in the conduct of motility and convection of lumen contents with villi. Fowl employ their extensive circular muscle to effect refluxive peristalsis that moves digesta back and forth over extensive distances. Such movements are greatest from gizzard to the end of the duodenum where alkaline fluid carrying bile and pancreatic juice enters for neutralization of lumen contents and initiation of digestion. Thereafter, reflux distances progressively decrease through to large intestine (Chawan *et al.*, 1978; Mueller *et al.*, 1990).

Swine combine peristalsis over short distances with segmentation to progressively move digesta through the intestine. Their *muscularis mucosae* is obvious and presented as two layers paralleling those 'above' by the major muscle layers. Longitudinal fibres within the mucosa are located towards the lumen with their contractions enhancing surface convection by rotating villi in place. Such villi movement also facilitates lymph conveyance and transfer of chylomicrons from absorbed fat to vena cava and direct use by the body at-large. Its adjacent circular layer transiently contracts during peristalsis–segmentation to super-impose Kerckring valves in the lumen that act by further expanding surface exposure (Fig. 13.2). *Muscularis mucosae* contractions are of particular importance in the duodenum by also 'forcing' release of alkaline fluid from Brunner's glands into the lumen.

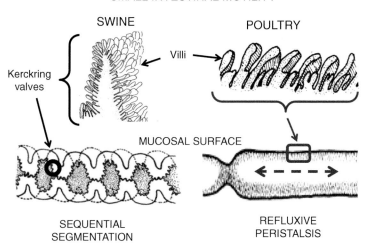

SMALL INTESTINAL MOTILITY

Fig. 13.2. Diagrammatic representation of motility and relative mucosal surface with fowl and swine. Fowl employ refluxive peristalsis to effect convection of lumen contents with a comparatively flat mucosa. Lumen nutrients released during digestion exist as laminar layers that progressively decrease in concentration from the core to mucosa. Resistance to laminar mixing seems to occur with viscosity to impair nutrient concentration at the surface and rate of absorption. Swine employ peristaltic segmentation that moves digesta in a slow progressive manner. Concurrently, transient contractions associated with the *muscularis mucosae* create Kerckring valves that increase surface exposure while rotating villi. The combination of actions with swine seems to be more effective in creating turbulence and realizing convection when encountering viscosity than occurs with fowl. (From Moran, 1982.)

13.3.2   Villi shape in fowl and swine

Villi shape as they protrude into the lumen is different between fowl and swine. Fowl generally express variations of leaf-shaped villi which optimize surface encounter during 'flow' with back-and-forth refluxive peristalsis (Bayer *et al.*, 1975; Bohórquez *et al.*, 2011). Swine largely present cylindrical villi which seem to be most appropriate for convection created by localized 'churning' when segmentation–peristalsis and Kerckring valves are combined (Yamauchi and Isshiki, 1991). Epithelial cells located on the top one-third of villi are represented as a mosaic of enterocytes and goblet cells with the unstirred water layer completely covering the surface. Enterocyte microvilli project attached mucin 'fibres' (glycocalyx) into the lumen while goblet cells release a soluble net-like mucin that becomes entangled with the glycocalyx to form the unstirred water layer (Moran, 2016a). Modified, unsulfated, sialylated and sulfated oligosaccharides that are associated with the mucin protein can be altered to maintain microclimate pH within the unstirred water layer as dietary conditions change (Shiau *et al.*, 1985; Moré *et al.*, 1987). Goblet cells producing the different oligosaccharides are histologically distinguishable by differential staining (Sharma *et al.*, 1997). Cellular details of the villi surface are superficially similar for both animals, but fowl do not have a lymphatic system within the core as do swine (Humphrey and Turk, 1974; Turk, 1982). Fowl form very-low-density lipoproteins during fat absorption that directly enter the vascular system for transit to the liver and facilitation of lipoprotein synthesis in support of yolk formation. Insignificance of the *muscularis mucosae* with fowl seems appropriate given the absence of lymph vessels within villi and reduced need for Kerckring valves during reflexive peristalsis.

13.3.3   Nutrient recovery from the lumen

A combination of several factors influences nutrient recovery from the lumen. Dispersion of pancreatic enzymes and fluidity of lumen contents are particularly important during motility. Released nutrients within the lumen must be conveyed to the unstirred water layer for absorption as generated. Trypsin, chymotrypsin and the carboxypeptidases 'collaborate' to yield free amino acids that are largely the essential ones along with short peptides dominated by the non-essentials (Moran, 2016b). Starch granules and remnants remaining after gastric residence continue into the small intestine then subsequently encounter pancreatic α-amylase. Structures that had been enhanced by annealing and retrogradation that occur during grain and feed heating remain resistant to digestion (Moran, 2019a). Although enzymes associated with feedstuffs and those supplemented to the diet are expected to largely bypass gastric destruction, their further viability in the small intestine is limited. Most are expected to succumb to pancreatic proteolysis unless stabilized. Pancreatic enzymes are all well stabilized by chelated calcium to defer autolysis until fulfilling their obligations before the end of the ileum (Caldwell, 1992). Supplemental amylase when fully loaded with calcium to provide a thermostable structure likely provides extended stability within the intestine (Ha *et al.*, 2000).

Dietary phytic acid is believed to impair structural stability of the pancreatic enzymes. Although dietary phytin is complexed with microminerals when in the feed, their dissociation during the low pH conditions of gastric digestion creates phytic acid that is subsequently in 'search' of divalents upon return to neutrality. While most dietary phytases pass through gastric digestion to appear in the duodenum, their activity upon approaching neutrality in the small intestine is of questionable significance. Amounts of phytase arriving at the ileum are very low to indicate that a proteolytic demise had occurred during the interim (Rapp *et al.*, 2001). Phytic acid prefers to sequester the first series transition elements, particularly zinc; however, having calcium at hand would seem to provide a favourable option (Schlegel *et al.*, 2010; Walk *et al.*, 2012). The carboxypeptidases require zinc as an essential cofactor which can easily be removed when faced with phytic acid to reduce their activities (Villegas *et al.*, 1995). Loss of pancreatic enzyme activity that occurs with removal of their chelated calcium essentially weakens their structural stability facilitating a premature autolysis. Reducing longevity of the pancreatic enzymes to effect digestion essentially provides an indirect means by which phytic acid could influence nutrient availability.

Phytic acid in 'need' to complex divalents may further damage nutrient recovery by disrupting the unstirred water layer. Associated mucins form a barrier to large molecules and microbes while the underlying space is buffered to optimize final digestion of nutrients for absorption (Moran, 2016b). Essentially, underlying goblet cells continually release gel-forming mucins as granules which had been packaged together with calcium (Paz *et al.*, 2003; Perez-Vilar, 2007). Ca^{2+} enables the negatively charged mucin chains to be tightly assembled into granules during their synthesis. Calcium progressively dissipates from the granule once released to allow the water-soluble mucin chains to slowly entangle with the membrane-bound mucin (glycocalyx). Granule release is viewed as being continual and necessary to replace surface losses from digestive dynamics and microbial action. Phytic acid is sufficiently small to readily enter the unstirred water layer then hypothetically increase the rate of calcium removal from the granule to accentuate mucin release. Attachment of *O*-linked oligosaccharides to the mucin protein chain sterically hinders lumen proteolysis and recovery of associated amino acids by the small intestine (Hansson *et al.*, 1991).

The amino acid composition of mucin corresponds to the increased endogenous losses created by phytic acid. These losses appear to be more extensive with fowl than observed with swine (Onyango *et al.*, 2009; Woyengo *et al.*, 2009). Such losses impair the overall efficiency of dietary protein utilisation (Cowieson *et al.*, 2008). As long as the increased phosphorus from phytin is contributing to the animal's requirement, response can be measured in terms of growth; however,

relief of impairments to pancreatic enzyme stability and excessive mucin loss are more likely to appear as improved feed conversion. These secondary improvements only become apparent with the superdosing of phytase that extends phosphorus release from dietary phytin beyond satisfying the animal's requirement (Cowieson *et al.*, 2011; Walk *et al.*, 2013).

13.3.4 Motility

Motility conveys digestion products that accumulate in the lumen core to the unstirred water layer for absorption. Convection is essential for rapid nutrient recovery as it increases the rate of absorption by 30–100% compared with a stationary system (Macagno *et al.*, 1982). Fowl and swine have similar neural systems within the small intestine to detect lumen and lamina propria nutrient levels enabling a synchronization of motility with nutrient recovery (Csoknya *et al.*, 1990; Brehmer *et al.*, 1997). Imposing viscosity has been shown to impair the absorption of water-soluble nutrients to a lesser extent than the much larger fat micelles (Huyghebaert, 1997; Dänicke *et al.*, 1999). In turn, fat soluble vitamins that are marginal during feed formulation may evolve into becoming deficient as lumen conditions thicken. Viscosity is also believed to impair recovery of lumen nutrients more so with fowl than swine. Nutrients arising during digestion occur as laminar layers that progressively decrease in concentration from the core to mucosa. Mixing to maximize exposure of lumen contents to the unstirred water layer would seem to suffer to a greater extent during refluxive peristalsis than occurs during localized turbulence created by peristalsis–segmentation (Lentle and Janssen, 2008). Increasing viscosity of intestinal contents has been shown to not only decrease convective efficiency but increase orocaecal transit with pigs (Cherbut *et al.*, 1990) that parallels similar effects with fowl (Palander *et al.*, 2010). The extent of difference that potentially exists between fowl and swine is open to question. Inability to impose definitive viscosities during experimentation hampers detecting differences in convection.

Just as viscosity reduces absorptive efficiency so also does oxygen transfer from mucosa to lumen decrease. This reduction becomes progressively extensive from duodenum through to ileum as intensity of motility and length of villi decrease. Hillman et al. (1993) observed a reduction of dissolved oxygen in the pig's lumen contents from duodenum to ileum, then a precipitous fall once in the colon. Such a reduction is considered to be a particularly important factor in determining activity and composition of lumen microflora. The increased concentration of lumen nutrients from impaired absorption readily aids expansion of the microbial population while lowering of oxygen modifies membership from aerobes to facultatives (Langhout et al., 2000). Having an escalating population of operational anaerobes also increases mucin-degrading abilities together with turnover of the villi epithelia (Morel et al., 2005; Cheled-Shoval et al., 2014). Understandably, supplemental broad-spectrum antibiotics can provide substantial relief from viscosity apart from the loss in convective efficiency (Moran and McGinnis, 1965). Broilers encountering intestinal viscosity without the benefit of supplemental antibiotics experience an increased incidence of subclinical infections from Clostridium perfringens, particularly when the mucosa is aggravated by coccidia (Moran, 2014).

13.4   Large Intestine

13.4.1   Gross anatomy

Gross anatomy presented by the large intestinal systems of fowl and swine differs extensively. Fowl have two large caeca and a short colon while swine present one short caecum and an extensive colon. The small intestine ends at the ileo-caeco-colonic valve in both animals, which is continuously closed except for the brief and forced entry of indigesta (Duke et al., 1975b). This valve separates aerobic conditions, extensive

villi and a minimal level of microbes existing in the small intestine from an extensive population of strict anaerobes and comparatively flat mucosa in the large intestine. These anaerobes play a major role in digesting cellulosic components with release of by-product VFAs that contribute to AME (Hartemink et al., 1996; Rinttilä and Apajalahti, 2013).

Absence of a 'functional' microbial population immediate to either hatching or parturition delays large intestinal 'operation'. Swine have less of a problem in establishing this population because piglet parturition is adjacent to the anal area with further faecal encounters upon nursing. Chicks hatching in the nest would have similar exposures with faeces originating from the setting hen. However, relative sterility exists in commercial hatcheries together with conditions at placement; thus, low as well as 'inappropriate' microbes delay formation of a 'competent' population (Moran, 2019b). Such impaired functionality is expected to decrease VFA contributions to AME. Yang et al. (2020) noted AME measurements with broilers to linearly increase from 7 to 28 days of age. Birds placed under commercial conditions can benefit from supplemental glucanase and xylanase when the small intestine is confronted with viscosity; however, caeca subsequently fail at generating VFAs while resulting excreta complicates litter management, regardless of xylanase (Moran et al., 1969).

13.4.2   Motility

Motility employed by fowl and swine in the large intestine differs by virtue of differences in anatomy. Motility by fowl, once indigesta enters the colon, again involves refluxive peristalsis (Fig. 13.3). As digesta is moved down the short colon, urine excreted into the urodeum returns to 'wash' lumen contents. Associated solutes, colloids and fines are transferred back and forced to enter the narrow caeca opening while coarse material is excluded to separately collect in the coprodeum. A more intensive microbial population exists in the caeca than colon

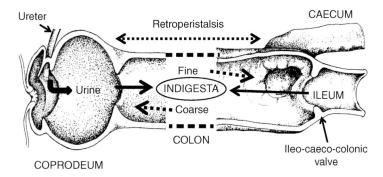

Fig. 13.3. Fowl thrust indigesta from the small intestine through the ileo-caeco-colonic valve into the colon. Refluxive peristalsis moves urine back from the urodeum to segregate indigesta. Caecal entry is small with villi projecting from the wall to limit entrance to solutes, colloids and fine materials. Coarse particulates are excluded to collect in the coprodeum until defecation. Caecal contents progressively accrue and rapidly ferment to release VFAs for use by the bird. A peristaltic 'rush' periodically eliminates the 'spent' contents as a separate dropping after the coprodeum is cleared. (From Moran, 1982.)

with both areas employing considerable mucin for surface protection (Suprasert et al., 1987). The chicken's caecal microbiome is extremely adaptable in its use of indigesta for its own development, with by-product VFAs arising because of anaerobic conditions (Sergeant et al., 2014). These VFAs are typically represented by acetic, butyric, propionic, isobutyric, isovaleric and isocaproic acids which can vary with bird age and differing sources of fermentable substrate (McCafferty et al., 2019). Each of the two caeca has motility patterns that facilitate mixing then evacuation of contents when spent (Janssen et al., 2009).

A large part of the soluble indigesta involves mucins corresponding to the endogenous losses from the small intestine, which phytic acid has been shown to accentuate (Onyango et al., 2009). These indigestible glycoproteins can now be used as microbial nutrients as can urinary nitrogen. Evacuation of caecal contents occurs as a peristaltic rush once the coprodeum is cleared to void a 'pasty' dropping that is distinctively different from the coarse faecal pellet. Inclusion of xylanase in maize–soybean meal feeds for broilers has been observed to increase size of caeca and amounts of contents (E.T. Moran Jr, 1987,

unpublished results) while differing feedstuffs alter the resulting proportions of VFAs (McCafferty et al., 2019). Differing grains and procedures in milling are prominent in creating an array of particulate types and sizes which could differentially enter the caeca. Subsequent feed manufacturing, carbohydrase action in the crop and gizzard maceration further influence caeca access and VFA production (Haberer et al., 1998; Amerah et al., 2009). Should viscosity issues exist, then combining supplemental carbohydrases not only relieves impaired nutrient absorption by the small intestine, but further modifies indigesta to improve AME recovery and excreta character.

The large intestine of swine initially presents a short caecum followed by long ascending, descending and transverse parts of the colon before ending at the rectal ampulla. Wall structure changes drastically from beginning to end. Caecum, ascending and descending colon have their longitudinal muscle fibres located towards the outside of the intestine that 'gather' into bands called taeniae coli, while circular muscle remains continuous (Fig. 13.4). Upon contraction of circular muscle, 'bulges' referred to as haustra form where longitudinal banding does not provide overhead stabilization.

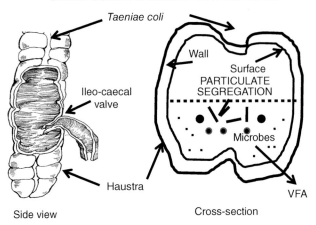

Fig. 13.4. An illustration of the swine's ileo-caeco-colonic junction. The ileo-caecal valve briefly opens to peristaltically move indigesta from the small intestine into the caecum. The helicoidal colon has its outside longitudinal muscle gathered into bands (*taeniae coli*) that enable the underlying circular muscle to form 'out-pocketings' (haustra) during contractions. Differential motility as effected by the circular and longitudinal muscles segregates indigesta such that large particulates gather in the core while smaller ones with colloids and solutes enter the haustra. An anaerobic microbial population is concentrated at the mucosal surface where ready fermentation forms VFAs for absorption. Microbes also engage core particulates, but their reduced surface area involving well-structured fibre resists rapid degradation and VFA production. (From Moran, 1982.)

Extent of out-pocketing decreases with progression to the transverse colon where they disappear upon return of a complete layer of longitudinal muscle that reforms a 'typical' intestinal wall.

Indigesta is directed into the caecum lumen by the ileo-caeco-colonic valve to initiate motility and move contents through the colon. Essentially, differential contractions of circular and longitudinal muscles create a separation of lumen indigesta. Solutes, colloids and small particulates accrue in the haustra 'out-pocketings' while coarse material collects in the core (Lentle and Janssen, 2008). This separation of small particulates and solutes into haustra with swine (Fig. 13.4) parallels their selective movement into caeca with fowl. Similarly, solutes and small particulates having an extensive surface are readily degraded by a concentrated microbial population located at the haustrum wall. Each haustrum slowly progresses along the colon while retaining its contents as the coarse particulates in the lumen proceed rectally at a more rapid rate. Upon return of

the longitudinal muscle 'covering', haustra contents have been microbiologically 'distilled' into a small pellet. This pellet is then 'pasted' on to the coarse core located in the lumen to create faeces having a nodular surface. Accrual in the rectal ampulla eventually leads to a 'critical mass' for defecation. Viscosity in the small intestine creates a converse situation with undigested nutrients concentrating in the core. Diminished recovery of nutrients from the duodenum–jejunum can be detected with indigesta arriving at the ileum; however, their microbial use in the large intestine 'corrects' this loss to 'distort' total digestibility measurements based on excreta.

13.4.3 Colonic mucosa of the pig

The swine colonic mucosa is well endowed with goblet cells that elaborate substantial mucus for protection. These mucins differ by producing acidic sulfo-glycoproteins as opposed to neural mucins that are prevalent in the jejunum (Moré et al., 1987). A relatively flat mucosa combined with an extensive mucus depth foster strict anaerobic conditions (Fogg et al., 1996; Johansson et al., 2011). Two mucus layers appear on the pig's mucosa with the outer one containing microbial representatives that 'seed' the lumen while excluding them from the inner layer (Janssen et al., 2009). Microbes that seed the lumen are continuously modified in membership to optimize 'talents' of the population at catabolizing an ever-changing indigesta. Resultant VFA proportions and quantity vary as a function of existing indigesta presented for fermentation. All VFAs readily enter the unstirred water layer where a pH approaching their pK exists. The non-dissociated forms now pass readily through cell membranes to be absorbed and used by the animal (Freeman et al., 1993).

While fermentation is prominent within haustra, core fibre encounters relatively less microbial activity. Reduced surface area presented by these large particulates together with a structural integrity representative of acid detergent fibre interfere with VFA production, but meaningful amounts still contribute to concurrent production in haustra (Russell, 1979). On the other hand, Bjornhag and Sperber (1977) noted the exclusion of large particulates from the caeca by turkeys which, combined with their short residence in the coprodeum, eliminates ready VFA contributions. A comparative use of peas and wheat supports the differential separation of particulates between animals. NSP particulates are substantial in the endosperm of pulses. Goodlad and Mathers (1991) reported the digestibility of dried field peas by pigs to be considerably greater than observed with wheat, whereas Longstaff and McNab (1987) found the converse to be true for chickens.

Duration of microbial encounter while indigesta is resident in each large intestinal system superimposes another variable. Food passage through the gastrointestinal system approximates 24 h with pigs (Entringer et al., 1975) compared with 2 h for chickens (Tuckey et al., 1958). Given a partial recovery of AME from coarse particulates over an extended period in the core of the pig's colon, then benefit from supplemental xylanase would be relatively less than derived with fowl. Essentially, imposing xylanase modifications to large particulates with fowl provides additional contributions to AME that would ordinarily have been recovered from the core of the pig's colon.

Protein entering the large intestine not only represents indigestible dietary protein, but also endogenous losses dominated by mucin. These sources of nitrogen are expected to be largely soluble and/or colloidal rather than associated with large particulates. Thus, the final location of most indigesta-nitrogen entering the large intestine would preferentially access caeca and haustra with fowl and swine, respectively. Experimentation relating equivalent digestibilities of CP between poultry and swine with the bulk of feedstuffs is rational given its similarity in final use while concurrently encountering frequent differences in AME recovery.

13.5   Overview

The gastrointestinal systems of fowl and swine differ in several aspects of anatomy and nutrient retrieval. Ingesta storage in either the crop of fowl or the stomach's cardiac region with swine is particularly important to the effectiveness of supplemental enzymes. A purposeful anaerobic population in both animals accrues lactic acid to decrease milieu pH. Supplemental amylase facilitates a further reduction in pH by microbes. Proteases indirectly contribute to this reduction in pH by availing starch entrapped in the flinty portions of grain. Reduction of pH is limited during ingesta storage by brevity of residence, but values approximating 5–6 can be expected. Concurrently, glucanases and xylanases relieve viscosity created by solubilized fibre while xylanases release nutrients and phytin encapsulated within resilient cell walls. Multiple approaches at reducing pH during this phase of digestion seem purposeful to emphasize phytase functioning that avails phosphorus while minimizing complications from dietary phytin.

HCl and pepsin combined with the physical forces encountered in either the gizzard or pyloric antrum dishevel food structure to improve nutrient accessibility during small intestinal digestion. Although improved nutrient availabilities can arise from earlier digestion of resistant starches by amylase as well as some structural proteins using supplemental chymotrypsin-like proteases, greater advantage is expected from the carbohydrases. Decreases in digesta viscosity and nutrient encapsulation can be substantial while altering physical characteristics of NSPs facilitates subsequent fermentation in the large intestine. Minimizing viscosity in the small intestine appears to be less advantageous with swine than poultry. Combining peristalsis with segmentation with the pig creates a lumen 'churning' that appears to be less influenced at conveying nutrients to the mucosa than occurs with fowl using refluxive peristalsis.

Providing phosphorus from phytin to meet the animal's requirement for growth is the most distinct advantage arising from phytase. Minimization of phytic acid may also extend the life of pancreatic enzymes by avoiding the removal of structural calcium and premature autolysis. Another indirect advantage seems to occur by minimizing the rate of calcium removal from mucin granules released from goblet cells to accentuate solubilization and lumen loss rather than retention by the unstirred water layer. Hyper-dosing of phytase can be credited for enabling these indirect advantages

that likely appear as subtle improvements in feed conversion.

The large intestinal systems capitalize on their strict anaerobe population to largely ferment NSPs and produce VFAs. Fowl use refluxive peristalsis to move solutes, fines and small particulates from colon into caeca for fermentation, while coarse material is conveyed to the coprodeum for excretion. Swine have a colon with haustra out-pocketings that collect these fermentable materials while coarse particulates concentrate in the core for movement to the rectal ampulla. Inadequate maturation of the microbial population following birth minimizes VFA yield and AME recovery, particularly with commercial fowl experiencing a relatively sterile environment.

Supplemental xylanases are also credited with modifying large particulates, enabling access to intensive microbial action. Although both animals benefit from these modifications, fowl seem to enjoy a greater advantage than swine. Large particulates normally voided by fowl may now enter the caeca and contribute AME. Prolonged residence of large particulates is ordinary within the pig's colon core to enable additional AME. In turn, fowl usually derive a greater relative benefit from xylanase than swine. Concurrently, undigested proteins and endogenous nitrogen are expected to be either soluble and/or colloidal in form. These nitrogen sources arising from most feedstuffs largely enter either the caeca of fowl or haustra of swine to favour equivalent CP utilization, regardless of microbial activity.

References

Al-Rabadi, G.J.S., Gilbert, R.G. and Gidley, M.J. (2009) Effect of particle size on kinetics of starch digestion in milled barley and sorghum grains by porcine alpha-amylase. *Journal of Cereal Science* 50, 198–204.

Amerah, A.M. and Ravindran, V. (2008) Influence of method of whole-wheat feeding on the performance, digestive tract development and carcass traits of broiler chickens. *Animal Feed Science and Technology* 147, 326–339.

Amerah, A.M., Ravindran, V. and Lentle, R.G. (2009) Influence of wheat hardness and xylanase supplementation on the performance, energy utilisation, digestive tract development and digesta parameters of broiler starters. *Animal Production Science* 49, 71–78.

Balance, G.M. and Manners, D.J. (1978) Structural analysis and enzymic solubilization of barley endosperm cell walls. *Carbohydrate Research* 61, 107–118.

Bamforth, C.W. and Kanauchi, M. (2001) A simple model for the cell wall of the starchy endosperm in barley. *Journal of the Institute of Brewing* 107, 235–240.

Barrow, P.A., Fuller, R. and Newport, M.J. (1971) Changes in the microflora and physiology of the anterior intestinal tract of pigs weaned at 2 days with special reference to the pathogenesis of diarrhea. *Infection and Immunity* 18, 586–595.

Bayer, R.C., Chawan, C.B. and Bird, F.H. (1975) Scanning electron microscopy of the chicken crop – the avian rumen? *Poultry Science* 54, 703–707.

Bedford, M.R., Walk, C.L. and Masey O'Neill, H.V. (2016) Assessing measurements in feed enzyme research: phytase evaluations in broilers. *Journal of Applied Poultry Research* 25, 305–314.

Bengtsson, S. (1991) Studies on cell structures and properties of soluble cell-wall polysaccharides in rye and barley. Dissertation, Swedish University of Agricultural Sciences, Uppsala, Sweden.

Bjornhag, G. and Sperber, I. (1977) Transport of various food components through the digestive tract of turkeys. *Swedish Journal of Agricultural Research* 7, 57–65.

Bohórquez, D.V., Bohórquez, N.E. and Ferket, P.R. (2011) Ultrastructural development of the small intestinal mucosa in the embryo and turkey poult: a light and electron microscopy study. *Poultry Science* 90, 842–855.

Brehmer, A., Schrödl, F. and Neuhuber, W. (1997) Mucosal innervations of the pig small intestine. A preliminary report. *Biogenic Amines* 13, 251–257.

Caldwell, R.A. (1992) Effect of calcium and phytic acid on the activation of trypsinogen and the stability of trypsin. *Journal of Agricultural and Food Chemistry* 40, 43–48.

Camus, M.-C. and Laporte, J.-C. (1976) Wheat as an *in vitro* inhibitor of peptic proteolysis. Role of phytic acid in by-products. *Annales de Biologie Animale, Biochemie, Biophysique* 16, 719–729.

Champ, M., Szylit, O., Raibaud, P. and Aït-Abdelkader, N. (1983) Amylase production by three *Lactobacillus* strains isolated from chicken crop. *Journal of Applied Bacteriology* 55, 487–493.

Chauncey, H.H., Henriques, B.L. and Tanzer, J.M. (1963) Comparative enzyme activity of saliva from the sheep, hog, dog, rabbit, rat, and human. *Archives of Oral Biology* 8, 615–627.

Chawan, F.H., Bird, F.H. and Gerry, R.W. (1978) Relationship between intestinal movements and pancreatic juice secretion in the domestic chicken. *Poultry Science* 57, 1084–1086.

Cheled-Shoval, S.L. Gamage, N.S.W., Amit-Robmach, E., Forder, R., Marshal, J., *et al.* (2014) Differences in intestinal mucin dynamics between germ-free and conventionally reared chickens after mannan-oligosaccharide supplementation. *Poultry Science* 93, 636–644.

Cherbut, C., Albina, E., Champ, M., Doublier, J.L. and Lecannu, G. (1990) Action of guar gums on the viscosity of digestive contents and on the gastrointestinal motor function in pigs. *Digestion* 46, 205–213.

Cowieson, A.J. (2010) Strategic selection of exogenous enzymes for corn/soy based poultry diets. *Japanese Journal of Poultry Science* 47, 1–7.

Cowieson, A.J. and Adeola, O. (2005) Carbohydrases, proteases, and phytase have an additive beneficial effect in nutritionally marginal diets for broiler chicks. *Poultry Science* 84, 1860–1867.

Cowieson, A.J. and Bedford, M.R. (2009) The effect of phytase and carbohydrase on ileal amino acid digestibility in monogastric diets: complimentary mode of action. *World's Poultry Science Journal* 65, 609–622.

Cowieson, A.J., Ravindran, V. and Selle, P.H. (2008) Influence of phytic acid and source of microbial phytase on ileal endogenous amino acid flows in broiler chickens. *Poultry Science* 87, 2287–2299.

Cowieson, A.J., Bedford, M.R. and Ravindran, V. (2010) Interactions between xylanase and glucanases in maize–soy diets for broilers. *British Poultry Science* 51, 246–257.

Cowieson, A.J., Toghyani, M., Kheravii, S.K., Wu, S.-B., Romero, L.F. and Choct, M. (2011) Super-dosing effects of phytase in poultry and other monogastrics. *World's Poultry Science Journal* 67, 225–235.

Cowieson, A.J., Toghyani, M., Kheravii, S.K., Wu, S.-B., Romero, L.F. and Choct, M. (2019) A mono-component microbial protease improves performance, net energy, and digestibility of amino acids and starch, and up regulates jejunal expression of genes responsible for peptide transport in broilers fed corn/wheat-based diets supplemented with xylanase and phytase. *Poultry Science* 98, 1321–1332.

Crea, F., Crea, P., De Robertis, A. and Sammartano, S. (2004) Speciation of phytate ion in aqueous solution. Characterization of Ca–phytate sparingly soluble species. *Chemical Speciation and Bioavailability* 16, 53–59.

Csoknya, M., Fekete, É., Gábriel, R., Halasy, K. and Benedeczky, I. (1990) Histochemical characterization of myenteric plexus in domestic fowl small intestine. *Zeitschrift für mikroskopisch-anatomische Forschung* 104, 625–638.

Dänicke, S., Vahjen, W., Simon, O. and Jeroch, H. (1999) Effects of dietary fat type and xylanase supplementation to rye-based broiler diets on selected bacterial groups adhering to the intestinal epithelium, on transit time of feed, and nutrient digestibility. *Poultry Science* 78, 1292–1299.

Duke, G.E. and Evanson, O.A. (1972) Inhibition of gastric motility by duodenal contents in turkeys. *Poultry Science* 51, 1625–1636.

Duke, G.E., Kostuch, T.E. and Evanson, O.A. (1975a) Gastroduodenal electrical activity in turkeys. *Digestive Diseases* 20, 1047–1058.

Duke, G.E., Kostuch, T.E. and Evanson, O.A. (1975b) Electrical activity and intraluminal pressures in the lower small intestine of turkeys. *Digestive Diseases* 20, 1040–1046.

Entringer, R.P., Plumlee, M.P., Conrad, J.H., Cline, T.R. and Wolfe, S. (1975) Influence of diet on passage rate and apparent digestibility of growing swine. *Journal of Animal Science* 40, 486–496.

Favero, A., Maiorka, A., Dahlke, F., Meurer, R.F.P., Oliveria, R.S. and Sens, R.F. (2009) Influence of feed form and corn particle size on the live performance and digestive tract development. *Journal of Applied Poultry Research* 18, 772–779.

Fogg, F.J.J., Hutton, D.A., Jumel, K., Pearson, J.P., Harding, S.E. and Allen, A. (1996) Characterization of pig colonic mucins. *Biochemistry Journal* 316, 937–942.

Freeman, K., Foy, T., Feste, S., Reeds, P.J. and Lifschitz, C.H. (1993) Colonic acetate in the circulating acetate pool of the infant pig. *Pediatric Research* 34, 318–322.

Furuichi, Y. and Takahashi, T. (1989) Purification and characterization of porcine salivary amylase. *Agricultural and Biological Chemistry* 53, 293–294.

Goodlad, J.S. and Mathers, J.C. (1991) Digestion by pigs of non-starch polysaccharides in wheat and raw peas (*Pisum sativum*) fed in mixed diets. *British Journal of Nutrition* 65, 259–270.

Ha, N.-C., Oh, B.-C., Shin, H.-J., Oh, T.-K., Kim, Y.-O., *et al.* (2000) Crystal structures of a novel, thermostable phytase in partially and fully calcium-loaded states. *Nature Structural Biology* 7, 147–153.

Haberer, B., Schultz, E. and Flachowsky, G. (1998) Effects of β-glucanase and xylanase supplementation in pigs fed a diet rich in nonstarch polysaccharides: disappearance and disappearance rate of nutrients including nonstarch polysaccharides in stomach and small intestine. *Journal of Animal Physiology and Animal Nutrition* 78, 95–103.

Hansson, G.C., Bouhours, J.-F., Karlsson, H. and Carlstedt, I. (1991) Analysis of sialic acid-containing oligosaccharides from porcine small intestine by high-temperature gas chromatography–mass spectrometry of their dimethyamides. *Carbohydrate Research* 221, 179–189.

Hartemink, R., Van Laere, K.M.J., Mertens, A.K.C. and Rombouts, F.M. (1996) Fermentation of xyloglucan by intestinal bacteria. *Anaerobe* 2, 223–230.

Henry, R.J. (1985) A comparison of the non-starch carbohydrates in cereal grains. *Journal of the Science of Food and Agriculture* 36, 1243–1253.

Hesselman, K. and Åman, P. (1985) A note on microscopy studies on water- and β-glucanase-treated barley. *Swedish Journal of Agricultural Research* 15, 139–143.

Hillman, K., Whyte, A.L. and Stewart, C.S. (1993) Dissolved oxygen in the porcine gastrointestinal tract. *Letters in Applied Microbiology* 16, 299–302.

Huber, K.C. and BeMiller, J.N. (1997) Visualization of channels and cavities of corn and sorghum starch granules. *Cereal Chemistry* 74, 537–541.

Humphrey, C.D. and Turk, D.E. (1974) The ultrastructure of normal chick intestinal epithelium. *Poultry Science* 53, 990–1000.

Huyghebaert, G. (1997) The effect of a wheat–fat-interaction on the efficacy of a multi-enzyme preparation in broiler chickens. *Animal Feed Science and Technology* 68, 55–66.

Janssen, P.W.M., Lentle, R.G., Hulls, C., Ravindran, V. and Amerah, A.M. (2009) Spatiotemporal mapping of the motility of the isolated chicken caecum. *Journal of Comparative Physiology B* 179, 593–604.

Johansson, M.E.V., Holmén, J.M. and Hansson, G.C. (2011) The two mucus layers of colon are organized by the MUC2 mucin, whereas the outer layer is a legislator of host–microbial interactions. *Proceedings of the National Academy of Sciences USA* 108, 4659–4665.

Kaczmarek, S.A., Rogiewicz, A., Moggielnicka, M., Rutkowski, A., Jones, R.O. and Slominski, B.A. (2014) The effect of protease, amylase, and nonstarch polysaccharide enzyme supplementation on nutrient utilization and growth performance of broiler chickens fed corn–soybean meal-based diets. *Poultry Science* 93, 1745–1753.

Kanauchi, M. and Bamforth, C.W. (2001) Release of β-glucan from cell walls of starchy endosperm of barley. *Cereal Chemistry* 78, 121–124.

Kaufman, H.W. and Kleinberg, I. (1971) Effect of pH on calcium binding by phytic acid and its inositol phosphoric acid derivatives and on the solubility of their calcium salts. *Archives of Oral Biology* 16, 445–460.

Knudsen, E.K.B. (2014) Fiber and nonstarch polysaccharide content and variation in common crops used in broiler diets. *Poultry Science* 93, 2380–2395.

Langhout, D.J., Schutte, J.B., de Jong, J., Sloetjes, H., Verstegen, M.W.A. and Tamminga, S. (2000) Effect of viscosity on digestion of nutrients in conventional and germ-free chicks. *British Journal of Nutrition* 83, 533–540.

Lee, S.A., Bedford, M.R. and Walk, C.L. (2018a) Meta-analysis: explicit value of mono-component protease in monogastric diets. *Poultry Science* 97, 2078–2085.

Lee, S.A., Dunne, J., Febery, E., Brearley, C.A., Mottram, T. and Bedford, M.R. (2018b) Exogenous phytase and xylanase exhibit opposing effects on real-time gizzard pH in broiler chickens. *British Poultry Science* 59, 568–578.

Lentle, R.G. and Janssen, P.W.M. (2008) Physical characteristics of digesta and their influence on flow and mixing in the mammalian intestine: a review. *Journal of Comparative Physiology B* 178, 673–690.

Liao, S.F., Kies, A.K., Sauer, W.C., Zhang, Y.C., Cervantes, M. and He, J.M. (2005) Effect of phytase supplementation to a low- and a high-phytate diet for growing pigs on the digestibilities of crude protein, amino acids, and energy. *Journal of Animal Science* 83, 2130–2136.

Liman, N., Alan, E. and Byram, G.K. (2010) The differences between the localizations of MUC1, MUC5AC, MUC6 and osteopontin in quail proventriculus and gizzard may be a reflection of functional differences in stomach parts. *Journal of Anatomy* 217, 57–66.

Longstaff, M. and McNab, J.M. (1987) Digestion of starch and fibre carbohydrates in peas by adult cockerels. *British Poultry Science* 28, 261–285.

Macagno, E.O., Christensen, J. and Lee, C.E. (1982) Modeling the effect of wall movement on absorption in the intestine. *American Journal of Physiology* 243, G541–G550.

McCafferty, K., Bedford, M.R., Kerr, B.J. and Dozier, W.A. (2019) Effects of age and supplemental xylanase in corn- and wheat-based diets on cecal volatile fatty acid concentrations of broilers. *Poultry Science* 98, 4787–4800.

McWorter, T.J., Caviedes-Vidal, E. and Karasov, W.H. (2009) The integration of digestion and osmoregulation in the avian gut. *Biological Reviews* 84, 533–563.

Meng, X., Slominski, B.A., Nyachoti, C.M., Campbell, L.D. and Guenter, W. (2005) Degradation of cell wall polysaccharides by combinations of carbohydrase enzymes and their effect on nutrient utilization and broiler chicken performance. *Poultry Science* 84, 37–47.

Moran, E.T. Jr (1982) *Comparative Nutrition of Fowl and Swine: The Gastrointestinal Systems*. University of Guelph, Guelph, Canada.

Moran, E.T. Jr (2014) Intestinal events and nutritional dynamics predispose *Clostridium perfringens* virulence in broilers. *Poultry Science* 93, 3028–3036.

Moran, E.T. Jr (2016a) Nutrients central to maintaining absorptive efficiency and barrier integrity with fowl. *Poultry Science* 96, 1348–1368.

Moran, E.T. Jr (2016b) Gastric digestion of protein through pancreozyme action optimizes intestinal forms for absorption, mucin formation and villus integrity. *Animal Feed Science and Technology* 221, 284–230.

Moran, E.T. Jr (2019a) Starch: granule, amylose-amylopectin, feed preparation, and recovery by the fowl's gastrointestinal tract. *Journal of Applied Poultry Research* 28, 566–586.

Moran, E.T. Jr (2019b) Clutch formation and nest activities by the setting hen synchronize chick emergence with intestinal development to foster viability. *Animal Feed Science and Technology* 250, 69–80.

Moran, E.T. Jr and McGinnis, J. (1965) The effects of cereal grain and energy level of the diet on the response of turkey poults to enzyme and antibiotic supplements. *Poultry Science* 44, 1253–1261.

Moran, E.T. Jr, Lall, S.P. and Summers, J.D. (1969) The feeding value of rye for the growing chick: effect of enzyme supplements, antibiotics, autoclaving, and geographical area of production. *Poultry Science* 48, 939–949.

Moré, J., Fioramonti, J., Bénazet, F. and Buéno, L. (1987) Histochemical characterization of glycoproteins present in jejunal and colonic goblet cells of pigs on different diets. A biopsy study using chemical methods and peroxidase-labeled lectins. *Histochemistry* 87, 189–194.

Morel, P.C.H., Melai, J., Eady, S.L. and Coles, G.D. (2005) Effect of non-starch polysaccharides and resistant starch on mucin secretion and endogenous amino acid losses in pigs. *Journal of Animal Science* 18, 1643–1641.

Mtei, A.W., Abdollahi, M.R., Schreurs, N.M. and Ravindran, V. (2019) Impact of corn particle size on nutrient digestibility values depending on bird type. *Poultry Science* 98, 5504–5513.

Mueller, L.R., Duke, G.E. and Evanson, O.A. (1990) Investigations of the migrating motor complex in domestic turkeys. *American Journal of Physiology* 259, G329–G333.

O'Dell, B.L. and Boland, A. (1976) Complexation of phytate with proteins and cations in corn germ and oilseed. *Agricultural and Food Chemistry* 24, 804–808.

Onyango, E.M., Bedford, M.R. and Adeola, O. (2005) Phytase activity along the digestive tract of the broiler chick: a comparative study of an *Escherichia coli*-derived and *Peniophora lycii* phytase. *Canadian Journal of Animal Science* 85, 61–68.

Onyango, E.M., Asem, E.K. and Adeola, O. (2009) Phytic acid increases mucin and endogenous amino acid losses from the gastrointestinal tract of chickens. *British Journal of Nutrition* 101, 836–842.

Öztürkcan, Ö. (1985) The determination of the presence of amylase enzyme in the crop of Golden Comet chickens. *Archive für Geflügelkunde* 49, 212–213.

Palander, S., Näsi, M. and Palander, P. (2010) Digestibility and energy value of cereal-based diets in relation to digesta viscosity and retention time in turkeys and chickens at different ages estimated with different markers. *Archives of Animal Nutrition* 64, 238–253.

Paz, H.B., Tisdale, A.S., Danjo, Y., Spurr-Michaud, S.J., Argüeso, P. and Gipson, I.K. (2003) The role of calcium in mucin packaging within goblet cells. *Experimental Eye Research* 77, 69–75.

Pearson, J., Allen, A. and Venables, C. (1980) Gastric mucus isolation and polymeric structure of the undegraded glycoprotein: its breakdown by pepsin. *Gastroenterology* 78, 709–715.

Perez-Vilar, J. (2007) Mucin granule intraluminal organization. *American Journal of Respiratory Cell and Molecular Biology* 36, 183–190.

Rapp, C., Lantzsch, H.-J. and Drochner, W. (2001) Hydrolysis of phytic acid by intrinsic plant and supplemented microbial phytase (*Aspergillus niger*) in the stomach and small intestine of minipigs fitted with re-entrant cannulas. *Journal of Animal Physiology and Animal Nutrition* 85, 414–419.

Ravindran, V. (2013) Feed enzymes: the science, practice, and metabolic realities. *Journal of Applied Poultry Research* 22, 628–636.

Regvar, M., Eichert, D., Kaulich, B., Gianoncelli, A., Pongrac, P., *et al.* (2011) New insights into globoids of protein storage vacuoles in wheat aleurone using synchrotron soft X-ray microscopy. *Journal of Experimental Botany* 62, 3929–3939.

Rhodes, D.I. and Stone, B.A. (2002) Proteins in walls of wheat aleurone cells. *Journal of Cereal Science* 36, 83–101.

Rinttilä, T. and Apajalahti, J. (2013) Intestinal microbiota and metabolites – implications for broiler chicken health and performance. *Journal of Applied Poultry Science* 22, 647–658.

Robertson, J.A., Majsak-Newman, G. and Ring, S.G. (1997) Release of mixed linkage $(1\rightarrow3)$, $(1\rightarrow4)$ β-D-glucans from barley by protease activity and effects on ileal effluent. *International Journal of Biological Macromolecules* 21, 57–60.

Rodrigues, I. and Choct, M. (2018) The foregut and its manipulation via feeding practices in the chicken. *Poultry Science* 97, 3188–3206.

Rostagno, H.S., Teixeira, A., Donzele, J.L., Gomes, P.C., De Oliveira, R.F.M., *et al.* (2005) *Brazilian Tables for Poultry and Swine: Composition of Feedstuffs and Nutritional Requirements.* Universidade Federal de Viçosa, Departamento de Zootecnia, Viçosa, Brazil.

Russell, E.G. (1979) Types and distribution of anaerobic bacteria in the large intestine of pigs. *Applied and Environmental Microbiology* 37, 187–196.

Schiffman, H.R. (1966) Textural preference and acuity in the domestic chick. *Journal of Comparative and Physiological Psychology* 67, 462–464.

Schlegel, P., Nys, Y.N. and Jondreville, C. (2010) Zinc availability and digestive zinc solubility in piglets and broilers fed diets varying in their phytate contents, phytase activity and supplemental zinc source. *Animal* 4, 200–209.

Sergeant, M.J., Constantinidou, C., Cogan, T.A., Bedford, M.R. and Penn, C.W. (2014) Extensive microbial and functional diversity within the chicken microbiome. *PLoS ONE* 9, e91941.

Sharma, R., Fernandez, F., Hinton, M. and Schumbacher, U. (1997) The influence of diet on the mucin carbohydrates in the chick intestinal tract. *Cellular and Molecular Life Sciences* 53, 935–942.

Shelton, J.L., Southern, L.L., Gaston, L.A. and Foster, A. (2004) Evaluation for the nutrient matrix values for phytase in broilers. *Journal of Applied Poultry Research* 13, 213–221.

Shiau, Y.-F., Fernandez, P., Jackson, M.J. and McMonagle, S. (1985) Mechanisms maintaining a low-pH microclimate in the intestine. *American Journal of Physiology* 248, G608–G617.

Slack, P.T., Baxter, E.D. and Wainwright, T. (1979) Inhibition by hordein of starch degradation. *Journal of the Institute of Brewing* 85, 112–114.

Steiner, T., Mosenthin, R., Zimmermann, B., Greiner, R. and Roth, S. (2007) Distribution of phytase activity, total phosphorus and phytate phosphorus in legume seeds, cereals and cereal by-products as influenced by harvest year and cultivar. *Animal Feed Science and Technology* 133, 320–334.

Suprasert, A., Fujioka, T. and Yamada, K. (1987) The histochemistry of glycoconjugates in the colonic epithelium of the chicken. *Histochemistry* 86, 491–497.

Szylit, O., Delort-Laval, J. and Borgida, L.P. (1974) Study of maize starches with different amylose levels; breakdown in the cock's crop and effect of chicken growth. *Annales de Zootechnie* 23, 253–265.

Tannock, G.W. and Smith, J.M.B. (1970) The microflora of the pig's stomach and its possible relationship to ulceration of the *pars oesophagea*. *Journal of Comparative Pathology* 80, 359–366.

Tester, R.F., Yousuf, R., Kettlitz, B. and Röper, H. (2007) Use of commercial protease preparations to reduce protein and lipid content of maize starch. *Food Chemistry* 105, 926–931.

Truong, H.H., Yu, S., Moss, A.F., Liu, S.Y. and Selle, P.H. (2016) Phytate degradation in the gizzard is pivotal to phytase responses in broiler chickens. *Proceedings of the Australian Poultry Science Symposium* 27, 174–177.

Tucker, A.L. and Widowski, T.M. (2009) Normal profiles for deciduous dental eruption in domestic piglets: effect of sow litter, and piglet characteristics. *Journal of Animal Science* 87, 2274–2281.

Tuckey, R., March, B.E. and Biely, J. (1958) Diet and rate of food passage in the growing chick. *Poultry Science* 37, 786–794.

Turk, D.E. (1982) The anatomy of the avian digestive tract as related to feed utilization. *Poultry Science* 61, 1225–1244.

Villegas, V., Vendrell, J. and Aviles, F.X. (1995) The activation pathway of procarboxypeptidase B from porcine pancreas: participation of the active enzyme in the proteolytic processing. *Protein Science* 4, 1792–1800.

Walk, C.L., Bedford, M.R. and McElroy, A.P. (2012) Influence of limestone and phytase on broiler performance, gastrointestinal tract pH and apparent ileal digestibility. *Poultry Science* 91, 1371–1378.

Walk, C.L., Bedford, M.R., Santos, T.S., Paiva, D., Bradley, J.R., *et al.* (2013) Extra-phosphoric effects of superdoses of a novel microbial phytase. *Poultry Science* 92, 719–725.

Walk, C.L., Santos, T.T. and Bedford, M.R. (2014) Influence of a novel microbial phytase on growth performance, tibia ash, and gizzard phytate and inositol in young broilers. *Poultry Science* 93, 1172–1177.

Walk, C.L., Juntunen, K., Paloheimo, M. and Ledoux, D.R. (2019) Evaluation of novel protease enzymes on growth performance and nutrient digestibility of poultry: enzyme dose response. *Poultry Science* 98, 5525–5532.

Wolf, P., Rust, P. and Kamphues, J. (2010) How to assess particle size distribution in diets for pigs? *Livestock Science* 133, 78–80.

Woyengo, T.A., Cowieson, A.J., Adeola, O. and Nyachoti, C.M. (2009) Ileal digestibility and endogenous flow of minerals and amino acids: responses to dietary phytic acid in piglets. *British Journal of Nutrition* 102, 428–433.

Yakubov, G.E., Papagiannopoulos, A., Rat, E. and Waigh, T.A. (2007) Charge and behavior of short-chain heavily glycosylated porcine stomach mucin. *Biomacromolecules* 8, 3791–3799.

Yamauchi, K.-E. and Isshiki, Y. (1991) Scanning electron microscopic observation on the intestinal villi in growing white leghorn and broiler chickens from 1 to 30 days of age. *British Poultry Science* 32, 67–78.

Yang, Z., Pirgozliev, V.R., Rose, S.P., Woods, S., Yang, H.M., *et al.* (2020) Effect of age on the relationship between metabolizable energy and digestible energy for broiler chickens. *Poultry Science* 99, 320–330.

Yi, Z. and Kornegay, E.T. (1996) Sites of phytase activity in the gastrointestinal tract of young pigs. *Animal Feed Science and Technology* 61, 361–368.

Yo, T., Siegel, P.B., Guerin, H. and Picard, M. (1997) Self-selection of dietary protein and energy by broilers grown under a tropic climate: effect of feed particle size on the feed choice. *Poultry Science* 76, 1467–1473.

14 The Influence of Feed Milling on the Stability of Feed Enzymes

Paul Steen*

AB Vista, Marlborough, UK

14.1 Introduction

The stability of exogenous feed enzymes, like other heat-labile feed additives, has been the focus of attention for the suppliers of these additives, nutritionists and feed manufacturers. Additionally, increasing attention is being drawn to the effect of processing on other nutrients such as lysine and more generally on protein digestion when using elevated processing temperatures. In their review, Boroojeni *et al.* (2016) summarized that the hydrothermal impact on macro components of the diet was minimal; however, vitamins, enzymes and antinutritional factors 'are prone to be reduced'. Feed additives such as exogenous enzymes play a pivotal role in the feed formulation both from an economic perspective and a nutritional aspect; for example, phytase supplementation has been shown to support broiler performance while reducing feed costs (Bedford, 2000). If the ascribed nutritional contribution from an enzyme is not achieved in the final composition of the formulation due to losses while processing, and subsequently fed to the targeted animal, the impact can be detrimental to both the feed producer and the animal.

There are differing ways to combat the impact of the thermal processes associated with feed production. Feed ingredient suppliers provide a range of different products with elevated thermal processing stability and alternative product forms such as liquids and coated products. Liquids have the clear advantage that they bypass the rigours of the hydrothermal and thermomechanical processes associated with the conditioning and the pelleting processes, as liquids are administered to the feed post-pelleting. Dry and coated products still have to navigate these processes and their ability to successfully traverse these conditions will be based on how robust the product is and how predictable and balanced that process is. These issues are discussed below.

14.2 The Pelleting Process

Pelleting and pellet quality have a huge impact on the value of the feed produced and the subsequent rearing of animals. The conditions employed influence many parameters of the end product and Moritz (2019) advocated that any improvement in bird performance, as a result of the pelleting

*Email: paul.steen@abvista.com

©CAB International 2022. *Enzymes in Farm Animal Nutrition, 3rd Edition* (M. Bedford *et al.* eds)
DOI: 10.1079/9781789241563.0014

process, is due to the relative effects this process has on pellet quality, feed hygienics and nutrient availability. However, pelleting and pellet quality differ dramatically between feed mills and geographical regions. The predominant influences on this are associated with how each feed plant is configured, the processing parameters adopted and the use of different raw materials.

The pelleting process can be described as a two-stage activity. The first is the conditioning of the feed, where saturated steam is applied in a conditioner to raise the temperature and moisture levels of the mash. The second phase is the compaction of the meal in a pellet press, extrusion through a die to mould and form the cylindrical shape we recognize as a pellet. The impact of the steam injected into the conditioner would be evident even to those who are not involved in the feed industry: that the meal will be subjected to a spike in temperature because of the steam (after all, steam is hot). What is less evident is the level of moisture imparted from the steam as it condenses after coming into contact with the meal. The level of moisture in the mash, preconditioning and from the conditioning process, will have a significant effect on the next stage of the process, extrusion through the pellet die. There are several other parameters which also have a bearing on the passage of the meal through the die, such as the rate of pelleting, the targeted conditioning temperature, the die thickness which governs the distance travelled by the pellet, the hole diameter and configuration, and the formulation which in turn can be affected by individual ingredient quality. These parameters then have a direct bearing on the frictional heat that the meal is subjected to during passage through the die, the consequence being that the hot pellet temperature will almost certainly be higher than the conditioning temperature. Truelock *et al.* (2019) observed that the hot pellet temperature increased as a consequence of pelleting with a thicker die (increase in length-to-diameter ratio; L:D) and by an increase in the conditioning temperature. Pope (2019) undertook a number of pelleting trials where it was

observed that the influence of the frictional heat of the pellet die, and the difference in temperature (delta) between the conditioned mash and the hot pellet, tend to be higher when the target conditioning temperature is lower. Pope (2019) also observed that the heat derived from friction at the die and the impact on the hot pellet temperature were diminished when fat or water was administered to the feed at the batch mixer. Corey (2013) found that the addition of mixer added fat (MAF) also decreased the hot pellet temperature. This is presumably due to the added level of moisture and the lubrication benefit the fat and the moisture would provide during the extrusion phase of the pelleting process.

14.3   Stress Points for Enzymes in Feed Manufacture

Historically, it has been thought that the main influence on feed additives has been the conditioning process, as this is the first point at which feed material is subjected to elevated temperatures and the combination of heat and moisture simultaneously. Although this holds true for some products, it is now becoming evident that the subordinate effect of the die configuration and the dwelled time of the meal in the die, as a function of the pelleting rate, has a significant outcome on the stability of additives, either as a primary consequence or as a secondary effect. This issue may well be overlooked when conducting stability trials with pilot-scale set-ups as the production rates fall far below the manufacturing rates associated with commercial feed production, although the processing parameters such as temperature and die L:D may well be comparable. Pope (2019) estimated that if the pellet L:D values between a pilot-scale and a commercial-scale pellet mill were constant, then the feed pelleted through the pilot-scale set-up would be retained within the die for approximately four times longer than in the commercial pellet mill configuration due to the slower rate of production in the former. An experiment undertaken was designed to look at different manufacturing rates combined with two different conditioning/pelleting temperatures to evaluate the in-feed recovery of a commercial xylanase and phytase which were supplemented to the mash as dry products. Each treatment was pelleted on a pilot-scale press with an L:D of 8 and with a calculated surface area of 548 cm². The feed production followed a logical process, starting with the lowest production rate and lowest conditioning temperature, collecting the necessary samples at predetermined intervals and then resetting the production rate for the desired capacity. This was repeated for the higher of the two conditioning temperatures. Samples of mash, conditioned mash and cooled pellets were collected and analysed for enzyme recovery. In addition to the monitoring of the conditioning temperature, the temperature of the hot pellets was also examined and recorded to establish the delta between these two observations. The xylanase product activity was not influenced by the conditioning temperature or the pellet mill capacity due to its extreme thermostability. Phytase recoveries were affected by an interaction between conditioning temperature and pellet mill capacity relative to the unconditioned mash. The poorest recovery was at the higher conditioning temperature and lower pelleting capacity, although for the treatments conditioned at the higher temperature and the higher pelleting rate the recovery for phytase was statistically equal to the treatments conditioned at the lower temperature. The phytase recovery in the conditioned mash was similar for both conditioning temperatures and at a level comparable to the unconditioned mash recovery, indicating that the phytase was stable during the conditioning phase regardless of temperature (Table 14.1). The delta between the conditioned mash and hot pellet was highest with the lower conditioning temperature and increased as a consequence of the pelleting capacity (Table 14.2). The author suggested that this

Table 14.1. Main effects of mash conditioning temperature (CT) and pellet mill throughput (PMT) on the relative activity of phytase and xylanase in conditioned mash compared with unconditioned mash (CM:UCM), pellets compared with conditioned mash (P:CM) and pellets compared with unconditioned mash (P:UCM). (From Pope, 2019.)

CT (°C)	PMT (kg/h)	n	Relative phytase recovery[a] (%)			Relative xylanase recovery[b] (%)		
			CM:UCM	P:CM	P:UCM	CM:UCM	P:CM	P:UCM
Main effects								
75		12	124.0[A]	95.4[A]	114.8[A]	81.0[A]	98.6[A]	79.2[A]
86		12	100.7[A]	55.8[B]	60.7[B]	86.8[A]	94.7[A]	81.9[A]
P value			0.069	0.001	0.001	0.134	0.461	0.469
SEM[c]			8.4	6.5	5.0	2.6	3.6	2.5
	227	6	87.7[A]	58.3[A]	52.8[C]	77.7[A]	96.1[A]	74.0[A]
	454	6	105.0[A]	76.9[A]	83.4[B]	86.7[A]	95.1[A]	81.4[A]
	908	6	127.1[A]	70.8[A]	90.3[B]	86.5[A]	95.3[A]	82.0[A]
	1816	6	129.4[A]	96.5[A]	124.5[A]	84.8[A]	100.1[A]	84.7[A]
	P value		0.079	0.067	0.001	0.300	0.885	0.223
	SEM[c]		11.8	9.2	7.1	3.7	5.0	3.6

SEM, standard error of the mean.
[a]Quantum® Blue 5G. Testing method was in accordance with ELISA specific for Quantum® Blue, ESC Standard Analytical Method, SAM099; AB Vista, Marlborough, UK.
[b]Econase® XT. Testing method was in accordance with ELISA specific for Econase® XT, ESC Standard Analytical Method, SAM115; AB Vista, Marlborough, UK.
[c]SEM for n = 12 samples for each CT and n = 6 samples for each PMT.
[A-C]In the separate CT and PMT comparisons, mean values within a column with unlike upper-case superscript letters are significantly different (P ≤ 0.01).

Table 14.2. Main effects of mash conditioning temperature (CT) and pellet mill throughput (PMT) on pellet durability index (PDI) as determined by the Holmen method for 30 s of testing and the change in temperature between hot pellets and conditioned mash (ΔT). (From Pope, 2019.)

CT (°C)	PMT (kg/h)	n	PDI (%)	ΔT (°C)
Main effects				
75		12	82.7[B]	6.7[A]
86		12	89.5[A]	2.5[B]
P value			0.001	0.001
SEM[a]			0.6	0.3
	227	6	94.9[A]	2.7[B]
	454	6	89.6[B]	4.7[A]
	908	6	84.5[C]	5.6[A]
	1816	6	75.6[D]	5.3[A]
	P value		0.001	0.001
	SEM[a]		0.7	0.3

SEM, standard error of the mean.
[a]SEM for $n = 12$ samples for each CT and $n = 6$ samples for each PMT.
[A-D]In the separate CT and PMT comparisons, mean values within a column with unlike upper-case superscript letters are significantly different ($P \leq 0.05$).

is likely due to the reduction in the steam volume to achieve the lower conditioning temperature and the resultant reduction in the moisture which would have condensed from the steam into the mash and ensuing deficiency in lubrication through the die while pelleting.

14.4 Commercial Pelleting Practice/Processes

14.4.1 Steam quality

Conditioning of feed prior to pelleting has long been an established practice; however, 'commercial practice as well as past research do not agree on one optimal setting for steam pressure or conditioning temperature' (Cutlip *et al.*, 2008). In its simplest terms, conditioning involves the injection of steam into the mash to raise its moisture and temperature and is the immediate pretreatment of the mash before it enters the pellet press for compaction and forming. An effective conditioning process will afford the best possible parameters for the pelleting process while maintaining the nutrient value of the feed. Boroojeni *et al.* (2016) concluded that

'hydrothermal processing improved the hygiene status of poultry feed, but the effect on nutrient availability is equivocal'. The balance between the requirements for the pellet press and the conditioning process is such that the efficiencies of the system rely on an optimum die thickness being employed in conjunction with the required manufacturing rates being attained, then pellet quality is met, and the key challenge of milling efficiency is achieved.

Feed is conditioned for multiple reasons but perhaps the primary reasons are associated with the preparation of feed material for the pelleting phase by adding heat and moisture to the mash, hygienization of the mash, starch gelatinization and in order to plasticize protein. With these conditions in mind and their importance and influence on the pelleting process, 'steam conditioning is likely the most important factor affecting pellet quality' (Fahrenholz, 2012). Indeed, steam conditioning influenced pellet quality by 20% (Reimer, 1992), and as a result it is essential to understand the properties of the steam and how best to accommodate these assets to ensure the best effective conditioning of the meal possible. Steam is produced in the feed mill in a boiler at high pressure. The reasons for producing steam at high pressure are so that a high volume of steam can be available for the processing of the mash. This ensures the steam can be efficiently distributed around the plant and that the energy from the steam is available at the point of use. Steam, when produced at a higher pressure, has a reduced volume and consequently occupies less space, therefore smaller-diameter pipework can be used. This concept is a very important consideration for when the steam pressure is reduced before it is injected into the conditioner.

Steam leaving the boiler should be as dry as possible to ensure it is carrying heat efficiently. Any condensate that occurs in the pipework should be removed using the appropriate trapping. The operating pressure of the boiler will be determined by the specifics of the boiler to ensure the operating efficiency and quality of the steam leaving the boiler. The effect of pressure is such that increasing the pressure at which the water transforms to steam makes the water more reluctant to change state, from liquid to gas (steam). As the pressure increases the more energy must be added to the water before it will boil, consequently the boiling temperature will be higher. Similar increases and decreases occur whenever the pressure is raised, and conversely when the pressure is decreased. This can be readily seen from steam tables (Table 14.3).

If the operating pressure of the boiler is 8 bar, then the properties of the steam will be as shown in Table 14.3. The three key parameters to observe are: temperature, 175°C; enthalpy of steam, 2774 kJ/kg; and the specific volume of the steam, 0.215 m³/kg. If the reduced steam pressure at which the steam is injected into the conditioner is 2 bar, the difference between the properties for the two pressures needs to be accommodated. If steam is distributed at high pressure, before it is injected into the conditioner, the pressure should first be reduced in order to allow the steam to be at a reduced temperature, closer to its saturation point as it enters the conditioner, when it will confer its energy, heat and moisture to the mash. This is achieved by the installation of a pressure-reducing valve (PRV) in the line to the conditioner. As alluded to earlier, understanding the parameters associated with steam at different pressures is key to having an effective steam line configuration for the reduced pressure. If the high-pressure steam is distributed around the feed mill via 50 mm diameter pipework, the velocity of the steam will be proportional to the volume of steam being conveyed and the cross-sectional area of the pipe. So, if we have the scenario that we require steam at 1300 kg/h, the velocity of the steam would be approximately 33 m/s. If

Table 14.3. The effect of pressure on the enthalpy of steam. (Author's own data, generated by sequential inputs of pressure data into https://www.spiraxsarco.com/resources-and-design-tools/steam-tables/dry-saturated-steam-line, accessed 29 June 2021.)

| Pressure (bar) (gauge) | Pressure (kPa) (gauge) | Temperature (°C) | Specific enthalpy (kJ/kg) | | | Specific volume of steam (m³/kg) |
			Water, h_f	Evaporation, h_{fg}	Steam, h_g	
0.00	00.0	99.97	418.9	2256.5	2675.5	1.673
1.00	100.0	120.42	505.6	2201.1	2706.7	0.881
2.00	200.0	133.69	562.2	2163.3	2725.5	0.603
3.00	300.0	143.75	605.3	2133.4	2738.7	0.461
4.00	400.0	151.96	640.7	2108.1	2748.8	0.374
5.00	500.0	158.92	670.9	2086.0	2756.9	0.315
6.00	600.0	165.04	697.5	2066.0	2763.5	0.272
7.00	700.0	170.50	721.4	2047.7	2769.1	0.240
8.00	800.0	175.43	743.1	2030.9	2774.0	0.215
9.00	900.0	179.97	763.0	2015.1	2778.1	0.194
10.00	1000.0	184.13	781.6	2000.1	2781.7	0.177

the steam is then reduced to 2 bar the main characteristic is the change in the steam volume, which is almost three times greater, in addition to the reduction in temperature and enthalpy of steam. If the post-PRV pipework diameter is maintained at the same diameter as the pre-PRV pipework diameter, the velocity of the steam would increase to approximately 90 m/s. However, the approach is to reduce the velocity to allow the steam to reach its saturation temperature for the reduced pressure, and to accomplish this it is necessary to increase the post-PRV pipework diameter. A lot of these aspects of the steam line are overlooked at a feed mill level. Often a new pelleting system, press and conditioner, would be installed without consideration for the steam configuration for the new set-up by employing the existing pipework. The fundamental outcome is that the conditioning and pelleting press are not balanced, and the risk is that the steam will transfer more energy in terms of temperature than moisture as the saturation conditions for the steam are not realized within the short time associated with the conditioning process. For steam to confer its energy, heat and moisture, it must first reach its saturation temperature for the corresponding pressure at which it exists. In feed production, although the pressure at which the steam is injected into the conditioner is above atmospheric pressure, the conditioner into which the steam enters is an atmospheric device. Therefore, the steam should now exist at atmospheric conditions, even though the temperature of the steam might be slightly higher than 100°C. When the steam meets the cooler mash, the temperature of the steam will begin to drop. When the steam reaches 100°C the steam will condense and will confer its moisture into the mash. Once all the steam is turned into water, its temperature will drop. This hydration process is time dependent and beyond the physical characteristics of the steam; the rate of diffusion will be further dependent on the set-up and operation of the conditioner and the formulation.

Cutlip *et al.* (2008) undertook an experiment to look at the influence of conditioning temperature and pressure on pellet quality and broiler performance. Two temperatures, 82.2 and 93.3°C, and two pressures, 138 and 552 kPa, were adopted. Increasing the processing temperature resulted in a higher production rate, a point Cutlip *et al.* (2008) assigned to an increase in moisture and heat, resulting in higher die lubrication and feed adhesion (Table 14.4). Moisture levels were highest for the high temperature treatments for both conditioned mash and hot pellets, which resulted in higher moisture level in the finished feed for the same treatments (Table 14.5). The higher conditioning temperature improved pellet durability index (PDI) and decreased the total quantity of fines, and the same was observed with the higher steam pressure, although the improvements obtained with the changes in steam pressure were not as dramatic as those attained with the increase in conditioning temperature. The pellets produced with the higher conditioning temperature decreased broiler feed intake and the feed conversion ratio (Table 14.6). For the two different steam pressures employed, the mass (kg) of steam required to achieve the targeted temperatures would be equal between temperatures, although for the higher temperatures a greater quantity of steam would be needed. If the parameters for the steam pipework were constant, then the properties of the steam, notably the velocity of the steam in the pipework post the PRV, will have been different between the two pressures and any consequential effect of this may have been overlooked. From Fig. 14.1 it can be calculated that the moisture transferred from the steam was 2.19% for the lower conditioning temperature and 2.74% for the higher temperature, the higher moisture level being attributable to the greater quantity of steam administered and condensation of the steam to the feed. If these values are equated to °C, then for a 1% increase in moisture, we can see that for the lower conditioning temperature the outcome was 26.1°C and for the higher temperature was 24.9°C (assuming the mean ambient mash temperature for the duration of the trial was 25°C). Both these

Table 14.4. Effect of steam conditioning feed on manufacturing variables and pellet quality (Latin square design using day and processing order for blocking). (From Cutlip et al., 2008.)

Treatment[a]	Production rate (ton/h)	PDI (%)	Modified PDI[b] (%)	Cooler fines[c] (%)	Bagged fines[d] (%)	Total fines[e] (%)	Bulk density (kg/m³)
LPLT	0.750[A]	89.59[C]	80.42[C]	48.20[A]	4.17[A]	8.92[A]	658.8[A]
LPHT	0.785[A]	93.33[B]	88.32[B]	38.54[A]	3.84[AB]	7.28[A]	659.3[A]
HPLT	0.756[A]	89.76[C]	81.14[C]	42.70[A]	4.81[A]	8.60[A]	657.9[A]
HPHT	0.791[A]	94.35[A]	90.50[A]	35.81[A]	2.07[B]	5.17[A]	651.9[A]
P value	0.2650	0.0001	0.0001	0.5196	0.0442	0.1115	0.4925
LSD[f]	—	0.99	1.77	—	1.81	—	—
P values for main effects and interaction							
Pressure	0.7128	0.0827	0.0299	0.5108	0.3183	0.2569	0.2912
Temperature	0.0676	0.0001	0.0001	0.2094	0.0260	0.0397	0.4697
Pressure × temperature	0.9915	0.1917	0.2061	0.8213	0.0602	0.3953	0.4119
SEM	0.016	0.287	0.512	5.887	0.522	0.971	0.227

SEM, standard error of the mean.
[a]Treatments are defined by steam conditioning pressure and temperature: LP = low pressure, 138 kPa; LT = low temperature, 82.2°C; HP = high pressure, 552 kPa; HT = high temperature, 93.3°C.
[b]Modified PDI completed utilizing five 13-mm hex nuts for added force on pellets.
[c]Percentage of fines associated with feed that fell through the horizontal cooler.
[d]Percentage of fines obtained from a sample of bagged feed collected at the sack off bin.
[e]The sum of fines collected from under the horizontal cooler and the sample bagged feed.
[f]Fisher's least significant difference test.
[A-C]Mean values within a column with unlike upper-case superscript letters are significantly different (P < 0.05).

Table 14.5. Effect of steam conditioning feed on moisture, protein and ash content (Latin square design using day and processing order for blocking). (From Cutlip et al., 2008.)

Treatment[a]	Moisture (%)			Crude protein (%)			Ash (%)		
	Dry mash	Sifted pellet	Sifted fines	Dry mash	Sifted pellet	Sifted fines	Dry mash	Sifted pellet	Sifted fines
LPLT	10.81[A]	12.86[C]	12.02[A]	22.11[A]	21.69[A]	20.67[A]	1.93[A]	1.94[A]	1.94[A]
LPHT	11.24[A]	13.96[A,B]	12.89[A]	21.09[A]	21.71[A]	19.66[A]	1.94[A]	1.94[A]	1.93[A]
HPLT	11.20[A]	13.34[B,C]	12.48[A]	20.12[A]	20.12[A]	20.14[A]	1.94[A]	1.94[A]	1.94[A]
HPHT	11.27[A]	14.18[A]	13.02[A]	22.16[A]	22.80[A]	20.28[A]	1.95[A]	1.94[A]	1.93[A]
P value	0.7026	0.0195	0.1954	0.5050	0.4025	0.7223	0.5910	0.8922	0.7801
LSD[b]	–	0.7651	–	–	–	–	–	–	–
P values for main effects and interaction									
Pressure	0.5230	0.1636	0.3701	0.6735	0.5355	0.9508	0.4961	0.8920	0.8281
Temperature	0.4495	0.0046	0.0623	0.6397	0.2616	0.5082	0.2703	0.4995	0.3605
Pressure × temperature	0.5744	0.5772	0.6172	0.1900	0.2690	0.3866	0.8025	0.8055	0.8020
SEM	0.22	0.16	0.22	0.73	0.59	0.44	0.007	0.006	0.006

SEM, standard error of the mean.

[a]Treatments are defined by steam conditioning pressure and temperature: LP = low pressure, 138 kPa; LT = low temperature, 82.2°C; HP = high pressure, 552 kPa; HT = high temperature, 93.3°C.

[b]Fisher's least significant difference test.

[A-C]Mean values within a column with unlike upper-case superscript letters are significantly different ($P < 0.05$).

Table 14.6. Effect of steam conditioning feed form on 21- to 39-day performance (randomized complete block design using ratio of females to males as a covariate). (From Cutlip et al., 2008).

Treatment[a]	Bird initial body weight (kg)	Pen feed intake (kg)	Bird live weight gain (kg)	Bird feed conversion ratio (kg/kg)	Bird ending body weight (kg)	Pen mortality (%)
LPLT	0.705[A]	45.76[A]	1.336[A]	2.16[A,B]	2.041[A]	1.56[C]
LPHT	0.705[A]	42.80[A]	1.376[A]	1.95[C]	2.081[A]	1.56[C]
HPLT	0.703[A]	45.43[A]	1.317[A]	2.19[A]	2.021[A]	3.90[B,C]
HPHT	0.704[A]	43.77[A]	1.400[A]	1.99[B,C]	2.101[A]	2.34[C]
UCM	0.703[A]	31.22[B]	0.925[B]	2.18[A,B]	1.628[B]	8.59[A,B]
HPHT reground	0.702[A]	33.95[B]	0.954[B]	2.28[A]	1.655[B]	5.47[B,C]
50% HPHT reground/50% HPHT pellets	0.705[A]	32.18[B]	0.956[B]	2.26[A]	1.661[B]	10.94[A]
P value	0.7458	0.0001	0.0001	0.0029	0.0001	0.0018
LSD[b]	—	3.34	0.09	0.19	0.09	5.28
P values for main effects and interaction						
Pressure	0.2438	0.5267	0.6028	0.8947	0.5095	0.6731
Temperature	0.5584	0.0586	0.2755	0.0319	0.2977	0.5992
Pressure × temperature	0.7746	0.4453	0.3924	0.8514	0.3692	0.6292
SEM	0.002	0.862	0.002	0.051	0.020	0.949
P values for feed form regression among reground mash, 50/50 reground mash and pellets, and all pellets (552 kPa, 93.3°C)						
Linear	0.0001	0.0002	0.0001	0.0023	0.0001	0.1307
Quadratic	0.8170	0.1307	0.2562	0.6559	0.3314	0.0610

SEM, standard error of the mean.

[a]Treatments are defined by steam conditioning pressure and temperature: LP = low pressure, 138 kPa; LT = low temperature, 82.2°C; HP = high pressure, 552 kPa; HT = high temperature, 93.3°C.

[b]Fisher's least significant difference test.

[A-C]Mean values within a column with unlike upper-case superscript letters are significantly different ($P < 0.05$).

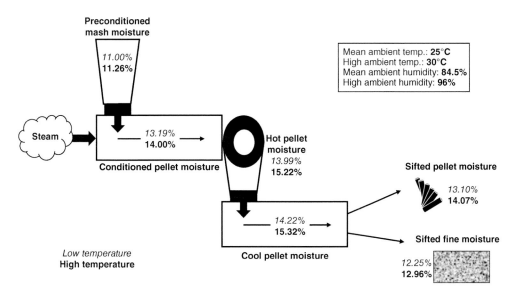

Fig. 14.1. Significant temperature effect on feed moisture. (Adapted from Cutlip *et al.*, 2008.)

figures are well above the anticipated level that is generally regarded as the norm of 13 to 16°C, the inference being that the steam is dry and not achieving its saturation temperature for the reduced pressure post the PRV. Although not a focus of the study, this could be associated with the properties of the steam and how able the steam was, given the set-up of the steam pipework configuration, to liberate both heat and moisture to the mash. Cutlip *et al.* (2008) remarked that the most implemented steam pressure ranged from 138 to 552 kPa and conditioning temperatures varied from 76.7 to 93.3°C, although 'past research has not accounted for these variables in a comprehensive manner'.

14.4.2 The influence of the die

Considering the stability of a commercial phytase during conditioning and pelleting, Truelock *et al.* (2019) investigated the interaction of conditioning temperature and die thickness in a factorial study incorporating three temperatures and two die thicknesses. The pelleting rate and the retention time within the conditioner were held constant for all treatments. Samples of the mash, conditioned mash and pellets were collected to determine enzyme activity. The temperature of the conditioned mash and hot pellets was monitored during the term of the experiment. The phytase product evaluated in this experiment had a loss of activity associated with the conditioning and the pelleting processes, respectively, even though there was no interaction between the die thickness and conditioning temperature (Table 14.7). The hot pellet temperature increased when pelleting with the thicker die presumably as a result of the dynamics of the frictional forces at the die. Additionally, the delta between the conditioned mash and the hot pellet was higher in all treatments for the thicker die. Across both die thicknesses, the delta was greater with the lower conditioning temperature, reducing as the condition temperature increased. The conclusion of the study was that phytase activity was reduced as a consequence of the increase in conditioning temperature and not the die thickness.

A series of experiments undertaken by Pope (2019) looked at factors to improve feed quality and nutritional quality and

Table 14.7. Effect of die thickness and conditioning temperature on pelleting characteristics and phytase stability of a finishing swine diet[a]. (From Truelock et al., 2019.)

Die L:D	5.6			8.0			SEM[b]	Probability[c]			
Conditioning temp. (°F)	165	175	185	165	175	185		Die	Linear	Quadratic	Die × temp.
Production rate (lb/min)	33.8	34.1	33.8	33.9	33.7	34.1	0.13	–	–	–	–
Conditioning temp. (°F)	165.1	175.3	185.2	165.3	175.5	184.3	0.19	–	–	–	–
Hot pellet temp. (°F)	176.6	181.8	189.2	178.6	184.1	190.5	0.80	<0.01	<0.01	0.16	0.73
PDI (%)	80.0	80.9	84.7	88.5	88.9	91.7	1.71	<0.01	0.03	0.39	0.91
Phytase (FYT/kg)											
Initial mash	772	772	772	743	743	743	141.1	0.74	1.00	1.00	1.00
Conditioned mash	1099	576	267	894	760	275	138.9	0.97	<0.01	0.74	0.28
Cooled pellet	603	329	166	538	292	206	42.6	0.54	<0.01	0.07	0.42
Phytase stability (%)											
Conditioned mash	102.8	61.0	35.4	91.4	77.5	36.2	8.14	0.72	<0.01	0.64	0.14
Cooled pellet	63.0	38.1	23.7	58.6	35.6	28.1	7.09	0.85	<0.01	0.19	0.70

SEM, standard error of the mean.

[a]Diets were steam-conditioned (10 in × 55 in Wenger twin staff preconditioner, model 150) for 30 s at 165, 175 or 185°F and pelleted (CPM, 1012-2 HD Master model) using a 5/32 in × 7/8 in (L:D = 5.6) or a 5/32 × 1/4 in (L:D = 8.0) pellet die.

[b]Pooled standard error of least-squares means (n = 3).

[c]Linear and quadratic contrasts were used to evaluate the effect of conditioning temperature.

used feed enzymes as a marker for protein denaturation. These experiments identified that the conditioning temperature was not the sole arbitrator in denaturing enzyme activity and a further detrimental loss of activity was associated with the pellet mill and the die: 'data indicated that the phytase utilized may have been stable to heat, but not to heat and pressure which would be experienced as the enzyme traversed the pellet mill die'. The author also alluded that past research had not sufficiently investigated the relationship between the effects of the conditioning process and the effects of the pelleting process by adequately separating the two. In an experiment investigating the percentage of MAF, enzyme recovery was greater with the treatment with the higher MAF inclusion, an indication that the additional lubricating value of fat is providing an advantageous benefit to enzyme recovery in-feed (Table 14.8). The paradox is that increasing levels of MAF also resulted in reducing PDI values and that increasing PDI correlated with decreasing enzyme (xylanase) recovery.

In an additional experiment, the benefit of adding water to the batch mixer was considered and the possible interaction the application of mixer added water (MAW) would have on enzyme recovery. The hypothesis was that water, like fat, would bring lubrication advantages in the pellet die as the meal is pressed through the die but also assist with the binding properties of the meal to improve pellet quality via starch gelatinization. The experiment consisted of three conditioning temperatures and two MAW levels. The treatments were conditioned for 30 s utilizing a steam pressure of 207 kPa and a production rate of 908 kg/h, die area of 548 cm^2 and L:D of 8 (Table 14.9).

There was no significant difference in the recovery of xylanase in the pellets relative to the conditioned mash irrespective of the conditioning temperature or the MAW level. For phytase, there were differences associated with the conditioning temperature but there was no benefit in the analytical recovery of the pelleted feeds in connection with any level of MAW. Both sets of data suggest that MAW is neither detrimental nor positive to the stability of the phytase or xylanase in this experiment.

14.5 Conclusion

Although feed processing techniques have advanced, they have not kept pace with the advances in nutrition. This has resulted in significant variation in feed processing methods and processing parameters. While the stability of key additives is a point of concern, other factors such as feed sanitation plus the demands on the feed mill to produce pellets of an acceptable quality also contribute to the abundance of variations in milling equipment and processing parameters that are experienced in the animal feed industry. In a review by Amerah et al. (2011), the authors suggested that for broiler performance, conditioning temperatures over 85°C should be avoided. In a more recent review by Moritz (2019), it was proposed that 'conditioning feed within the range of 80 to 82°C from 10 to 60 seconds without excessive throughput may produce pellets of adequate physical quality to improve bird performance', plus 'this temperature and time range combination should support a feed Salmonella control program, maintain amino acid digestibility and support exogenous enzyme activity'.

It is apparent that enzyme stability is not solely related to the conditioning temperature as activity can be denatured due to other aspects of the feed manufacturing process and specifically in the formation of the pellet. The variation of conditioning methods and the use of steam deviate significantly with no apparent industrial standard. The pellet press poses varied facets that can impact enzyme stability such as pressure and frictional heat encountered within it. Understanding each of these intricacies and balancing the thermodynamic properties are essential for enzyme stability.

Table 14.8. Effect of percentage mixer added fat (MAF) on the relative activity of xylanase in conditioned mash compared with unconditioned mash (CM:UCM), pellets compared with conditioned mash (P:CM) and pellets compared with unconditioned mash (P:UCM). (From Pope, 2019.)

MAF (%)	n	Relative xylanase activity (%)		
		CM:UCM	P:CM	P:UCM
1.00	3	36.7	66.4	24.0
3.00	3	42.6	60.6	25.7
5.00	3	28.1	111.6	30.4
Linear P value		0.337	0.027	0.302
Quadratic P value		0.291	0.006	0.593
SEM[a]		5.8	6.6	4.1

SEM, standard error of the mean.
[a]SEM for $n = 3$ samples for each percentage MAF.

Table 14.9. Effect of mash conditioning temperature (CT) and level of mixer added water (MAW) on the relative activity of phytase and xylanase in conditioned mash compared with unconditioned mash (CM:UCM), pellets compared with conditioned mash (P:CM) and pellets compared with unconditioned mash (P:UCM). (From Pope, 2019.)

CT (°C)	MAW (%)	n	Relative phytase recovery[a] (%)			Relative xylanase recovery[b] (%)		
			CM:UCM	P:CM	P:UCM	CM:UCM	P:CM	P:UCM
Main effects								
80		9	104.4[A]	76.4[A]	77.1[A]	87.2[A]	108.8[A]	94.7[A]
86		9	100.1[A]	35.8[B]	33.8[B]	91.0[A]	112.1[A]	101.3[A]
92		9	81.9[B]	6.3[C]	5.2[C]	90.1[A]	107.6[A]	96.7[A]
P value			0.006	0.001	0.001	0.430	0.654	0.091
	0.0	9	95.8[A,B]	42.0[A,B]	40.8[A]	90.9[A]	108.8[A]	98.2[A]
	1.0	9	85.1[B]	44.9[A]	40.3[A]	91.3[A]	109.4[A]	99.7[A]
	2.0	9	105.6[A]	31.7[B]	35.1[A]	86.2[A]	110.4[A]	94.8[A]
	P value		0.018	0.042	0.480	0.185	0.946	0.240
	SEM[c]		4.4	3.5	3.6	2.0	3.5	2.1

SEM, standard error of the mean.
[a]Quantum Blue® 5G. Testing method was in accordance with ELISA specific for Quantum® Blue, ESC Standard Analytical Method, SAM099; AB Vista, Marlborough, UK.
[b]Econase® XT. Testing method was in accordance with ELISA specific for Econase® XT, ESC Standard Analytical Method, SAM115; AB Vista, Marlborough, UK.
[c]SEM for $n = 9$ samples for each CT and $n = 9$ samples for each level of MAW.
[A–C]In the separate CT and MAW comparisons, mean values within a column with unlike upper-case superscript letters are significantly different at $P \leq 0.05$ (CT) or $P \leq 0.01$ (MAW).

References

Amerah, A.M., Gilbert, C., Simmins, P.H. and Ravindran, V. (2011) Influence of feed processing on the efficacy of exogenous enzymes in broiler diets. *World's Poultry Science Journal* 67, 29–46.

Bedford, M.R. (2000) Exogenous enzymes in monogastric nutrition – their current value and future benefits. *Animal Feed Science and Technology* 86, 1–13.

Boroojeni, F.G., Svihus, B., von Reichenbach, H.G. and Zentek, J. (2016) The effects of hydrothermal processing on feed hygiene, nutrient availability, intestinal microbiota and morphology in poultry – a review. *Animal Feed Science and Technology* 220, 187–215.

Corey, A.M. (2013) Effects of varying levels of calcium lignosulfonate, mixer-added fat and feed form on feed manufacture and broiler performance. MSc thesis, West Virginia University, Morgantown, West Virginia.

Cutlip, S.E., Hott, J.M., Buchanan, N.P., Rack, A.L., Latshaw, J.D. and Moritz, J.S. (2008) The effect of steam-conditioning practices on pellet quality and growing broiler nutritional value. *Journal of Applied Poultry Research* 17, 249–261.

Fahrenholz, A.C. (2012) Evaluating factors affecting pellet durability and energy consumption in a pilot feed mill and comparing methods for evaluating pellet durability. PhD thesis, Kansas State University, Manhattan, Kansas.

Moritz, J.S. (2019) Feed manufacture effects on pellet quality, hygienics, and nutrient availability. Presented at the Multi-State Feeding and Nutrition Conference and Silvateam's Technical Symposium, Indianapolis, Indiana, USA, 21–23 May 2019.

Pope, J.T. (2019) Non-conditioning factors affecting enzyme thermostability during feed processing. PhD thesis, North Carolina State University, Raleigh, North Carolina.

Reimer, L. (1992) Conditioning. In: *Proceedings of the Northern Crops Institute Feed Mill Management and Feed Manufacturing Technology Short Course*. California Pellet Mill Co., Crawfordsville, Indiana, p. 7.

Truelock, C.N., Ward, N.E., Wilson, J.W., Stark, C.R. and Paulk, C.B. (2019) Effect of pellet die thickness and conditioning temperature during the pelleting process on phytase stability. *Kansas Agricultural Experiment Station Research Reports* 5.

15 Enzymes and the Microbiome in the Post-Antibiotic Era

Richard Ducatelle*, Filip Van Immerseel, Venessa Eeckhaut and Evy Goossens
Ghent University, Merelbeke, Belgium

15.1 Introduction

The commercial application of enzymes in monogastric farm animal nutrition developed only in the late 1980s. In the early days enzymes were added to animal feed with the aim to compensate for deficiencies in the host enzyme arsenal, allowing, among others, a more complete breakdown of certain digestible components of the feed such as starch, protein and fat, but above all allowing the breakdown of fractions that are not attacked by the host enzymes at all, in essence the non-starch polysaccharides (NSPs) that make up the cell walls of plants. More recently, these enzymes have been proposed as alternatives to the in-feed antibiotics which were banned in 2006 in the EU, a process that is ongoing to various degrees of implementation in other markets (Yang *et al.*, 2009; Cowieson and Kluenter, 2019). This association refers only to the effects on performance, not to the modes of action, which in both cases still are under investigation. Indeed, even if growth-promoting antibiotics have been used in animal feed for almost half a century, the modes of action of these low concentrations of antibiotics included in feed are still being investigated today (Robinson *et al.*, 2019).

Reports from the field claim that banning of antibiotic growth promotors has compromised control of coccidiosis, necrotic enteritis and other gut health issues associated with wet litter (Smith, 2019). Gut health issues at the level of the individual bird are characterized by intestinal inflammation, gut barrier leakage and shifts in the composition of the intestinal microbiome (for a review, see Ducatelle *et al.*, 2018). In line with this recent evolution, in-feed enzymes, especially the carbohydrate-degrading enzymes, are now claimed to promote intestinal health in pigs and in poultry (for a review, see Kiarie *et al.*, 2013). The gut-health-promoting effects of NSP-degrading enzymes (NSPases) are believed to result from the decrease in digesta viscosity, the rupture of the plant cell walls releasing nutrients present inside plant cells (the so-called 'cage release effect'), and the solubilization and partial hydrolysis of NSPs, generating prebiotic oligosaccharides (Courtin *et al.*, 2008; Aftab and Bedford, 2018). It is well documented that the intestinal microbiota interacts with prebiotic oligosaccharides, as was shown recently again for the arabinoxylo-oligosaccharides (AXOS) (Bautil *et al.*, 2019). It is, however, unclear to what

---

*Email: Richard.Ducatelle@UGent.be

©CAB International 2022. *Enzymes in Farm Animal Nutrition, 3rd Edition* (M. Bedford *et al.* eds)
DOI: 10.1079/9781789241563.0015

extent the beneficial effects of NSPases on intestinal health and on performance in broilers and pigs may be through their positive steering effect on the intestinal microbiota. Moreover, there is some controversy in the literature whether other feed enzymes also modulate the intestinal microbiota and whether or not this may be beneficial to the health of the animals. The purpose of this chapter is to critically review the literature on these topics in order to give some cues that may help to clarify, at least partially, the aforementioned issues. This is challenging because the available scientific information on the interactions between feed enzymes and the intestinal microbiota is fragmentary and often preliminary, even if such interactions have been assumed already many years ago (Choct, 2006). Prior to examining the effects of exogenous enzymes on the microbiota, some information on the establishment and composition of the microbiota is needed.

15.2   The Microbiome

The intestinal ecosystem is shaped by the interactions between three factors: (i) the feed; (ii) the host intestinal mucosa; and (iii) the microbiota. Along the intestinal tract, the microbiome is geographically specific, forming a dynamic equilibrium with a remarkable robustness and resilience. In the duodenum and jejunum, the bacterial density is very low due to the secretion of powerful antimicrobial substances and the diffusion of oxygen from the host mucosa. In contrast, the density of the intestinal microbiome is much higher in the caecum and colon in pigs and in the ileum and caeca in chickens.

Groundbreaking studies on the composition of the intestinal microbiota in broilers were compiled by the group of Lee and Hofacre back in 2003 (Lu *et al.*, 2003). They clearly established the extreme difference in composition between the microbiota of the ileum and that of the caeca, two organs that are directly connected to each other. Indeed, the ileal microbiota is dominated by members of the Lactobacillaceae

family, whereas the caecal microbiota is dominated by what was later renamed as Ruminococcaceae and Lachnospiraceae families. These studies for the first time showed that in the chicken, as opposed to the pig (and other mammals), there is, to some extent, a spatial separation between two major steps in the fermentation process of NSPs from fibre. Indeed, in chickens, there is a large population of lactobacilli in the ileum which can hydrolyse the plant cell wall NSPs, generating lactic acid as an intermediate metabolite. The conversion of lactic acid into butyric acid is mainly done by members of the Lachnospiraceae family in the caeca. Only some members of the Ruminococcaceae family (e.g. *Faecalibacterium prausnitzii*) residing predominantly in the caeca can take care of the entire cascade of the breakdown of the NSP macromolecular complexes into butyrate. This topographical differentiation seems to be less pronounced in the pig (Crespo-Piazuelo *et al.*, 2018), except under pathological conditions (Pollock *et al.*, 2019). Butyrate appears to be a very important end product of bacterial metabolism in the lower intestinal tract of many different animal species. It is not only an important energy source for the epithelial cells lining the lower intestinal tract, but also an important 'interkingdom' messenger, generating a wide range of beneficial responses in the host (for a review, see Guilloteau *et al.*, 2010).

All of the above-mentioned observations suggest that, in a healthy intestine, the entire digestible fraction of the feed is completely absorbed by the time the gut content reaches the ileum (in the chicken) or the ileo-caecal valve (in the pig). This means that the lower intestinal microbiota should live to some extent on host secretions (including sloughed-off epithelial cells, mucins and enzymes), but most importantly on the remaining indigestible fibre fraction, composed essentially of NSPs. The role of dietary fibre NSPs as a critically important substrate for the gut microbiota is recognized not only in monogastric farm animals but also in humans (Hills *et al.*, 2019). The NSPs in feed mostly come from cereal grain hulls and soybean hulls, where they are present as large macromolecular structures composed of interconnected long branched chains of different sugar polymers. Depending on the source of the feed ingredients, the chemical composition of the NSPs can vary considerably. In most cases, however, arabinoxylans and β-glucans make up the dominant fractions of the NSPs. Therefore, one should expect that these will predominantly fuel the expansion and metabolic activity of the above-mentioned dominant families in the ileum and caeca. Other NSP fractions may, however, support other members of the ileal and/or caecal microbiome. One way to investigate this is by supplying an additional amount of one specific NSP fraction (on top of what is already present in the ingredients of the feed) and check for specific changes in the microbiome. We recently used this approach to identify the members of the microbiota which are responsible for cellulose breakdown (De Maesschalck *et al.*, 2019). In these studies in broilers, it was shown that cellulose could be hydrolysed by genus *Alistipes*, belonging to the Rikenellaceae family. Metagenomic analysis of a single caecal microbiota from a broiler, however, has shown that a number of other bacteria in the caeca also carry genes coding for cellulases, but it is not known to what extent they contribute to cellulose breakdown (Sergeant *et al.*, 2014).

Another approach to identify members of the intestinal microbiota with beneficial functions is by comparing the microbiota of broiler flocks with high versus low performance. Using this approach, Torok *et al.* (2011) found performance-related operational taxonomic units in the ileum and caeca of broilers fed different feed formulas.

Finally, meta-analyses of large numbers of studies investigating human gut microbiota composition have allowed identification of categories of bacteria associated with poor (gut) health. Using this approach, Shin *et al.* (2015) found Proteobacteria (including the family Enterobacteriaceae) as a 'microbial signature of dysbiosis'. Expansion of the phylum Proteobacteria is also seen in poultry and swine under various conditions of poor intestinal health. The Proteobacteria, however, seem to show like two sides of

a coin. *Escherichia coli* and some other members of the family Enterobacteriaceae, phylum Proteobacteria, appear to be among the very first colonizers of the lower intestinal tract in chickens (Videnska *et al.*, 2014), playing a crucial role in the reduction of the oxygen tension in the caeca, which is a prerequisite for the colonization by Lachnospiraceae and Ruminococcaceae. Proteobacteria also have been suggested to play a role in training the intestinal immune system in pigs (Zwiritz *et al.*, 2019). On the other hand, in laboratory animal models and in humans it was found that excessive expansion at a later age of Proteobacteria in general is a microbial signature of dysbiosis (Shin *et al.*, 2015). *E. coli* and other members of the Proteobacteria tend to use oxygen as terminal electron acceptor in their energy production, generating oxygen radicals which are powerful triggers of inflammation in the intestinal mucosa (Hughes *et al.*, 2017). A similar ambiguous role probably can be attributed to the *Lactobacillus* genus. Expansion of lactobacilli in the caeca was associated with better feed conversion in laying hens (Yan *et al.*, 2017) and in broilers (Torok *et al.*, 2011). In contrast, Torok *et al.* (2013) found the *Lactobacillus* genus to be significantly decreased in the ileum of broilers that were more feed efficient, using qPCR. These seemingly controversial findings might suggest that lactobacilli are beneficial as they fuel butyrate production through cross-feeding, but their excessive expansion in the small intestine (especially when expanding into the proximal segment) may be harmful due to competition with the host for the digestible fraction of the diet.

Exogenous enzymes may beneficially shift this delicate equilibrium of the feed, the host mucosa and the microbiota in many different ways. Since enzymes can become active as soon as they have passed the stomach/proventriculus, they may exert their effects at different levels of the intestinal tract. Unfortunately, many of the studies examining the effects of in-feed enzymes on the microbiome have used enzyme blends, making it impossible to draw conclusions about the effect of specific single enzymes.

15.3 Non-Starch Polysaccharide (NSP)-Degrading Enzymes (NSPases)

As the NSPs from plant cell walls make up the bulk of the substrate available for the microbes that live in the lower gastrointestinal tract, and NSPases can be active all along the small intestine, it seems logical to assume that in-feed NSPases may make the NSPs more readily available for the microbiota, especially in very young animals, when the intestinal microbiome is still immature.

15.3.1 Xylanases and the microbiome

The effects of added β-1,4-xylanases on performance are well documented. Among other factors (e.g. reducing viscosity in the small intestine in broilers), the mechanism of action may involve an effect on the microbiota through the generation of prebiotic oligosaccharides from the arabinoxylans present in the cereal hulls in feed. Enzymatic degradation of cereal-derived arabinoxylans has indeed been shown to generate both AXOS and xylo-oligosaccharides (XOS) (Broekaert et al., 2011).

The first reports on the interaction between in-feed xylanases and intestinal microbes looked at effects on culturable bacteria. Hubener et al. (2002) found that xylanase supplementation to a wheat–rye-based diet for broilers led to lower colony-forming units in the small intestine while the capacity of bacteria cultured from ileal samples to utilize NSPs was enhanced. Hirsch et al. (2006) found a shift in Lactobacillus spp. in the terminal jejunum in piglets on a diet supplemented with a xylanase, whereas in the study of Li et al. (2019) the supplementation of xylanase resulted in lower ileal Lactobacillus counts in piglets. Thus, xylanases may to some extent prevent excessive expansion of the microbiome upstream in the small intestine and protect against what is called in human medicine 'small intestinal bacterial overgrowth' (SIBO) (Aziz et al., 2017). De Maesschalck et al. (2015) investigated the effects of supplementing low-molecular-weight XOS on the caecum and colon microbiota of broilers on a wheat- and rye-based diet using 16S rRNA gene sequencing. Supplementation of XOS to a wheat- and rye-based diet significantly increased the relative abundance of Lactobacillaceae family in the colon and the butyrate-producing family Clostridium cluster XIVa (Lachnospiraceae) in the caeca of broilers. Furthermore, cross-feeding between two species belonging to these families (Lactobacillus crispatus and Anaerostipes butyraticus) was shown in vitro, generating high amounts of butyrate. McCafferty et al. (2019), however, found inconsistent effects of xylanase supplements on short-chain fatty acid (SCFA) concentrations in the caeca. Nevertheless, one should take into account that concentrations of SCFAs in the lumen are the result of production by the bacteria and receptor-mediated uptake by the mucosa.

Ribeiro et al. (2018) supplemented broiler feed with either XOS or a β-1,4-xylanase. They confirmed the changes in the microbiota observed by De Maesschalck et al. (2015) in both groups. To further understand the mode of action of the xylanases, Ravn et al. (2017) incubated wheat bran with a xylanase in vitro and analysed the AXOS that were released. AXOS with an average degree of polymerization (aDP) of 10 were generated. Increasing the enzyme concentration could further lower the aDP to 4–8. These prebiotic AXOS supported the expansion of butyrate-producing genera in an in vitro fermentation experiment with broiler caecal microbiota (Ravn et al., 2017).

It is well established that increased arabinose to xylose ratio and glucuronation of arabinoxylans may greatly hinder the activity of many β-1,4-xylanases especially on specific substrates such as maize (Bach Knudsen, 1997). Therefore, Ravn et al. (2018) investigated the combination of a xylanase and a debranching α-L-arabinofuranosidase, showing beneficial effects on intestinal health and an increase in caecal butyrate but no significant effects on the caecal microbiota in broilers.

15.3.2 β-Glucanases + xylanases and the microbiome

β-Glucans usually represent the second most abundant fraction of the NSPs in monogastric animal diets, after the arabinox-ylans. Nevertheless, to the best of our know-ledge, there are no studies examining the effects of single glucanases on the microbiome.

Many enzyme blends, however, contain both an endo-β-1,4-xylanase and an endo-1,3-β-glucanase, aiming to degrade the bulk of the NSPs in the feed. Yacoubi *et al.* (2016) fermented whole wheat grains *in vitro* with such an enzyme blend. The enzyme treat-ment increased the water-soluble fraction of the arabinoxylans and it decreased the aDP of the xylan backbone, without formation of oligosaccharides with an aDP < 10. The low-molecular-weight fraction of the solubilized arabinoxylans obtained after enzymatic treatment of wheat significantly increased SCFA and lactate production when incu-bated with caecal microbiota from broilers. Solubilized arabinoxylans from *in vitro* en-zymatically treated wheat (compared with non-enzymatically treated wheat) were sub-sequently added to the feed of broilers at a concentration of 0.1%. At day 14 post-hatch, the solubilized arabinoxylans significantly increased the abundance of *Enterococcus durans* and *Candidatus arthromitus* in the ileum. It also increased the abundance of several butyrate-producing members of the Lachnospiraceae and Ruminococcaceae fam-ilies in the caeca (Yacoubi *et al.*, 2017). These changes were associated with re-duced inflammation and increased SCFA concentration in the caecal content. The most remarkable finding in this study, how-ever, was the increased density of L-cells in the ileal epithelium. L-cells are butyrate-responsive endocrine cells producing glucagon-like peptide 2, which supports the replication and the differentiation of intes-tinal epithelial cells. This observation may explain the beneficial effects on small intes-tinal morphology and function of butyrate production in the caeca.

In a study comparing wheat- versus maize-based diets with and without endo-β-1, 4-xylanase and endo-1,3-β-glucanase, Munyaka *et al.* (2016) showed more viscosity reduction in the jejunal content on the wheat-based diet. The enzyme blend also improved starch digestibility on the wheat-based diet, indicating that the enzymes were active in the small intestine. On the maize-based diet,

the enzyme blend increased the abundance of families Lactobacillaceae, Lachnospiraceae and Peptostreptococcaceae as well as some genera belonging to the Ruminococcaceae in the ileum. A similar shift was observed on the wheat-based diet but this time in the caeca. Combined endo-β-1,4-xylanases and endo-1,3-β-glucanases also have been used in pig diets. In pigs fed an oats-based diet, the inclusion of such enzyme blend was as-sociated with higher numbers of lactobacilli in the caecum and colon and *Bifidobacteri-um* in the ileum using a microbial plate count method (Murphy *et al.*, 2012). These observations suggest a similar effect of the enzyme blend on lactate producers in the proximal part of the lower intestine in pigs as in poultry.

All of these data indicate that com-bined endo-β-1,4-xylanases and endo-1,3-β-glucanases are associated with changes in the microbiota that are remarkably similar to those observed with endo-β-1,4-xylanas-es only. It is unclear whether the additional inclusion of the endo-1,3-β-glucanases is a bonus or not.

15.3.3   Mannanases and the microbiome

Mannans of plant cell wall origin are β-1,4 linked, and thus different from the mannans present in yeast cell walls which are β-1,3 linked. Depending on the source, plant mannans can have glucose and/or galactose residues on the backbone chain, which may affect their enzymatic hydrolysis (Shastak *et al.*, 2015). Plant-derived mannans are considered one of the major antinutritional components in monogastric nutrition, even if mannans represent only a minor fraction of the NSPs in most common feed ingredi-ents for poultry and pigs. Soybean meal, for example, may contain β-mannans up to 16 g/kg (Hsiao *et al.*, 2006). Some uncommon feed ingredients, such as guar meal, coconut meal, palm kernel meal and copra meal, however, contain much larger amounts of mannans (Shastak *et al.*, 2015). The hy-drolysis of plant mannans by β-mannanases *in vitro* releases manno-oligosaccharides (MOS) (Nopvichai *et al.*, 2019). Unfortunately, *in vivo* studies investigating the effects of

MOS on the intestinal microbiota in poultry and pigs almost exclusively used MOS from yeast cell walls. It is uncertain whether MOS enzymatically generated from plant cell walls will yield similar results, so these studies will not be discussed here.

Direct supplementation of β-mannanases in feed has been shown to reduce the feed conversion ratio in fattening pigs (Rychen et al., 2018). Similarly, β-mannanase supplementation to a maize–soy-based diet improves performance in broilers, especially under challenge (Eimeria) conditions (Jackson et al., 2003). In a similar experimental set-up (maize–soy and Eimeria challenge), Bortoluzzi et al. (2019) investigated the effects on ileal and caecal microbiota. At family level, β-mannanase supplementation was associated with expansion of the Ruminococcaceae in the caeca. At genus level, there was an expansion of Lactobacillus in the ileum. In the caeca, a reduction in Bacteroides and an increase in Akkermansia was observed. Akkermansia can utilize mucus as a carbon and nitrogen source, producing acetate and propionate (Fujio-Vejar et al., 2017). These limited observations regarding the effects of β-mannanase on the intestinal microbiota are a first indication that this category of enzymes may also support SCFA production in the caeca.

15.3.4 Other NSPases and the microbiome

For a number of NSP-hydrolysing enzymes the effects on the microbiome have not been investigated yet. This is the case for galactosidases, cellulases and pectinases, for instance. They are mostly designed to improve digestibility and to reduce viscosity of the small intestinal content in poultry (Tahir et al., 2008). Cellulase has been used in enzyme blends but not separately and the effects on the microbiota are unknown.

15.4 Enzymes Hydrolysing Non-NSP Feed Components

Effects of this category of enzymes on the microbiota can be expected when the host enzymes are not capable of completely hydrolysing the digestible fraction. In this case nutrients other than NSPs become available to the microbiota, eventually leading to dysbiosis.

15.4.1 Amylases and the microbiome

Animals and humans produce starch-hydrolysing amylases in the salivary glands and in the pancreas. Plants store starch in tightly packed granules, consisting of layers of amylose and amylopectin. These granules may have different structure and shape characteristics which may affect digestion. Larger starch granules are less available to host enzyme digestion because the lower percentage of surface area reduces the enzyme binding rate. Resistant starch is inaccessible to enzymes due to starch granule conformation or cannot be hydrolysed by the host amylases. This resistant starch reaches the lower intestinal tract where it is fermented by the microbiota to form SCFA (Warren et al., 2018).

The effects of supplementation of exogenous α-amylase on starch digestibility, performance and the microbiota were investigated by Yin et al. (2018). They added α-amylase to a diet formulated with newly harvested maize for broilers. Newly harvested maize is known to be incompletely digested in the small intestine (Yin et al., 2018). Adding the enzyme did not significantly increase total starch digestibility in the small intestine. It did, however, significantly increase villus length and villus to crypt ratio in the duodenum at day 16. This was associated with enrichment of the Lactobacillaceae family in the caeca. At genus level, there was an expansion of Lactobacillus, Coprobacter (belonging to the family Porphyromonadaceae) and Parasutterella (belonging to the family Sutterellaceae) in the caeca. Surprisingly, this was not accompanied by a significant expansion of the Lachnospiraceae family in this case.

15.4.2 Proteases and the microbiome

Proteins escaping digestion and absorption in the duodenum and jejunum of the chicken or in the small intestine of the pig mostly include proteins secreted by the host mucosa which are resistant to proteolytic degradation (host proteases, peptidases, IgA, etc.) as well as remnants of sloughed epithelial cells and mucins. These are classified under the heading of 'endogenous nitrogen'. Additionally, some proteins from the feed that are masked from the host enzymes also may escape digestion in the small intestine (so-called 'ileal bypass'). These proteins constitute important nutrient sources for the lactobacilli in the caecum of pigs and in the ileum of chickens, as lactobacilli are unable to synthesize many of their own amino acids (Morishita *et al.*, 1981). Ileal protein bypass can be increased by excessive protein levels in feed or by a reduction in the digestion and absorption of feed protein in the small intestine (e.g. due to *Eimeria* infection). Increased ileal bypass supports expansion of protein-fermenting bacteria in the ileum and the caeca of chickens and in the caecum and colon of pigs. Expansion of protein-fermenting bacteria in the small intestine may increase microbial competition for dietary protein, which has been associated with SIBO (for a review, see Rodriguez *et al.*, 2019) or, in the case of expansion of *Clostridium perfringens*, may lead to necrotic enteritis in broilers. Protein fermentation is characterized by the release of branched-chain fatty acids and biogenic amines (Apajalahti and Vienola, 2016).

Adding an exogenous protease to the diet upregulates the expression of genes responsible for peptide transport in the jejunum of broilers, which explains the improved pre-ileal amino acid absorption (Cowieson *et al.*, 2019). Borda-Molina *et al.* (2019) investigated the effects of different proteases on the microbiota of the terminal ileum in broilers. One protease, supplemented at 1600 mg/kg and an activity of 75,000 U/g, was associated with enrichment of the *Lactobacillus* genus and the *Peptoclostridium* genus (formerly genus *Clostridium* XI, belonging to the Peptostreptococcaceae family), when added at this high concentration. Lactobacilli require many different amino acids in their environment, and Peptostreptococcaceae are known to use mostly peptides as their sole nutrient source.

In accordance with these findings, Park and Kim (2018) found no difference in *Lactobacillus* counts in the ileum of broilers when the diet was supplemented or not with the same enzyme at 200 mg/kg. The protease at the high concentration thus may itself be the substrate for the growth of the microorganisms in the small intestine. To the best of our knowledge, there are no studies examining the effects of exogenous protease on the caecal microbiota of chickens or the caecum and colon microbiota of pigs.

15.4.3   Phytases and the microbiome

Phytase is commonly used in monogastric animal diets to improve phosphorus availability and reduce phosphorus loss by excretion. It has also been shown to moderately increase amino acid digestibility in the small intestine (Siegert *et al.*, 2019). Borda-Molina *et al.* (2016) studied the effects of adding phytase to a maize–soy-based diet for broilers on both the luminal and the mucosa-associated microbiota in different segments of the intestine. The effects of the phytase on the microbiota were limited. In another study from the same group with a similar experimental set-up, supplementation of phytase was associated with a shift in the species composition of the *Lactobacillus* genus in the ileum: increased abundance of *Lactobacillus salivarius* and *Lactobacillus taiwanensis*, and decreased abundance of *L. crispatus* (Witzig *et al.*, 2015). The functional significance of this shift is unclear, however.

15.5   Enzymes Interacting Directly with the Microbiota

The number of bacterial cells present in the gastrointestinal tract is estimated to outnumber the total number of cells in the entire body of the host. These bacteria replicate continuously, yet the total remains relatively constant. This means that numerous bacteria die all along the gastrointestinal tract, leaving remnants composed predominantly of peptidoglycan and lipopolysaccharide from the bacterial cell walls. The epithelial cells and other cells in the intestinal mucosa carry Toll-like receptors that recognize these so-called 'danger-associated molecular patterns' (DAMP) and may trigger an immune response. Enzymes have been described that interfere with this complex interplay between the microbiota and the host. Enzymes designed to kill bacteria, however, should be considered as antibiotics and thus cannot be used in animal feed according to European legislation. Lysozyme is an enzyme that naturally occurs in various bodily secretions and in egg white. Although it has documented antibacterial activity (Ellison and Giehl, 1991), it is used in diets of pigs and poultry. Oxidoreductases are enzymes that use different substrates to generate hydrogen peroxide. The latter is a powerful broad-spectrum bactericidal substance. Other enzymes attacking the bacterial cell components are alkaline phosphatase, which can inactivate lipopolysaccharide, and non-lysozyme muramidases, which can break down peptidoglycan. However, to the best of our knowledge, no effects on the gut microbiota have been reported for these two at the time of writing.

The activity of these enzymes in the small intestine may contribute to the natural antibacterial resistance mechanisms already in place in this intestinal segment, preventing SIBO and avoiding competition between the microbiota and the host for the nutrients in feed.

15.5.1 Lysozyme and the microbiome

Lysozyme is a 1,4-β-N-acetylmuramidase that cleaves the glycosidic bond between N-acetylglucosamine and N-acetylmuramic acid in the peptidoglycan of all bacterial cell walls. Supplementation of lysozyme in the feed has been shown to improve performance and intestinal health in growing pigs (for a review, see Oliver and Wells, 2015) and in broilers (Abdel-Latif et al., 2017). Zou et al. (2019) examined the effect of two different levels of lysozyme in the diet (50 and 100 mg/kg) on caecal microbiota

of growing pigs. No effects were found at phylum level. The high lysozyme level, however, was associated with a lower α-diversity of the caecal microbiota.

15.5.2 Oxidoreductases and the microbiome

Glucose oxidase catalyses the oxidation of glucose to gluconic acid, with host-derived molecular oxygen (reaching the intestinal lumen by diffusion from the capillaries of the host mucosa) as an electron acceptor and simultaneous production of hydrogen peroxide. Wu et al. (2018) showed beneficial effects on performance of broilers from adding small amounts of glucose oxidase (up to 60 U/kg) to the diet. The glucose oxidase supplementation was associated with increased abundance of Faecalibacterium and Coprobacillus genera and reduced abundance of Brenneria in the caeca at 21 days, whereas at 42 days there was increased abundance of Clostridium and decreased abundance of Sutterella in the caeca.

15.6 Conclusion

The commercial lines of chickens and pigs used in intensive animal production have been selected for rapid growth and high feed intake. This high feed intake puts a lot of pressure on the delicate interactions between the feed, the host mucosa and the microbes present in the gastrointestinal tract. Any disturbances of these interactions will lead to deterioration of intestinal health, characterized by inflammation, a shift in the microbiota composition and leakage at tight junctions between the intestinal epithelial cells (Ducatelle et al., 2018). These phenomena are often referred to as dysbiosis. Exogenous enzymes added to the feed can help to prevent dysbiosis. They support or compensate for deficiencies in the endogenous enzymes, which are naturally derived from the feed (mostly plant enzymes), the host and the microbes. In order to choose the right enzymes as feed supplements, the critical factors that trigger the dysbiosis need to be identified. Effects of exogenous enzymes on intestinal health and performance may, in many cases, at least in part be attributed to direct or indirect effects on the intestinal microbiota. The enzymes may either boost beneficial microbes in specific segments of the gastrointestinal tract or they may protect from expansion of microbiota in regions where absorption of nutrients is the priority.

The available data on the interactions between exogenous enzymes and the intestinal microbiota are still fragmentary. Future research should focus on the effects of the enzymes on the microbiota present in the different geographical locations within the digestive system, considering the source of enzyme and preferably using pure enzymes rather than blends.

References

Abdel-Latif, M.A., El-Far, A.H., Elbestawy, A.R., Ghanem, R., Mousa, S.A. and Abd El-Hamid, H.S. (2017) Exogenous dietary lysozyme improves the growth performance and gut microbiota in broiler chickens targeting the antioxidant and non-specific immunity mRNA expression. *PLoS ONE* 12, e0185153.

Aftab, U. and Bedford, M.R. (2018) The use of NSP enzymes in poultry nutrition: myths and realities. *World's Poultry Science Journal* 74, 277–286.

Apajalahti, J. and Vienola, K. (2016) Interaction between chicken intestinal microbiota and protein digestion. *Animal Feed Science and Technology* 221, 323–330.

Aziz, I., Tornblom, H. and Simren, M. (2017) Small intestinal bacterial overgrowth as a cause for irritable bowel syndrome: guilty or not guilty? *Current Opinion in Gastroenterology* 33, 196–202.

Bach Knudsen, K.E. (1997) Carbohydrate and lignin contents of plant materials used in animal feeding. *Animal Feed Science and Technology* 67, 319–338.

Bautil, A., Verspreet, J., Buyse, J., Goos, P., Bedford, M.R. and Courtin, C.M. (2019) Age-related arabinoxylan hydrolysis and fermentation in the gastrointestinal tract of broilers fed wheat-based diets. *Poultry Science* 98, 4606–4621.

Borda-Molina, D., Vital, M., Sommerfeld, V., Rodehutscord, M. and Camarinha-Silva, A. (2016) Insights into broilers' gut microbiota fed with phosphorus, calcium and phytase supplemented diets. *Frontiers in Microbiology* 7, 2033.

Borda-Molina, D., Zuber, T., Siegert, W., Camarinha-Silva, A., Feuerstein, D. and Rodehutscord, M. (2019) Effects of protease and phytase supplements on small intestinal microbiota and amino acid digestibility in broiler chickens. *Poultry Science* 98, 2906–2918.

Bortoluzzi, C., Scapini, L.B., Ribeiro, M.V., Pivetta, M.R., Buzim, R. and Fernandes, J.I.M. (2019) Effects of β-mannanase supplementation in the intestinal microbiota composition of broiler chickens challenged with a coccidiosis vaccine. *Livestock Science* 228, 187–194.

Broekaert, W.F., Courtin, C.M., Verbeke, K., Van De Wiele, T., Verstraete, W. and Delcour, J. (2011) Prebiotic and other health-related effects of cereal-derived arabinoxylans, arabinoxylan-oligosaccharides, and xylo-oligosaccharides. *Critical Reviews in Food Science and Nutrition* 51, 178–194.

Choct, M. (2006) Enzymes and the feed industry: past, present and future. *World's Poultry Science Journal* 62, 5–15.

Courtin, C.M., Broekaert, W.F., Swennen, K., Lescroart, O., Anagbesan, O., *et al.* (2008) Dietary inclusion of wheat bran arabinoxylooligosaccharides induces beneficial nutritional effects in chickens. *Cereal Chemistry* 85, 607–613.

Cowieson, A.J. and Kluenter, A.M. (2019) Contribution of exogenous enzymes to potentiate the removal of antibiotic growth promoters in poultry production. *Animal Feed Science and Technology* 250, 81–92.

Cowieson, A.J., Toghyani, M., Kheravii, S.K., Wu, S.B., Romero, L.F. and Choct, M. (2019) A mono-component microbial protease improves performance, net energy, and digestibility of amino acids and starch, and upregulates jejunal expression of genes responsible for peptide transport in broilers fed corn/wheat-based diets supplemented with xylanase and phytase. *Poultry Science* 98, 1321–1332.

Crespo-Piazuelo, D., Estellé, J., Revilla, M., Criado-Mesas, L., Ramayo-Caldas, Y., *et al.* (2018) Characterization of bacterial microbiota compositions along the intestinal tract in pigs and their interactions and functions. *Scientific Reports* 8, 12727.

De Maesschalck, C., Eeckhaut, V., Maertens, L., De Lange, L., Marchal, L., *et al.* (2015) Effects of xylo-oligosaccharides on broiler chicken performance and microbiota. *Applied and Environmental Microbiology* 81, 5880–5888.

De Maesschalck, C., Eeckhaut, V., Maertens, L., De Lange, L., Marchal, L., *et al.* (2019) Amorphous cellulose feed supplement alters the broiler caecal microbiome. *Poultry Science* 98, 3811–3817.

Ducatelle, R., Goossens, E., De Meyer, F., Eeckhaut, V., Antonissen, G., *et al.* (2018) Biomarkers for monitoring intestinal health in poultry: present status and future perspectives. *Veterinary Research* 49, 43.

Ellison, R.T. and Giehl, T. (1991) Killing of Gram-negative bacteria by lactoferrin and lysozyme. *Journal of Clinical Investigation* 88, 1080–1091.

Fujio-Vejar, S., Yessania, V., Morales, P., Magne, F., Vera-Wolf, P., *et al.* (2017) The gut microbiota of healthy Chilean subjects reveals a high abundance of the phylum Verrucomicrobia. *Frontiers in Microbiology* 8, 1221.

Guilloteau, P., Martin, L., Eeckhaut, V., Ducatelle, R., Zabielski, R. and Van Immerseel, F. (2010) From the gut to the peripheral tissues: the multiple effects of butyrate. *Nutrition Research Reviews* 23, 366–384.

Hills, R.D., Pontefract, B.A., Mishcon, H.R., Black, C.A., Sutton, S.C. and Theberge, C.R. (2019) Gut microbiome: profound implications for diet and disease. *Nutrients* 11, 1613.

Hirsch, K., Simon, O. and Vahjen, W. (2006) Influence of a xylanase feed additive on *Lactobacillus* species in the jejunum of piglets. *Berliner und Munchener Tierarztliche Wochenschrift* 119, 486–492.

Hsiao, H.Y., Anderson, D.M. and Dale, N.M. (2006) Levels of β-mannan in soybean meal. *Poultry Science* 85, 1430–1432.

Hubener, K., Vahjen, W. and Simon, O. (2002) Bacterial responses to different dietary cereal types and xylanase supplementation in the intestine of broiler chicken. *Archives of Animal Nutrition* 56, 167–187.

Hughes, E.R., Winter, M.G., Duerkop, B.A., Spiga, L., Furtado de Carvalho, T., *et al.* (2017) Microbial respiration and formate oxidation as metabolic signatures of inflammation-associated dysbiosis. *Cell, Host & Microbe* 21, 208–219.

Jackson, M.E., Anderson, D.M., Hsiao, H.Y., Mathis, G.F. and Fodge, D.W. (2003) Beneficial effects of β-mannanase feed enzyme on performance of chicks challenged with *Eimeria* sp. and *Clostridium perfringens*. *Avian Diseases* 47, 759–763.

Kiarie, E., Romero, L.F. and Nyachoti, C.M. (2013) The role of added feed enzymes in promoting gut health in swine and poultry. *Nutrition Research Reviews* 26, 71–88.

Li, Q., Schmitz-Esser, S., Loving, C.L., Gabler, N.K., Gould, S.A. and Patience, J. (2019) Exogenous carbohydrases added to a starter diet reduced markers of systemic immune activation and decreased *Lactobacillus* in weaned pigs. *Journal of Animal Science* 97, 1242–1253.

Lu, J., Idris, U., Harmon, B., Hofacre, C., Maurer, J.J. and Lee, M.D. (2003) Diversity and succession of the intestinal bacterial community of the maturing broiler chicken. *Applied and Environmental Microbiology* 69, 6816–6824.

McCafferty, K.W., Bedford, M.R., Kerr, B.J. and Dozier, W.A. (2019) Effects of age and supplemental xylanase in corn- and wheat-based diets on cecal volatile fatty acid concentrations of broilers. *Poultry Science* 98, 4787–4800.

Morishita, T., Degushi, Y., Yajima, M., Sakurai, T. and Yura, T. (1981) Multiple nutritional requirements of lactobacilli: genetic lesions affecting amino acid biosynthetic pathways. *Journal of Bacteriology* 148, 64–71.

Munyaka, P.M., Nandha, N.K., Kiarie, E., Nyachoti, C.M. and Khafpour, E. (2016) Impact of combined β-glucanase and xylanase enzymes on growth performance, nutrients utilization and gut microbiota in broiler chickens fed corn or wheat-based diets. *Poultry Science* 95, 528–540.

Murphy, P., Dal Bello, F., O'Doherty, J.V. and Arendt, E.K. (2012) Effects of cereal β-glucans and enzyme inclusion on the porcine gastrointestinal tract microbiota. *Anaerobe* 18, 557–565.

Nopvichai, C., Charoenwongpaiboon, T., Luengluepunya, N., Ito, K., Muanprasat, C. and Pichyangkura, R. (2019) Production and purification of mannan oligosaccharide with epithelial tight junction enhancing activity. *PeerJ* 7, 7206.

Oliver, W.T. and Wells, J.E. (2015) Lysozyme as an alternative to growth promoting antibiotics in swine production. *Journal of Animal Science and Biotechnology* 6, 35.

Park, J.H. and Kim, I.H. (2018) Effects of a protease and essential oils on growth performance, blood cell profiles, nutrient retention, ileal microbiota, excreta gas emission, and breast meat quality in broiler chicks. *Poultry Science* 97, 2854–2860.

Pollock, J., Hutchings, M.R., Hutchings, K.E.K., Gally, D.L. and Houdijk, J.G.M. (2019) Changes in the ileal, but not fecal, microbiome in response to increased dietary protein level and enterotoxigenic *Escherichia coli* in pigs. *Applied and Environmental Microbiology* 85, e01252-19.

Ravn, J.L., Thogersen, J.C., Eklof, J., Pettersson, D., Ducatelle, R., *et al.* (2017) GH11 xylanase increases pre-biotic oligosaccharides from wheat bran favouring butyrate-producing bacteria *in vitro*. *Animal Feed Science and Technology* 226, 113–123.

Ravn, J.L., Glitso, V., Pettersson, D., Ducatelle, R. and Van Immerseel, F. (2018) Combined endo-β-1,4-xylanase and α-1-arabinofuranosidase increases butyrate concentration during broiler cecal fermentation of maize glucurono-arabinoxylan. *Animal Feed Science and Technology* 236, 159–169.

Ribeiro, T., Cardoso, V., Ferreira, L.M.A., Lordelo, M.M.S., Coelho, E., *et al.* (2018) Xylo-oligosaccharides display a prebiotic activity when used to supplement wheat or corn-based diets for broilers. *Poultry Science* 97, 4330–4341.

Robinson, K., Becker, S., Xiao, Y., Lyu, W., Yang, Q., *et al.* (2019) Differential impact of subtherapeutic anti-biotics and ionophores on intestinal microbiota of broilers. *Microorganisms* 7, 282.

Rodriguez, D., MacDaragh Ryan, P., Monjaraz, E., Mayans, J. and Quigley, E. (2019) Small intestinal bacterial overgrowth in children: a state-of-the-art review. *Frontiers in Pediatrics* 7, 363.

Rychen, G., Aquilina, G., Azimonti, G., Bampidis, V., de Lourdes Bastos, M., *et al.* (2018) Safety and efficacy of Hemicell® HT (endo-1,4-β-mannanase) as a feed additive for chickens for fattening, chickens reared for laying, turkey for fattening, turkeys reared for breeding, weaned piglets, pigs for fattening and minor poultry and porcine species. *EFSA Journal* 16, 5270.

Sergeant, M., Constantinidou, C., Cogan, T.A., Bedford, M.R., Penn, C.W. and Pallen, M.J. (2014) Extensive microbial and functional diversity within the chicken cecal microbiome. *PLoS ONE* 9, e91941.

Shastak, Y., Ader, P., Feuerstein, D., Ruehle, R. and Matuschek, M. (2015) β-Mannan and mannanase in poultry nutrition. *World's Poultry Science Journal* 71, 161–173.

Shin, N.R., Whon, T.W. and Bae, J.W. (2015) Proteobacteria: microbial signature of dysbiosis in gut micro-biota. *Trends in Biotechnology* 33, 496–503.

Siegert, W., Zuber, T., Sommerfeld, V., Krieg, J., Feuerstein, D., *et al.* (2019) Prececal amino acid digestibility and phytate degradation in broiler chickens when using different oilseed meals, phytase and protease supplements in the feed. *Poultry Science* 98, 5700–5713.

Smith, J.A. (2019) Broiler production without antibiotics: United States field perspectives. *Animal Feed Science and Technology* 250, 93–98.

Tahir, M., Saleh, F., Ohtsuka, A. and Hayashi, K. (2008) An effective combination of carbohydrases that en-ables reduction of dietary protein in broilers: importance of hemicellulose. *Poultry Science* 87, 713–718.

Torok, V.A., Hughes, R.J., Mikkelsen, L.L., Perez-Maldonado, R., Balding, K., *et al.* (2011) Identification and characterization of potential performance-related gut microbiotas in broiler chickens across various feeding trials. *Applied and Environmental Microbiology* 77, 5867–5878.

Torok, V.A., Dyson, C., McKay, A. and Ophel-Keller, K. (2013) Quantitative molecular assays for evaluating changes in broiler gut microbiota linked with diet and performance. *Animal Production Science* 53, 1260–1268.

Videnska, P., Sedlar, K., Lukac, M., Faldynova, M., Gerzova, L., *et al.* (2014) Succession and replacement of bacterial populations in the caecum of egg laying hens over their whole life. *PLoS ONE* 9, e115142.

Warren, F.J., Fukuma, N.M., Mikkelsen, D., Flanagan, B.M., Williams, B.A., *et al.* (2018) Food starch structure impacts gut microbiome composition. *mSphere* 3, 00086.

Witzig, M., Camarinha da Silva, A., Green-Engert, R., Hoelzle, K., Zeller, E., *et al.* (2015) Spatial variation of the gut microbiota in broiler chickens as affected by dietary available phosphorus and assessed by T-RFLP analysis and 454 pyrosequencing. *PLoS ONE* 10, e0143442.

Wu, S., Li, T., Niu, H., Zhu, Y., Liu, Y., *et al.* (2018) Effects of glucose oxidase on growth performance, gut function, and cecal microbiota of broiler chickens. *Poultry Science* 98, 828–841.

Yacoubi, N., Van Immerseel, F., Ducatelle, R., Rhayat, L., Bonnin, E. and Saulnier, L. (2016) Water-soluble fractions obtained by enzymatic treatment of wheat grains promote short chain fatty acids production by broiler cecal microbiota. *Animal Feed Science and Technology* 218, 110–119.

Yacoubi, N., Saulnier, L., Bonnin, E., Devillard, E., Eeckhaut, V., *et al.* (2017) Short-chain arabinoxylans pre-pared from enzymatically treated wheat grain exert prebiotic effects during the broiler starter period. *Poultry Science* 97, 412–424.

Yan, W., Sun, C., Yuan, J. and Yang, N. (2017) Gut metagenomics analysis reveals prominent roles of *Lactoba-cillus* and cecal microbiota in chicken feed efficiency. *Scientific Reports* 7, 45308.

Yang, Y., Iji, P.A. and Choct, M. (2009) Dietary modulation of gut microflora in broiler chickens: a review of the role of six kinds of alternatives to in-feed antibiotics. *World's Poultry Science Journal* 65, 97–114.

Yin, D., Yin, X., Lei, Z., Wang, M., Guo, Y., *et al.* (2018) Supplementation of amylase combined with gluco-amylase or protease changes intestinal microbiota diversity and benefits for broilers fed a diet of newly harvested corn. *Journal of Animal Science and Biotechnology* 9, 24.

Zou, L., Xiong, X., Liu, H., Zhou, J., Liu, Y. and Yin, Y. (2019) Effects of dietary lysozyme levels on growth performance, intestinal morphology, immunity response and microbiota community of growing pigs. *Journal of the Science of Food and Agriculture* 99, 1643–1650.

Zwiritz, B., Pinior, B., Metzler-Zebeli, B., Handler, M., Gense, K., *et al.* (2019) Microbiota of the gut–lymph node axis: depletion of mucosa-associated segmented filamentous bacteria and enrichment of *Methano-brevibacter* by colistin sulfate and linco-spectin in pigs. *Frontiers in Microbiology* 10, 599.

16 Parameters Impacting Responses in Animal Feed Enzyme Trials

Carrie L. Walk[1]* and Milan Hruby[2]

[1]*DSM Nutritional Products, Heanor, UK;* [2]*ADM, Decatur, Illinois, USA*

16.1 Introduction

In his review, Ravindran (2013) commented that responses to enzyme supplementation are often variable and there are many factors contributing to that observed variability. The objective of this chapter is to evaluate parameters likely impacting the response to feed enzymes as a guide for those designing feed enzyme studies. The authors of this chapter were also interested, based on their own experience from conducting feed enzyme research and from feed enzyme users' feedback, to provide guidance on how to reduce variability in measured responses in feed enzyme studies. This is done by listing potential parameters to consider when designing and executing feed enzyme research. Furthermore, Bedford (2018) identified the lack of standardization of details presented in materials and methods of research studies with enzymes as a significant barrier to a meaningful retrospective data analysis and thus limiting advances in the understanding of the mode of action of feed enzymes. For the authors, the key objective was to identify all potentially relevant parameters which could impact the response in enzyme studies. Such parameters should be considered when designing enzyme research and specified when findings of enzyme research are published. Implementing such a strategy should enable construction of more meaningful and complete retrospective statistical models, repetition of past experiments and comparison of results. Retrospective modelling, such as holo-analysis or meta-analysis using large literature data sets, further improves our understanding of the mode of action of enzyme(s) and their true value in commercial practice.

16.2 How to Measure Enzyme Efficacy in Animal Trials

Prior to starting any experiment, particularly one with novel enzymes or unknown outcomes, a clear objective and simple experimental design are key to interpretation and discovery. Statistical models and methods of means separation, the number of replicates employed and the selected response variables can all influence the results and conclusions. For more information on methods of means separation, number of replicates, experimental power and best-fit models, the reader is encouraged to study

---

*Email: carrie.walk@dsm.com

Kaps and Lamberson (2004), Pesti *et al.* (2009), Bedford *et al.* (2016) and the University of Georgia Extension website (Pesti *et al.*, 2018).

When considering the efficacy of enzymes, or any product for use in animal feed, Rosen (2004a) summarized the seven key questions to answer or ask. These questions apply to suppliers, consumers and academics. They are especially relevant when deciding which enzymes to develop as novel or next-generation products, the enzymes to utilize in animal production diets and/or the enzymes that require further discovery or evaluations under various trial conditions.

1. How many properly controlled feeding tests are available on the efficacy of the product?
2. How many of these tests have no negative control?
3. Can a bibliography be supplied for questions 1 and 2?
4. How many times out of ten does the product improve live weight gain and feed conversion ratio (FCR)?
5. What are the coefficients of variation in live weight gain and FCR?
6. What dosage of the product will maximize the return on investment?
7. Can a model be supplied to predict the product response under my conditions?

In addition to the factors above and below, when designing experiments, the test diets and conditions of the experiment should reflect the conditions to which the enzymes will be exposed, and the correct statistical model and response variables employed to adequately interpret the data (Bedford, 2016). For example, adequate determination of P-releasing curves by a phytase requires a measured response to graded levels of inorganic phosphate and phytase dose. To adequately calculate the phytate-P released by each dose of phytase, the measured response should fall within the measured response of graded dose of inorganic P (Bedford *et al.*, 2016); anything above will overestimate the P-releasing value beyond that of the parameters of the test, as highlighted by Fernandez *et al.* (2019). Another example is the use of fully factorial experiments to test the

products and doses alone and in combination. This allows for accurate determination of the effects of the individual products, their interaction and the inference of any antagonistic, additive or synergistic influences on efficacy in the animal (Masey O'Neill, 2016). Numerous other factors to consider when designing and reporting enzyme experiments are highlighted in the following sections.

16.3 Factors That Can Influence Enzyme Response

Table 16.1 summarizes key parameters which can play a role in responses to feed enzymes in various studies and should be considered when designing experiments to evaluate enzyme efficacy in animals. It is not surprising that, for some parameters, enzyme effects provide different and/or opposite results between published studies, while for others only a very limited amount of data exists.

16.3.1 Animal

16.3.1.1 Age and sex

According to research by Olukosi *et al.* (2007), chicks benefited more from exogenous enzyme addition (a mixture of non-starch polysaccharide (NSP)-degrading enzymes, amylase, protease and phytase) at 1 and 2 weeks of age and the enzymes' contribution to nutrient retention decreased with age. On the other hand, Vieira *et al.* (2007) reported the efficacy of amylase and β-glucanase supplementation to a maize–soy broiler diet gave most benefit after 21 days of age. Protease (pepsin, pancreatin and papain) supplementation into nutrient-adequate diets fed to 6- to 10-day-old weaned piglets improved relative gain by 19 to 29% due to compensation for endogenous enzyme insufficiency (Lewis *et al.*, 1955). However, more recently, amino acid digestibility was improved with exogenous protease supplementation in pigs at 28 days post-weaning with no effect reported at 14 days post-weaning (Guggenbuhl

Table 16.1. The impact of various parameters relevant to responses to enzymes.

Parameter	Potential impact on enzyme response	Reference examples
Animal		
Age	Magnitude of response was reduced by age; there could be differences due to a diet type, enzyme and response variables	Lewis *et al.* (1955); Olukosi *et al.* (2007); Vieira *et al.* (2007); Guggenbuhl *et al.* (2012); Sang (2014); Babatunde *et al.* (2019); Craig *et al.* (2020a)
Sex	Response to NSP-degrading enzymes was comparable for females and males. A better improvement in uniformity for males	Hadorn *et al.* (2001)
Animal production/ health status	Magnitude of response for some enzymes, such as protease, appears greater in challenged animals, but this is not the case for phytases	Peek *et al.* (2009); Shaw *et al.* (2011); Amerah *et al.* (2012); Waititu *et al.* (2016); Adedokun and Adeola (2017); Lee *et al.* (2018b)
	Phytase efficacy was greater in growing pigs compared with gestating sows	
Intestinal section studied	Greater magnitude of response for nutrient digestibility in the jejunum compared with the ileum	Meng *et al.* (2004); Moss *et al.* (2017)
Control bird performance	In a suboptimal-performing animal, the magnitude of response will be likely greater	Rosen (2010); Ravindran (2013)
Feed form/diet		
Feed form; processing conditions	Likely dependent on ingredients used	Cowieson *et al.* (2005); Attia *et al.* (2014)
	Significant interaction between pelleting temperature and xylanase addition	
Particle size/whole grains	Improved response in diets containing whole grains or coarse particle size; response might be age-dependent	Mavromichalis *et al.* (2000); Wu and Ravindran (2004)
Response on top of other enzymes	Magnitude influenced likely by target animal, diet type, enzyme combination and dose	Cowieson and Bedford (2009); Rosen (2010); Kalmendal and Tauson (2012); Yan *et al.* (2017); Zeng *et al.* (2018)
Substrate	Protease efficacy on growth performance greater in diets containing soybean meal, but diet mix did not influence efficacy of amino acid digestibility	Leske and Coon (1999); Cowieson *et al.* (2006); Ravindran *et al.* (2006); Cowieson and Roos (2014); Santos *et al.* (2014); Cowieson *et al.* (2016); Bedford (2018); Walk and Rama Rao (2020)
	Effect of substrate on fibre-degrading enzyme efficacy is much less consistent due to substrate complexity (soluble and insoluble), mistaken enzymatic identity and inferred mode of action	
	Phytase efficacy is often dependent on phytate concentration, phytate source, phytase dose and phytase source	
Minerals	Excess dietary Ca, Fe, P or Zn reduces phytase efficacy	Augspurger *et al.* (2004); Banks *et al.* (2004); Santos *et al.* (2015); Zeller *et al.* (2015); Akter *et al.* (2017); Li *et al.* (2017)
	Magnitude of response is dependent on phytase dose and mineral concentration	
	No effect of Cu on phytase efficacy	
	Relationship between phytase inhibition and trace mineral source	
Presence of natural enzyme inhibitors in diet	Reduced efficacy, especially if feeds are not heat-treated	Ponte *et al.* (2004); Brufau *et al.* (2006)

Continued

Table 16.1. Continued.

Parameter	Potential impact on enzyme response	Reference examples
Organic acids	No effect, sub-additive or additive effect on phytase or fibre-degrading enzyme efficacy; magnitude of the effect depends on the response variable, organic acid and animal species Too high dietary inclusion of organic acids can significantly reduce growth performance and this negative effect can be partially mitigated with enzyme supplementation	Rice *et al.* (2002); Omogbenigun *et al.* (2003); Snow *et al.* (2004); Ao *et al.* (2009); Esmaeilipour *et al.* (2011); Nourmohammadi *et al.* (2012); Ghanaatparast-Rashti *et al.* (2016); Roofchaei *et al.* (2019)
Added fat and type of fat	Greater effect of fibre-degrading enzymes on nutrient digestibility when supplemented in diets containing animal fat compared with diets containing vegetable fat Greater response to phytase on growth performance in low-P diets as the concentration of vegetable fat increased in the diet	Meng *et al.* (2004); Samat *et al.* (2013); Tancharoenrat *et al.* (2014)
Antibiotics/ coccidiostats	Sub-additive effect of enzymes and antibiotics on gain, feed conversion and mortality No effect on specific efficacy of phytase Removal of antimicrobials increased magnitude of response to fibre-degrading or multi-enzymes on fibre digestibility with no benefits reported on growth performance. Since control performance can be reduced in diets without antibiotics, there is a greater likelihood for a positive response with feed enzymes	Rosen (2003a); Han *et al.* (2017); McCormick *et al.* (2017)
Prebiotics (β-glucans, MOS, FOS, GOS, XOS)	No effect on phytase efficacy or a negative effect on β-mannanase efficacy in broilers reported No effect of XOS on xylanase efficacy	Barros *et al.* (2015); Shang *et al.* (2015); Craig *et al.* (2020a)
Essential oils	Greater effect of enzymes on nutrient retention in broilers with no effect on growth performance Reduced xylanase efficacy in piglets, a reduction in average daily feed intake by 12%	Basmacioglu Malayoglu *et al.* (2010); Cao *et al.* (2010); Amerah *et al.* (2012); Jiang *et al.* (2015); Park and Kim (2018)
Probiotics	Limited data on the efficacy of exogenous enzymes with probiotics; improvements in digestible energy observed, but no effect or a muted effect on growth performance with the combination	Wealleans *et al.* (2017); Konieczka *et al.* (2018)
Pellet binders, silicates or preservatives	Adsorb or bind to enzymes during the assay extraction process which can result in lower-than-expected recoveries in the diet but no effect of preservatives *in vivo*	Sheehan (2010); Santos *et al.* (2013)
Vitamin and mineral premixes	Storage in premixes reduced enzymatic activity over time compared with the enzymes stored as pure products	Sulabo *et al.* (2011); El-Sherbiny *et al.* (2016)
Initial diet/ ingredient value/ quality	Magnitude of response (AME) was greater with xylanase addition for wheat samples with lower starting energy value	Ravindran (2013)
Environment/husbandry		
Housing type – cage, floor, bedding type, research versus commercial farm	Significant effect of a multi-enzyme on apparent ileal digestibility in birds raised on floor pens, but no effect in birds raised in cages	Madrid *et al.* (2010)

Continued

Table 16.1. Continued.

Parameter	Potential impact on enzyme response	Reference examples
Length of time on experimental diets	Optimum days on trial to result in maximum enzyme response depends on the enzyme, animal species, trial objective and response variable	Bedford and Walk (2017); Bedford (2018); Li *et al.* (2018); Babatunde *et al.* (2019); Fernandez *et al.* (2019)
Intermittent feeding programmes	Limited data. Magnitude of the response dependent on response variable: i.e. no improvement in phytase efficacy as measured with growth performance, but improvement in phytate degradation	Svihus *et al.* (2013); Sacranie *et al.* (2017)
Heat stress	Magnitude of the response increased during heat stress	Kidd *et al.* (2001)
Enzyme storage conditions – humidity, temperature, time	Enzymatic activity was reduced as storage time (days), temperature and/or humidity increased	Sulabo *et al.* (2011); El-Sherbiny *et al.* (2016)

MOS, manno-oligosaccharides; GOS, gluco-oligosaccharides; FOS; fructo-oligosaccharides; NSP, non-starch polysaccharide; AME, apparent metabolizable energy; XOS, xylo-oligosaccharides.

et al., 2012). The authors suggested the lack of an effect of protease on amino acid digestibility at day 14 could be due to the increased capacity of the animals' own endogenous proteolytic enzymes at 14 days post-weaning. On the other hand, for phytase supplementation, Babatunde *et al.* (2019) suggested the greatest impact of phytase on P digestibility was observed in 14-day-old broilers but when growth rate was the response, the greatest effect was in 22-day-old broilers. The lack of consistent recommendations for the effect of age on enzyme efficacy has been recently confirmed in a review article (Sang, 2014). The author collected a number of references evaluating animal age and feed enzyme response and did not observe consistency among diet substrates, enzyme types and efficacy in younger versus older animals. Differences in feed enzyme responses between males and females are not clearly reported.

16.3.1.2 Animal health status

It is well known that intestinal diseases or pathogens will negatively influence nutrient digestibility, feed intake, body weight gain and feed efficiency in pigs and chickens. The benefit of exogenous enzymes to partially improve nutrient utilization and growth performance during an intestinal challenge has been observed. Amerah *et al.* (2012) reported a significant decrease in *Salmonella* prevalence in the caeca of 42-day-old broilers fed xylanase. Supplementation of piglet diets with a multi-carbohydrase enzyme improved body weight and average daily gain comparable to piglets fed an antibiotic when challenged with lipopolysaccharide (Waititu *et al.*, 2016). The objective of the former experiment was to determine the influence of exogenous enzymes on growth performance, nutrient utilization and markers of gut health during an intestinal challenge, rather than the influence of intestinal challenges on enzyme efficacy. To prove that intestinal challenges influence enzyme efficacy, the same dietary treatments must be fed to non-challenged and challenged animals. For example, there was no effect of protease supplementation on body weight gain of broilers (+1%) except when challenged with *Eimeria maxima*, in which protease improved gain by +15% (Peek *et al.*, 2009). Others have observed no effect of coccidia challenge on phytase efficacy (Shaw *et al.*, 2011). However, Adedokun and Adeola (2017) reported the effect of phytase on N or energy digestibility in the jejunum was greater in non-coccidia-vaccinated broilers when compared with coccidia-vaccinated birds fed the same diets.

From the limited data mentioned above, it could be concluded that exogenous enzymes will partially alleviate the negative impact of the intestinal challenge on growth performance or nutrient digestibility, particularly protein or amino acid utilization. The magnitude of the response for some enzymes, such as protease, appears greater in challenged animals, but this is not the case for phytases. However, in general and in challenged animals, enzyme supplementation was not able to improve growth or nutrient digestibility comparable to animals exposed to the non-challenged, nutrient-adequate control treatments. The lack of a full recovery from the challenge due to enzyme supplementation may be due to the enzyme's effect on nutrient utilization, rather than a direct effect of the enzyme on the pathogen.

16.3.1.3   Evaluated intestinal section (digestibility studies)

Meng *et al.* (2004) reported an improvement in fat, starch or N digestibility with supplementation of a multi-carbohydrase enzyme in wheat-based broiler diets. However, when comparing the magnitude of improvement, the enzyme response was approximately 4 percentage units greater in the jejunum than in the ileum. This may be the result of lower digestibility in the jejunum when compared with the ileum allowing for a greater observed effect of the enzyme. Selle *et al.* (2013) reported that a protease significantly increased starch digestibility in the distal jejunum by 13.6% and by 4.8% in the proximal ileum in broilers offered sorghum-based diets. For phytase, the effect of intestinal section seems inconsistent. For example, Moss *et al.* (2017) reported that phytase improved protein (N) digestibility to the greatest degree in the proximal jejunum, followed by the distal ileum, proximal ileum and then proximal jejunum. For starch, the effect was greater in proximal and distal ileum than in the other sections.

16.3.1.4   Control bird performance

It is generally accepted that in poorly performing birds, due to various factors including

substandard nutrition, health, antibiotic growth promoter-free nutrition, stress, etc., the magnitude of an enzyme treatment response will be likely greater, as noted by Rosen (2003b) and Ravindran (2013).

16.3.2   Feed form/diet

16.3.2.1   Feed form

In their research, Cowieson *et al.* (2005) observed that increasing conditioning temperature from 80 to 90°C increased viscosity in a wheat-based diet and reduced broiler body weight gain by 7%. The authors observed a significant interaction between temperature and the addition of exogenous xylanase, with a proportionately greater positive response in diets that were pelleted at higher temperatures. Attia *et al.* (2014) observed a lack of significant interaction between feed form (mash versus pellets) and enzyme supplementation (phytase plus amylase, xylanase and protease) on broiler performance and nutrient digestibility for the whole study period, indicating that the effects of multi-enzyme plus phytase or phytase alone supplemented to mash or pellet diets were independent of feed type. It is likely that the effect of feed form on feed enzyme response will also be dependent on type of diet, since a wheat-based diet in mash form might contain natural inhibitors to reduce efficacy of xylanases (Ponte *et al.*, 2004).

16.3.2.2   Particle size/whole grain feeding

Based on their research with various forms of viscous grains, Jones and Taylor (2001) suggested that the use of exogenous enzyme additions to broiler diets may be reduced by incorporating whole grains into pelleted diets for broiler chickens. On the other hand, Wu and Ravindran (2004) indicated that gizzard development, possibly associated with increased retention time, may improve the efficacy of exogenous enzymes as the magnitude of the enzyme response (FCR) was improved in diets where a portion of ground wheat was replaced by whole wheat in the complete diet. Svihus (2010) reviewed this parameter's effect in his comprehensive manuscript. In swine, Mavromichalis *et al.* (2000) reported that weaned pigs fed diets of various particle sizes and supplemented with or without xylanase enzymes showed improved gain to feed when enzyme supplementation was combined with the coarse particle size (1300 μm), but not when the wheat was ground to 600 and 400 μm. However, responses in grower and finisher pigs were less clear, suggesting that age may interact with different particle size with regard to enzyme response.

16.3.2.3   Response on top of other enzymes

The review conducted by Rosen (2004b) suggested a full additivity between carbohydrases and phytase in broiler diets, but the data evaluated were heavily biased towards wheat-based diets. Cowieson and Bedford (2009) also revealed that xylanases and phytases may be considered broadly additive in effect; however, on an individual amino acid basis this effect ranged from sub-additive (e.g. threonine) to synergistic (e.g. arginine). In other cases, the response to additional enzymes resulted in no further beneficial effects on growth performance or nutrient digestibility. For example, supplementing broiler diets with a monocomponent xylanase or protease improved FCR and nutrient digestibility, but there were no further benefits reported with the combination of both enzymes (Kalmendal and Tauson, 2012). Similarly, Yan *et al.* (2017) reported that protease alone or a multifibre-degrading enzyme improved body weight gain or FCR of broilers with no further benefits observed when the combination was fed. In contrast, pectinases and α-galactosidases are only reported to be beneficial when fed in combination with other enzymes (see Lee and Brown, Chapter 5, this volume, 2022). The responses to additional exogenous enzymes other than phytase and fibre-degrading enzymes are less clear, have been much less researched and will be highly dependent on other factors described in this chapter, such as the nutrient sufficiency of the diet, substrate

concentration in the diet, assay-ability of the enzymes, interactions with other enzymes and adequate design of experiments, to name but a few.

16.3.2.4   Substrate

The influence of phytate on phytase efficacy has received considerable attention over the past 30 years. In general, increasing dietary phytate results in significant reductions in growth performance and nutrient digestibility. This negative effect on performance and nutrient utilization creates room for observed and measured responses of phytase efficacy, often dependent on phytate concentration, phytase dose and phytase source (Cowieson *et al.*, 2006; Ravindran *et al.*, 2006; Santos *et al.*, 2014; Walk and Rama Rao, 2020).

The effect of substrate on fibre-degrading enzyme efficacy is considerably less consistent. This may be due to numerous substrates and complexity in their composition, mistaken enzymatic identity and inferred mode of action (Bedford, 2018). Recently, Wang *et al.* (2019) determined that the efficacy of xylanase on energy and nutrient digestibility was influenced by the feed formulation, specifically the ingredient used to restrict or dilute energy in the diet of both pigs and poultry. The authors tested wheat bran, diatomaceous earth and sand, reporting significant improvements in xylanase efficacy on nutrient digestibility when wheat bran was used compared with efficacy of xylanase in the diet diluted with diatomaceous earth (which was decreased) due to the increase in substrate for the enzyme with wheat bran. On the other hand, Amerah *et al.* (2015) reported that xylanase and β-glucanase supplementation into broiler diets containing increasing concentrations of fibre from sunflower and canola meal improved FCR by 1, 3 and 9 points as fibre concentration in the diet increased. A large portion of this response may be related to the inherent digestibility of the diet. Generally, the inclusion of excess substrate, whether it is phytate or fibre, has a detrimental influence on inherent digestibility and growth performance, thereby allowing greater space for an observed enzymatic response.

Exogenous enzymes are utilized to degrade antinutritional substrates, such as phytate, and facilitate nutrient digestion by aiding endogenous enzymes and microbes to degrade protein, lipids, peptides, and poly- or oligosaccharides. The quality and quantity of substrate may be important factors impacting the response observed in enzyme studies. For example, a monocomponent protease significantly improved body weight gain (+5%) when supplemented into broiler diets containing 38% soybean meal. However, this effect of protease on gain was reduced to +1.5% when supplemented into diets containing canola meal, maize gluten and dried distillers' grains as the protein source (Cowieson *et al.*, 2016). This was despite the fact that the diet mix did not appear to influence the efficacy of proteases on amino acid digestibility, which was largely influenced by inherent diet digestibility (Cowieson and Roos, 2014; Lee *et al.*, 2018a).

16.3.2.5   Minerals

Ca, P, Fe, Zn and Cu are important minerals in pig and poultry nutrition. Their impact on enzyme efficacy (predominantly phytase) largely depends on the enzyme, the dose, the response variable used to measure enzyme efficacy and the dietary mineral concentration. For example, excess dietary Ca, Fe, P or Zn has been reported to reduce phytase efficacy as measured by bone ash or phytate degradation in pigs and poultry (Augspurger *et al.*, 2004; Zeller *et al.*, 2015; Akter *et al.*, 2017; Li *et al.*, 2017). Others have reported no effect of Cu or Zn on phytase efficacy while reporting reductions in P retention due to excess minerals in the diets fed to pigs or chickens in the absence of phytase (Banks *et al.*, 2004; Walk *et al.*, 2015). Very little information is available comparing the potential antagonisms which can occur between different mineral sources and enzymes within premixes as well as the repercussions that this might have in terms of lost enzyme efficacy. A recent study (Santos *et al.*, 2015) demonstrated a significant

effect of a trace mineral source on phytase inhibition. Organic mineral proteinates were significantly less inhibitory than most other mineral sources evaluated. Further understanding and characterization of mineral interactions within the gastrointestinal tract may provide useful information in describing the influences of these minerals on enzyme efficacy.

16.3.2.6   Presence of natural enzyme inhibitors in a diet

Brufau *et al.* (2006) discussed enzyme inhibitors present in cereal grains as a potential cause of inefficiency of added NSP-degrading enzymes, particularly xylanases. The authors pointed out that all the inhibitory compounds are inactivated by heat treatment as also supported by Ponte *et al.* (2004), although those present in bran fractions could be more resistant to heat. The presence of natural inhibitors indicates that they may affect the efficacy of enzyme supplementation and thus in some cases a lack of response to xylanase supplementation, particularly in wheat-based diets.

16.3.2.7   Organic acids

Organic acids are included in pig or poultry diets to improve growth performance, nutrient digestibility and promote beneficial bacterial growth in the gastrointestinal tract through a reduction in gastrointestinal pH and an increase in mineral solubility. Phytase efficacy and phytate susceptibility to degradation occur at the pH encountered in the stomach of pigs or the crop, proventriculus and gizzard of poultry. It has been hypothesized that addition of organic acids in poultry or pig diets may decrease gastrointestinal pH and provide a more optimal environment for phytase. Previous authors have reported improvements in P or phytate-P retention of broilers fed low-P diets containing organic acids (Liem *et al.*, 2008; Esmaeilipour *et al.*, 2011) or reduced P excretion from pigs fed phytase plus an organic acid mix (Omogbenigun *et al.*, 2003). Snow *et al.* (2004) reported no effect (experiment 1) or a significant effect of citric acid and phytase (experiment 2) on broiler growth performance and tibia ash, indicting a possible additive effect of organic acids on phytase efficacy. Others have reported significant and additive effects of sodium citrate, but no effect of propionic acid, on phytase efficacy as measured by broiler growth performance, bone ash and P digestibility in low-P diets (Ghanaatparast-Rashti *et al.*, 2016). However, Rice *et al.* (2002) reported no beneficial effects of supplementing citric acid at 3% on phytase efficacy in pig diets. Likewise, Omogbenigun *et al.* (2003) reported no additional benefits of supplementing an organic acid mix in diets containing phytase on piglet growth performance, gastrointestinal pH, bone ash or amino acid digestibility. Finally, Nourmohammadi *et al.* (2012) reported no beneficial effects of citric acid on phytase efficacy in broilers; however, feeding 6% citric acid significantly reduced 21-day-old broiler daily feed intake and gain, as well as protein, Ca and P digestibility, and this negative effect of citric acid was partially mitigated with phytase supplementation.

Similarly, others have evaluated the influence of organic acids on the efficacy of fibre-degrading enzymes with inconsistent results. For example, Esmaeilipour *et al.* (2011) reported no benefit of feeding 2 or 4% citric acid on xylanase efficacy in broilers fed low-P, wheat-based diets. However, Roofchaei *et al.* (2019) reported that broiler FCR from hatch to day 35 was improved by 7 or 10 points with dietary supplementation of a carbohydrate (xylanase and glucanase) or the carbohydrate plus an organic acid mix, respectively, when compared with a non-supplemented control diet. Ao *et al.* (2009) also reported significant and synergistic effects of feeding 2% citric acid with an α-galactosidase on neutral detergent fibre retention in broilers; with improvements of 3.2, 1.4 or 11.4 percentage points in broilers fed citric acid, α-galactosidase or the combination, respectively, above that of the low energy control. In the same experiment, apparent metabolizable energy (AME_n) retention was improved with the combination of citric acid and α-galactosidase enzyme in a sub-additive manner, with no benefit reported on AME_n re-

tention from the additives alone and 100 kcal improvement with the combination. However, there was no beneficial effect of the combination on growth performance (Ao *et al.*, 2009).

In general, organic acid supplementation reduced stomach or crop pH and influenced P retention and excretion and phytate degradation. However, the additive effects of organic acids on exogenous enzyme efficacy are inconsistent and appear dependent on the organic acid, response variable and animal species, with some benefits noted in broilers but none reported in pigs. It could be concluded that organic acids do not appear to influence the efficacy of exogenous enzymes on growth performance, bone ash or nutrient digestibility in pigs, while inconsistent, sub- or additive effects of organic acids on exogenous enzyme efficacy were reported in broilers.

16.3.2.8 Added fats and type of fat

Meng *et al.* (2004) reported a multicarbohydrase enzyme improved fat digestibility by 8.1 versus 2.3 percentage units when supplemented in wheat-based diets containing beef tallow compared with canola oil, respectively, in 18-day-old broilers. Additionally, Tancharoenrat *et al.* (2014) reported xylanase supplementation improved AME in wheat-based diets, but only when supplemented in diets containing tallow compared with diets containing soy oil. Tallow contains long chains of saturated fatty acids and digestibility is dependent on bile salts for emulsification, which may be particularly relevant in young broilers with limited digestive enzyme secretion capabilities. Therefore, the magnitude of the response to fibre-degrading enzyme supplementation was greater in diets containing tallow due to the known poor digestibility of this fat source compared with vegetable oils.

Other authors have suggested that feeding greater concentrations of dietary fat will increase gastrointestinal tract retention time and promote phytate degradation by phytase. Samat *et al.* (2013) reported a greater and significant impact of phytase on 3-week-old broiler body weight gain, feed intake, and phytate degradation (Samat, 2015) when supplemented in isocaloric diets containing 5% soy oil compared with diets containing 1% soy oil.

16.3.2.9 Antibiotics, coccidiostats or ionophores

Due to concerns over antibiotic resistance and the use of antibiotics in animal feed, numerous studies have evaluated feed enzymes as antibiotic, ionophore or coccidiostat replacements. Very few studies have specifically evaluated the effect of these antimicrobials on exogenous feed enzyme efficacy. Rosen (2003a) reported sub-additive effects of antimicrobials and enzymes on broiler gain, feed efficiency and mortality. Antimicrobials have been reported to improve N and energy utilization in pigs (McCormick et al., 2017) and similarly supplementation of diets with enzymes is known to improve nutrient utilization. Therefore, would the combination of antimicrobials and enzymes result in further improvements in nutrient utilization? In a study by McCormick et al. (2017), three different antimicrobials and three doses of phytase were evaluated in pig and poultry diets as a factorial arrangement of treatments. The authors reported phytase supplementation improved growth performance and nutrient digestibility, regardless of the use of antimicrobials. Han et al. (2017) reported no effect of a multi-enzyme or antibiotic on growth performance or apparent total tract digestibility of protein, ash or dry matter in 21 to 40 kg pigs. However, in the same experiment, in the absence of antibiotics, supplementation of the diets with the multi-enzyme significantly improved apparent total tract digestibility of crude fibre by 4 percentage units above that of pigs fed the multi-enzyme diet in the presence of antibiotics. Therefore, albeit with limited data, it could be concluded that antimicrobials do not influence the efficacy of phytase. However, the removal of antimicrobials allows for a greater influence of multi- or fibre-degrading enzymes on nutrient digestibility (Yin et al., 2001a; Bedford and Walk, 2017).

16.3.2.10 Prebiotics and mycotoxin binders (β-glucans, yeast cell walls, clays or oligosaccharides)

Prebiotics can be defined as non-digestible feed ingredients or additives observed to modulate the gastrointestinal environment, stimulate or 'prime' the immune cells, bind to and eliminate pathogenic bacteria, and 'feed' or promote beneficial bacteria. Some examples of prebiotics include β-glucans, yeast cell walls and manno- (MOS), fructo- (FOS) and xylo-oligosaccharides (XOS). Data evaluating the effect of prebiotics on exogenous enzymes are limited and may indicate further evaluations are required to justify the need for prebiotics and enzymes in monogastric nutrition. For example, Barros et al. (2015) observed a 4 to 5% reduction in body weight gain and 4- to 7-point increase in FCR of broilers fed a combination of β-mannanase and MOS compared with broilers fed β-mannanase or MOS individually. Similarly, Waititu et al. (2016) reported a significant reduction in average daily feed intake of piglets fed a yeast extract and multi-carbohydrase enzyme on day 11 post-weaning. Shang et al. (2015) reported no benefits of FOS supplementation on phytase activity in broilers. Craig et al. (2020a) reported improvements in broiler growth performance with xylanase supplementation at day 14 and increases in caeca total short-chain fatty acids (SCFAs) with XOS supplementation, with no interactive effects of xylanase plus XOS on performance, nutrient digestibility, caeca SCFAs or total soluble or non-soluble NSPs in the ileum. Other authors have reported XOS (Craig et al., 2020b) or arabinoxylan plus xylanase (Morgan et al., 2019) supplementation to improve growth performance in young broilers when compared with xylanase or arabinoxylan supplementation, respectively, alone. However, these trials did not evaluate the full factorial effects of the enzymes plus oligosaccharides or NSPs, and therefore conclusions about the efficacy of the combination cannot be determined. In other cases, the lack of a beneficial response or even negative effects of prebiotic supplementation in the presence of enzymes may be due to the nature of the prebiotic and its effect on the microbial population in the gastrointestinal tract, stimulation of an immune response, or the exogenous enzyme degrading the oligosaccharide into monosaccharides. The above factors can reduce feed intake and growth performance. Definitive characterization of the prebiotic, such as composition, structure and degree of polymerization, will enable better use of the combination of exogenous enzymes and prebiotics in monogastric production.

16.3.2.11   Essential oils

An essential oil blend of cinnamaldehyde and thymol improved the response noted in young broilers fed a diet containing phytase and xylanase on FCR by 3 points ($P = 0.09$) and AME retention by 0.35 MJ/kg ($P = 0.02$) (Cao *et al.*, 2010). However, there was no further benefit on broiler performance by combining an essential oil blend of cinnamaldehyde and thymol with xylanase supplementation, except the combination resulted in a reduction in *Salmonella*-positive caecal samples by 25 percentage units (Amerah *et al.*, 2012). Similarly, the magnitude of the effect of protease (Park and Kim, 2018) or multi-fibre-degrading enzyme (Basmacioglu Malayoglu *et al.*, 2010) on broiler growth performance was not improved with the addition of an essential oil blend. However, N retention was improved ($P < 0.05$) by 5% (Park and Kim, 2018) or 10% (Basmacioglu Malayoglu *et al.*, 2010) and ammonia emissions were reduced ($P < 0.05$) by 15% (Park and Kim, 2018) with the combination, and this was greater than the effect of the individual additives. Conversely, in piglets, feeding an essential oil blend of thymol and cinnamaldehyde in combination with a xylanase significantly reduced average daily feed intake by approximately 12% when compared with feeding the xylanase alone (Jiang *et al.*, 2015).

16.3.2.12   Probiotics

Probiotics or direct-fed microbials (DFMs) are defined as live microorganisms and are observed to modulate the gastrointestinal environment, stimulate the gut-associated immune system, reduce pathogenic bacteria and promote beneficial bacteria. When fed in combination with exogenous enzymes, the influence of DFMs on the enzymatic response will depend on the microbial fed, the nature of the exogenous enzyme and the response variable. For example, there was no further benefit on growth performance of broilers fed a DFM without or with a multi-enzyme containing xylanase, amylase or protease (Wealleans *et al.*, 2017). However, the combination of multi-enzyme and DFM reduced the flow of total soluble and insoluble NSPs in the ileum and total tract and improved ileal digestible energy above that of the individual additives (Wealleans *et al.*, 2017). Konieczka *et al.* (2018) observed no additional benefits of feeding a probiotic in broiler diets containing xylanase and β-glucanase on growth performance, endogenous enzymes or SCFAs. And in some instances, the authors observed a muted response with the enzyme and DFM combination compared with the response to the individual additives alone (Konieczka *et al.*, 2018). Other experiments have evaluated the combination of DFMs and enzymes on various response variables in broilers, layers and pigs. However, the absence of a treatment with the enzyme or DFM alone limits the ability to determine the influence of the DFM on the enzyme efficacy and therefore these experiments are not described.

16.3.2.13   Pellet binders, silicates or preservatives

Sheehan (2010) suggested that insoluble ingredients, such as silicates or pellet binders, may non-specifically adsorb enzymes, thereby blocking their activity during the extraction process of the *in vitro* assay. The adsorption can be prevented with the addition of a non-specific blocking protein, such as bovine serum albumin, during the extraction stage (Sheehan, 2010). Furthermore, the use of formaldehyde-based products in the diet may reduce phytase activity recovered during the in-feed assay but will have no impact on the efficacy in the animal (Santos *et al.*, 2013). This is due to the binding of formaldehyde to the enzyme protein, thereby reducing the enzyme solubility and extractability during the in-feed assay with no impact on *in vivo* efficacy.

16.3.2.14   Vitamins or trace mineral premixes

Inclusion of enzymes into diets as part of the vitamin or vitamin and trace mineral premix can provide an advantage in feed mixing, cost and ease of handling. However, storage of phytase (Sulabo *et al.*, 2011) or xylanase (El-Sherbiny *et al.*, 2016) in vitamin and trace mineral premixes reduced their activity over time when compared with the enzymes stored as pure products. The loss of phytase or xylanase activity was greater when stored with trace mineral premixes or vitamin and trace mineral premixes than with vitamin premixes (Sulabo *et al.*, 2011; El-Sherbiny *et al.*, 2016), therefore it is thought that ionic charges in the mineral salts can act as oxidizing agents and denature enzyme activity.

16.3.2.15   Enzyme storage conditions – humidity, temperature and time

Sulabo *et al.* (2011) determined that retained phytase activity was reduced as storage time (days), temperature and humidity were increased. Storage of samples at room temperature or less resulted in the most stable products over time. However, increasing humidity, even at room temperature (23°C) or 5°C, promoted mould growth and reduced phytase activity and storage stability over time. Similarly, El-Sherbiny *et al.* (2016) reported a reduction in xylanase activity over time (days) when stored at 35°C compared with the same enzyme stored at 4°C. Therefore, storing enzymes in their pure form (rather than in premixes, see above), at room temperature or lower, and with less than 40% humidity, may have advantages in retaining original enzymatic activity over time.

16.3.3   Environment/husbandry

16.3.3.1   Housing type – cage, floor, bedding, research versus commercial farm

Housing conditions may have a significant impact on nutrient requirements and this in turn may impact the magnitude of the response noted with exogenous enzyme supplementation. For example, gilts housed in groups showed higher metabolizable energy and a significantly lower energy requirement for maintenance compared with gilts housed in individual stalls (Geverink *et al.*, 2004). Housing conditions (cages, aviaries or floor pens) and litter quality also influence the microbial population in chickens (Nordentoft *et al.*, 2011; Kers *et al.*, 2018), all of which can influence nutrient digestibility and ultimately enzyme efficacy. Significant effects of a multi-enzyme on apparent ileal digestibility in birds raised on floor pens was noted but no effect in birds raised in cages was reported by Madrid *et al.* (2010). However, such papers evaluating the effect of housing type or conditions on enzyme efficacy in poultry or pigs are sparse.

16.3.3.2   Length of time on experimental diets

Recent research indicates that 'days on trial' can impact the magnitude of the response noted with exogenous enzymes. In some instances, this is due to the nutrient requirements of the animal and their ability to adapt to dietary deficiencies through changes in feed intake and nutrient metabolism. For example, it could take 8 to 12 weeks to note a significant decrease in egg production of laying hens fed P-deficient diets and this will impact the calculated P equivalency values of phytase (Fernandez *et al.*, 2019). In broiler chickens, diets deficient in Ca or P should be fed for longer than 2 days and in birds less than 20 days post-hatch to result in significant reductions in growth rate or bone ash (Babatunde *et al.*, 2019), allowing for determination of phytase efficacy. For example, the average effect of phytase on broiler body weight gain was +2 or +25% in broilers weighed at day 22 when on trial for 2 or 16 days, respectively (Babatunde *et al.*, 2019). Conversely, when considering the effects of phytase on Ca or P digestibility, Ca- or P-deficient diets should be fed for less than 30 h (Li *et al.*, 2018) and at day 14 post-hatch in broilers (Babatunde *et al.*, 2019). This will limit physiological adaptations of the bird to the nutrient-deficient diets and enable determination of the inherent effects of the diet or phytase on digestibility. Trials determining the optimum 'days on trial' and phytase efficacy in pigs are limited. However, a recent meta-analysis evaluating P intake and utilization determined that P retention in soft tissues was prioritized over bones, suggesting bone ash (rather than body weight gain) would be a more appropriate response variable in pigs when evaluating phytase efficacy (Misiura *et al.*, 2020).

When considering fibre-degrading, multior protease enzymes, the adaptation period and magnitude of the exogenous enzyme response may be partially dependent on the maturity of the gut, specifically the endogenous enzyme secretions (age effect noted above) and microbial populations. In this regard, the response to fibre-degrading enzymes on growth performance and nutrient digestibility may require full grow-out trials in both pigs and poultry due to the prebiotic-like effect of the end products and the adaptation period of the gut microbes to those same end products (Bedford and Walk, 2017; Bedford, 2018). Unfortunately, when describing the optimum days on trial to determine enzyme efficacy, there is no 'one size fits all' recommendation. However, the above information provides a range of trial days to consider when designing experiments or interpreting results, which will be different depending on the trial objective, response variables, animal species and enzyme under evaluation.

16.3.3.3   Feeding programmes

Phytase efficacy, measured by growth performance, was not improved with intermittent feeding of broilers when compared with those fed continuously (Svihus *et al.*, 2013). However, phytate degradation by phytase was greater in broilers exposed to intermittent feeding compared with those fed *ad libitum* (Sacranie *et al.*, 2017).

16.3.3.4   Heat stress

Kidd *et al.* (2001) observed improved feed conversion and lower mortality in broilers fed enzyme-supplemented maize/soybean diets, especially during periods of heat stress.

16.4   Conclusion: Parameters for Consideration in Enzyme Research

The impact of feed enzymes on performance, nutrient and energy digestibility is well accepted. For phytase, the improvement in digestibility of various nutrients such as P, Ca, Na, amino acids, trace minerals and energy can be supported by numerous studies (Kies *et al.*, 2001; Cowieson *et al.*, 2017). Similarly, the effect of NSP-degrading enzymes, namely xylanase (Yin *et al.*, 2000) and β-glucanase, but also of other enzymes like amylases (Gracia *et al.*, 2003) and proteases (Zuo *et al.*, 2015) on nutrient digestibility has been reported in both swine and poultry research. For some enzyme activities like amylase, a variable nutrient digestibility response has been observed (Ritz *et al.*, 1995; Shapiro and Nir, 1995). In fact, publications indicating positive response, no response or even negative response to various measured parameters are available, if not for all, then for most studied enzymes to date. Phytase, on the other hand, is likely one exogenous enzyme which has a high rate of research with positive responses reported. According to Selle and Ravindran (2007), phytase has a more general application as its substrate is invariably present in pig and poultry diets and its dietary inclusion economically generates bioavailable P and reduces P load on the environment.

Commercially, a combination of two or more feed enzymes will be more typically used and there is research available supporting combinations of various enzymes as contributors to improvements in nutrient digestibility (Yin *et al.*, 2001b; Lee and Brown, Chapter 5, this volume). In his review, Rosen (2004b) suggested existence of a full additivity between carbohydrases and phytase in broiler diets mainly based on wheat. As concluded by Zeng *et al.* (2018), the magnitude of nutrient digestibility response to phytase and carbohydrase supplementation in pigs may be influenced by the addition of wheat bran to a diet. That would suggest that both substrates for enzymes and potentially target animals will determine the magnitude of response to various feed enzyme combinations. Other parameters such as gastrointestinal health have also been impacted by the application of feed enzymes. Employing a necrotic enteritis disease challenge model where oral inoculation of *Eimeria* sp. and *Clostridium perfringens* was incorporated, Jackson *et al.* (2003) reported that β-mannanase was as effective as antibiotics in mitigating the disease effects as measured by growth performance and the incidence of coccidial lesion scores compared with the control. An opportunity for enzymes to help during coccidial challenge was raised a quarter of a century ago by Morgan and Bedford (1995), who demonstrated that enzyme supplementation in wheat diets reduced growth depression due to coccidiosis in pullets. Furthermore, enzyme supplementation reduced intestinal viscosity and improved feed efficiency in broilers fed wheat diets, in both normal and coccidiosis-challenged birds. In young pigs, Chen *et al.* (2017) reported that protease supplementation improved protein digestion and maintained gut health, irrespective of whether used in sorghum- or maize-based diets. Similarly, Borda-Molina

et al. (2019) reported that addition of protease but also phytase contributed to changes in gut microflora and these responses differed between the commercial protease sources studied. On top of these less typically evaluated parameters in enzyme trials, we have started to see other measures being assessed, such as expression of nutrient transport and absorption genes, production of specific endogenous enzymes and evaluation of various blood biomarkers (Jiang *et al.*, 2008; Zuo *et al.*, 2015). Impact of enzymes on gut morphology has also been increasingly included, with the production of tight junction proteins such as claudin, occludin, zonula occludens and β-actin being measured as parameters in enzyme studies (Tiwari *et al.*, 2018).

The enzyme research of today encompasses the investigation of many parameters including performance, digestibility, carcass quality, gut histology, changes in gut microbiome, immune status, gene expression and hormonal changes. Studying all these factors can be extremely helpful in providing greater understanding of a specific enzyme mode of action. Practically, that knowledge can support a more targeted use of feed enzymes in commercial practice, their more frequent use and consistent response benefit.

References

Adedokun, S.A. and Adeola, O. (2017) The response in jejunal and ileal nutrient and energy digestibility and the expression of markers of intestinal inflammation in broiler chickens to coccidial vaccine challenge and phytase supplementation. *Canadian Journal of Animal Science* 97, 258–267.

Akter, M., Iji, P.A. and Graham, H. (2017) Increased iron level in phytase-supplemented diets reduces performance and nutrient utilization in broiler chickens. *British Poultry Science* 58, 409–417.

Amerah, A.M., Mathis, G. and Hofacre, C.L. (2012) Effect of xylanase and a blend of essential oils on performance and *Salmonella* colonization of broiler chickens challenged with *Salmonella* Heidelberg. *Poultry Science* 91, 943–947.

Amerah, A.M., van de Belt, K. and van der Klis, J.D. (2015) Effect of different levels of rapeseed meal and sunflower meal and enzyme combination on the performance, digesta viscosity and carcass traits of broiler chickens fed wheat-based diets. *Animal* 9, 1131–1137.

Ao, T., Cantor, A.H., Pescatore, A.J., Ford, M.J., Pierce, J.L. and Dawson, K.A. (2009) Effect of enzyme supplementation and acidification of diets on nutrient digestibility and growth performance of broiler chicks. *Poultry Science* 88, 111–117.

Attia, Y.A., El-Tahawy, W.S., Abd El-Hamid, A.E., Nizza, A., Bovera, F., *et al.* (2014) Effect of feed form, pellet diameter and enzymes supplementation on growth performance and nutrient digestibility of broiler during days 21–37 of age. *Archiv für Tierzucht* 57, 34, 1–11.

Augspurger, N.R., Spencer, J.D., Webel, D.M. and Baker, D.H. (2004) Pharmacological zinc levels reduce the phosphorus-releasing efficacy of phytase in young pigs and chickens. *Journal of Animal Science* 82, 1732–1739.

Babatunde, O.O., Cowieson, A.J., Wilson, J.W. and Adeola, O. (2019) Influence of age and duration of feeding low-phosphorus diet on phytase efficacy in broiler chickens during the starter phase. *Poultry Science* 98, 2588–2597.

Banks, K.M., Thompson, K.L., Jaynes, P. and Applegate, T.J. (2004) The effects of copper on the efficacy of phytase, growth and phosphorus retention in broiler chicks. *Poultry Science* 83, 1335–1341.

Barros, V.R.S.M., Lana, G.R.Q., Lana, S.R.V., Lana, A.M.Q., Cunha, F.S.A. and Neto, J.V.E. (2015) β-Mannanase and mannan oligosaccharides in broiler chicken feed. *Ciência Rural* 45, 111–117.

Basmacioglu Malayoglu, H., Baysal, S., Misirlioglu, Z., Polat, M., Yilmaz, H. and Turan, N. (2010) Effects of oregano essential oil with or without feed enzymes on growth performance, digestive enzyme, nutrient digestibility, lipid metabolism and immune response of broilers fed on wheat–soybean meal diets. *British Poultry Science* 51, 67–80.

Bedford, M.R. (2016) General principles of designing a nutrition experiment. In: Bedford, M.R., Choct, M. and Masey O'Neill, H.V. (eds) *Nutrition Experiments in Pigs and Poultry: A Practical Guide*. CAB International, Wallingford, UK, pp. 1–20.

Bedford, M.R. (2018) The evolution and application of enzymes in the animal feed industry: the role of data interpretation. *British Poultry Science* 59, 486–493.

Bedford, M.R and Walk, C.L. (2017) The use of exogenous enzymes to improve feed efficiency in pigs. In: Wiseman, J. (ed.) *Achieving Sustainable Production of Pig Meat*. Vol. 2: *Animal Breeding and Nutrition*. Burleigh Dodds Science Publishing, Cambridge, pp. 1–21.

Bedford, M.R., Walk, C.L. and Masey O'Neill, H.V. (2016) Assessing measurements in feed enzyme research: phytase evaluation in broilers. *Journal of Applied Poultry Research* 25, 305–314.

Borda-Molina, D., Zuber, T., Siegert, W., Camarinha-Silva, A., Feuerstein, D. and Rodehutscord, M. (2019) Effects of protease and phytase supplements on small intestinal microbiota and amino acid digestibility in broiler chickens. *Poultry Science* 98, 2906–2918.

Brufau, J., Francesch, M. and Pérez-Vendrell, A.M. (2006) The use of enzymes to improve cereal diets for animal feeding. *Journal of the Science of Food and Agriculture* 86, 1705–1713.

Cao, P.H., Li, F.D., Li, Y.F., Ru, Y.J., Peron, A., *et al.* (2010) Effect of essential oils and feed enzymes on performance and nutrient utilization in broilers fed a corn/soy-based diet. *International Journal of Poultry Science* 9, 749–755.

Chen, H., Zhang, S., Park, I. and Kim, S.W. (2017) Impacts of energy feeds and supplemental protease on growth performance, nutrient digestibility, and gut health of pigs from 18 to 45 kg body weight. *Animal Nutrition* 3, 359–365.

Cowieson, A.J. and Bedford, M.R. (2009) The effect of phytase and carbohydrase on ileal amino acid digestibility in monogastric diets: complimentary mode of action? *World's Poultry Science Journal* 65, 609–624.

Cowieson, A.J. and Roos, F.F. (2014) Bioefficacy of a mono-component protease in diets of pigs and poultry: a meta-analysis of effect on ileal amino acid digestibility. *Journal of Applied Animal Nutrition* 2, 1–8.

Cowieson, A.J., Hruby, M. and Isaksen, M.F. (2005) The effect of conditioning temperature and exogenous xylanase addition on the viscosity of wheat-based diets and the performance of broiler chickens. *British Poultry Science* 46, 717–724.

Cowieson, A.J., Acamovic, T. and Bedford, M.R. (2006) Phytic acid and phytase: implications for protein utilization by poultry. *Poultry Science* 85, 878–885.

Cowieson, A.J., Lu, H., Ajuwon, K.M., Knap, I. and Adeola, O. (2016) Interactive effects of dietary protein source and exogenous protease on growth performance, immune competence and jejunal health of broiler chickens. *Animal Production Science* 57, 252–261.

Cowieson, A.J., Ruckebusch, J.-P., Sorbara, J.O.B., Wilson, J.W., Guggenbuhl, P., *et al.* (2017) A systematic view on the effect of microbial phytase on ileal amino acid digestibility in pigs. *Animal Feed Science and Technology* 231, 138–149.

Craig, A.D., Khattak, F., Hastie, P., Bedford, M.R. and Olukosi, O.A. (2020a) Xylanase and xylo-oligosaccharide prebiotic improve the growth performance and concentration of potentially prebiotic oligosaccharides in the ileum of broiler chickens. *British Poultry Science* 61, 70–78.

Craig, A.D., Khattak, F., Hastie, P., Bedford, M.R. and Olukosi, O.A. (2020b) Similarity of the effect of carbohydrase or prebiotic supplementation in broilers aged 21 days, fed mixed cereal diets and challenged with coccidiosis infection. *PLoS ONE* 15, e0229281.

El-Sherbiny, M.A., Abdel-Moneim, M.A., El-Shinnawy, A.M., Hamady, G.A.A. and El-Chaghaby, G.A. (2016) Stability of commercial xylanases stored singly or combined with vitamins and/or minerals premix at different temperatures. *Journal of Animal Health and Production* 4, 111–117.

Esmaeilipour, O., Shivazad, M., Moravej, H., Aminzadeh, S., Rezaian, M. and van Krimpen, M.M. (2011) Effects of xylanase and citric acid on the performance, nutrient retention, and characteristics of gastro-intestinal tract of broilers fed low-phosphorus wheat-based diets. *Poultry Science* 90, 1975–1982.

Fernandez, S.R., Charraga, S. and Avila-Gonzalez, E. (2019) Evaluation of a new generation phytase on phytate phosphorus release for egg production and tibia strength in hens fed a corn–soybean meal diet. *Poultry Science* 98, 2087–2093.

Geverink, N.A., Heetkamp, M.J.W., Schouten, W.G.P., Wiegant, V.M. and Schrama, J.W. (2004) Backtest type and housing conditions of pigs influence energy metabolism. *Journal of Animal Science* 82, 1227–1233.

Ghanaatparast-Rashti, M., Shariatmadari, F., Karimi-Torshizi, M.A. and Mohiti-Asli, M. (2016) Effects of pro-pionic acid, sodium citrate, and phytase on growth performance, mineral digestibility and tibia proper-ties in broilers. *Journal of Applied Animal Research* 44, 370–375.

Gracia, M.I., Aranibar, M.J., Lazaro, R., Medel, P. and Mateos, G.G. (2003) α-Amylase supplementation of broiler diets based on corn. *Poultry Science* 82, 436–442.

Guggenbuhl, P., Wache, Y. and Wilson, J.W. (2012) Effects of dietary supplementation with a protease on the apparent ileal digestibility of the weaned piglet. *Journal of Animal Science* 90, 152–154.

Hadorn, R., Wiedmer, H. and Broz, J. (2001) Effect of an enzyme complex in a wheat-based diet on perform-ance of male and female broilers. *Journal of Applied Poultry Research* 10, 340–346.

Han, X.-Y., Yan, F.-Y., Nie, X.-Z., Xia, W., Chen, S., *et al.* (2017) Effect of replacing antibiotics using multi-enzyme preparations on production performance and antioxidant activity in piglets. *Journal of Integra-tive Agriculture* 16, 640–647.

Jackson, M.E., Anderson, D.M., Hsiao, H.Y., Mathis, G.F. and Fodge, D.W. (2003) Beneficial effect of beta-mannanase feed enzyme on performance of chicks challenged with *Eimeria* sp. and *Clostridium perfrin-gens*. *Avian Diseases* 47, 759–763.

Jiang, X.R., Awati, A., Agazzi, A., Vitari, F., Ferrari, A., *et al.* (2015) Effects of a blend of essential oils and an enzyme combination on nutrient digestibility, ileum histology and expression of inflammatory mediators in weaned piglets. *Animal* 9, 417–426.

Jiang, Z., Zhou, Y., Lu, F., Han, Z. and Wang, T. (2008) Effects of different levels of supplementary alpha-amylase on digestive enzyme activities and pancreatic amylase mRNA expression of young broilers. *Asian-Australasian Journal of Animal Sciences* 21, 97–102.

Jones, G.P.D. and Taylor, R.D. (2001) The incorporation of whole grain into pelleted broiler chicken diets: production and physiological responses. *British Poultry Science* 42, 477–483.

Kalmendal, R. and Tauson, R. (2012) Effects of xylanase and protease, individually or in combination, and an ionophore coccidiostat on performance, nutrient utilization, and intestinal morphology in broiler chick-ens fed a wheat–soybean meal-based diet. *Poultry Science* 91, 1387–1393.

Kaps, M. and Lamberson, W.R. (2004) *Biostatistics for Animal Science*. CAB International, Wallingford, UK.

Kers, J.G., Velkers, F.C., Fischer, E.A.J., Hermes, G.D.A., Stegeman, J.A. and Smidt, H. (2018) Host and envir-onmental factors affecting the intestinal microbiota in chickens. *Frontiers in Microbiology* 9, 235.

Kidd, M.T., Morgan, G.W., Price, C.J., Welch, P.A. and Fontana, E.A. (2001) Enzyme supplementation to corn and soybean meal diets for broilers. *Journal of Applied Poultry Research* 10, 65–70.

Kies, A.K., Van Hemert, K.H.F. and Sauer, W.C. (2001) Effect of phytase on protein and amino acid digestibil-ity and energy utilization. *World's Poultry Science Journal* 57, 109–126.

Konieczka, P., Nowicka, K., Madar, M., Taciak, M. and Smulikowska, S. (2018) Effects of pea extrusion and enzyme and probiotic supplementation on performance, microbiota activity and biofilm formation in the broiler gastrointestinal tract. *British Poultry Science* 59, 654–662.

Lee, J.T. and Brown, K.D. (2022) Mannanase, α-galactosidase and pectinase: minor players or yet to be ex-ploited? In: Bedford, M.R., Partridge, G.G., Hruby, M. and Walk, C.L. (eds) *Enzymes in Farm Animal Nutrition*, 3rd edn. CAB International, Wallingford, UK, pp. 70–88.

Lee, S.A., Bedford, M.R. and Walk, C.L. (2018a) Meta-analysis: explicit value of mono-component protease in monogastric diets. *Poultry Science* 97, 2078–2085.

Lee, S.A., Walk, C.L. and Stein, H.H. (2018b) Comparative digestibility and retention of calcium and phos-phorus by gestating sows and growing pigs fed low- and high-phytate diets without or with microbial phytase. *Journal of Animal Science* 96(Suppl. 2), 83.

Leske, K.L. and Coon, C.N. (1999) A bioassay to determine the effect of phytase on phytate phosphorus hy-drolysis and total phosphorus retention of feed ingredients as determined with broilers and laying hens. *Poultry Science* 78, 1151–1157.

Lewis, C.J., Catron, D.V., Liu, C.H., Speer, V.C. and Ashton, G.C. (1955) Enzyme supplementation of baby pig diets. *Journal of the Science of Food and Agriculture* 3, 1047–1050.

Li, W., Angel, R., Kim, S.W., Brady, K., Yu, S. and Plumstead, P.W. (2017) Impacts of dietary calcium, phytate, and phytase on inositol hexakisphosphate degradation and inositol phosphate release in different segments of the digestive tract of broilers. *Poultry Science* 96, 3626–3637.

Li, W., Angel, R., Kim, S.-W., Jiménez-Moreno, E., Proszkowiec-Weglarz, M. and Plumstead, P.W. (2018) Impacts of age and calcium on phytase efficacy in broiler chickens. *Animal Feed Science and Technology* 238, 9–17.

Liem, A., Pesti, G.M. and Edwards, H.M. Jr (2008) The effect of several organic acids on phytate phosphorus hydrolysis in broiler chicks. *Poultry Science* 87, 689–693.

Madrid, J., Catala-Gregori, P., Garcia, V. and Hernandez, F. (2010) Effect of a multienzyme complex in wheat–soybean meal diet on digestibility of broiler chickens under different rearing conditions. *Italian Journal of Animal Science* 9, e1.

Masey O'Neill, H.V. (2016) Characterization of the experimental diets. In: Bedford, M.R., Choct, M. and Masey O'Neill, H.V. (eds) *Nutrition Experiments in Pigs and Poultry: A Practical Guide*. CABI International, Wallingford, UK, pp. 62–73.

Mavromichalis, I., Hancock, J.D., Senne, B.W., Gugle, T.L., Kennedy, G.A., *et al.* (2000) Enzyme supplementation and particle size of wheat in diets for nursery and finishing pigs. *Journal of Animal Science* 78, 3086–3095.

McCormick, K., Walk, C.L., Wyatt, C.L. and Adeola, O. (2017) Phosphorus utilization response of pigs and broiler chickens to diets supplemented with antimicrobials and phytase. *Animal Nutrition* 3, 77–84.

Meng, X., Slominski, B.A. and Guenter, W. (2004) The effect of fat type, carbohydrase, and lipase addition on growth performance and nutrient utilization of young broilers fed wheat-based diets. *Poultry Science* 83, 1718–1727.

Misiura, M.M., Filipe, J.A.N., Walk, C.L. and Kyriazakis, I. (2020) How do pigs deal with dietary phosphorus deficiency? *British Journal of Nutrition* 124, 256–272.

Morgan, A.J. and Bedford, M.R. (1995) Advances in the development and application of feed enzymes. *Australian Poultry Science Symposium* 7, 109–115.

Morgan, N.K., Keerqin, C., Wallace, A., Wu, S.-B. and Choct, M. (2019) Effect of arabinoxylo-oligosaccharide and arabinoxylans on net energy and nutrient utilization in broilers. *Animal Nutrition* 5, 56–62.

Moss, A.F., Chrystal, P.V., Truong, H.H., Liu, S.Y. and Selle, P.H. (2017) Effects of phytase inclusions in diets containing ground wheat or 12.5% whole wheat (pre- and post-pellet) and phytase and protease additions, individually and in combination, to diets containing 12.5% pre-pellet whole wheat on the performance of broiler chickens. *Animal Science and Technology* 234, 139–150.

Nordentoft, S., Molbak, L., Bjerrum, L., De Vylder, J., Immerseel, F.V. and Pedersen, K. (2011) The influence of the cage system and colonization of *Salmonella* Enteritidis on the microbial gut flora of laying hens studied by T-RFLP and 454 pyrosequencing. *BMC Microbiology* 11, 187.

Nourmohammadi, R., Hosseini, M.S., Farhangfar, H. and Bashtani, M. (2012) Effect of citric acid and microbial phytase enzyme on ileal digestibility of some nutrients in broiler chicks fed corn–soybean meal diets. *Italian Journal of Animal Science* 11, 36–40.

Olukosi, O.A., Cowieson, A.J. and Adeola, O. (2007) Age-related influence of a cocktail of xylanase, amylase, and protease or phytase individually or in combination in broilers. *Poultry Science* 86, 77–86.

Omogbenigun, F.O., Nyachoti, C.M. and Slominski, B.A. (2003) The effect of supplementing microbial phytase and organic acids to a corn–soybean based diet fed to early-weaned pigs. *Journal of Animal Science* 81, 1806–1813.

Park, J.H. and Kim, I.H. (2018) Effects of a protease and essential oils on growth performance, blood cell profiles, nutrient retention, ileal microbiota, excreta gas emission, and breast meat quality in broiler chicks. *Poultry Science* 97, 2854–2860.

Peek, H.W., van der Klis, J.D., Vermeulen, B. and Landman, W.J.M. (2009) Dietary protease can alleviate negative effects of a coccidiosis infection on production performance in broiler chickens. *Animal Feed Science and Technology* 150, 151–159.

Pesti, G.M., Vedenov, D., Cason, J.A. and Billard, L. (2009) A comparison of methods to estimate nutritional requirements from experimental data. *British Poultry Science* 50, 16–32.

Pesti, G.M., Vedenov, D., Nunes, R. and Alhotan, R. (2018) *Three Workbooks to Help Estimate Experimental Power and Normalize Experimental Data*. Bulletin No. 1491. University of Georgina Extension, Athens, Georgia. Available at: https://extension.uga.edu/publications/detail.html?number=B1491&title=Three%20Workbooks%20to%20Help%20Estimate%20Experimental%20Power (accessed 25 June 2019).

Ponte, P.I.P., Ferreira, L.M.A., Soares, M.A.C., Gama, L.T. and Fontes, C.M.G.A. (2004) Xylanase inhibitors affect the action of exogenous enzymes used to supplement *Triticum durum*-based diets for broiler chicks. *Journal of Applied Poultry Research* 13, 660–666.

Ravindran, V. (2013) Feed enzymes: the science, practice, and metabolic realities. *Journal of Applied Poultry Research* 22, 628–636.

Ravindran, V., Morel, P.C.H., Partridge, G.G., Hruby, M. and Sands, J.S. (2006) Influence of an *Escherichia coli*-derived phytase on nutrient utilization in broiler starters fed diets containing varying concentrations of phytic acid. *Poultry Science* 85, 82–89.

Rice, J.P., Pleasant, R.S. and Radcliffe, J.S. (2002) The effect of citric acid, phytase and their interaction on gastric pH, and Ca, P and dry matter digestibilities. In: *Purdue University Swine Research Report*. Purdue University, West Lafayette, Indiana, pp. 36–42.

Ritz, C.W., Hulet, R.M., Self, B.B. and Denbow, D.M. (1995) Endogenous amylase levels and response to supplemental feed enzymes in male turkeys from hatch to eight weeks of age. *Poultry Science* 74, 1317–1322.

Roofchaei, A., Rezaeipour, V., Vatandour, S. and Zaefarian, F. (2019) Influence of dietary carbohydrases, individually or in combination with phytase or an acidifier, on performance, gut morphology and microbial population in broiler chickens fed a wheat-based diet. *Animal Nutrition* 5, 63–67.

Rosen, G.D. (2003a) Setting and meeting standards for the efficient replacement of pronutrient antibiotics in broiler, turkey, and pig nutrition. In: Kreuzer, M., Wenk, C. and Lanzini, T. (eds) *Gesunde Nutztiere: heutiger Stellewert der Futterzusatzstoffe in der Tierernährung*. Tagungsbericht, Band 24: *Schriftenreihe aus den Institut für Nutztierwissenschaften Gruppe Ernährung, ETH Zürich*. ETH-Zentrum, Zurich, pp. 72–88.

Rosen, G. (2003b) Effects of genetic, managemental and dietary factors on the efficacy of exogenous microbial phytase in broiler nutrition. *British Poultry Science* 44(Suppl. 1), 25–26.

Rosen, G. (2004a) Optimizing the replacement of pronutrient antibiotics in poultry nutrition. In: Lyons, T.P. and Jacques, K.A. (eds) *Nutritional Biotechnology in the Feed and Food Industries*. Nottingham University Press, Nottingham, UK, pp. 93–101.

Rosen, G. (2004b) *Admixture of exogenous phytases and xylanases in broiler nutrition*. Presented at *XXII World's Poultry Congress, Istanbul, Turkey, 8–13 June 2004*.

Rosen, G. (2010) Holo-analysis of the efficacy of exogenous enzyme performance in farm animal nutrition. In: Bedford, M.R. and Partridge, G.G. (eds) *Enzymes in Farm Animal Nutrition*, 2nd edn. CAB International, Wallingford, UK, pp. 273–303.

Sacranie, A., Adiya, X., Mydland, L.T. and Svihus, B. (2017) Effect of intermittent feeding and oat hulls to improve phytase efficacy and digestive function in broiler chickens. *British Poultry Science* 58, 442–451.

Sang, J.O. (2014) Meta-analysis to draw the appropriate regimen of enzyme and probiotic supplementation to pigs and chicken diets. *Asian-Australasian Journal of Animal Sciences* 24, 573–586.

Samat, N. (2015) Improvement of phytase efficacy in poultry through dietary fat supplementation. PhD thesis, University of Leeds, Leeds, UK.

Samat, N., Kuehn, I., Walk, C. and Miller, H. (2013) Effects of fat and phytase supplementation on growth performance of young broiler chickens. *Abstracts 2013, British Poultry Abstracts* 9, 19–20.

Santos, T.T., Gomes, G.A., Walk, C.L., Freitas, B.V. and Araujo, L.F. (2013) Effect of formaldehyde inclusion on phytase efficiency in broilers. *Journal of Applied Poultry Research* 22, 204–210.

Santos, T.T., Walk, C.L. and Srinongkote, S. (2014) Influence of phytate level on broiler performance and the efficacy of 2 microbial phytases from 0 to 21 days of age. *Journal of Applied Poultry Research* 23, 181–187.

Santos, T.T., Connolly, C. and Murphy, R. (2015) Trace element inhibition of phytase activity. *Biological Trace Element Research* 163, 255–265.

Selle, P.H. and Ravindran, V. (2007) Microbial phytase in poultry nutrition. *Animal Feed Science and Technology* 135, 1–41.

Selle, P.H., Liu, S.Y., Cai, J. and Cowieson, A.J. (2013) Steam-pelleting temperatures, grain variety, feed form and protease supplementation of mediumly ground, sorghum-based broiler diets: influences on growth performance, relative gizzard weights, nutrient utilisation, starch and nitrogen digestibility. *Animal Production Science* 53, 378–387.

Shang, Y., Rogiewicz, A., Patterson, R., Slominski, B.A. and Kim, W.K. (2015) The effect of phytase and fructooligosaccharide supplementation on growth performance, bone quality, and phosphorus utilization in broiler chickens. *Poultry Science* 94, 955–964.

Shapiro, F. and Nir, I. (1995) Stunting syndrome in broilers: effect of age and exogenous amylase and protease on performance, development of the digestive tract, digestive enzyme activity, and apparent digestibility. *Poultry Science* 74, 2019–2028.

Shaw, A.L., van Ginkel, F.W., Macklin, K.S. and Blake, J.P. (2011) Effects of phytase supplementation in broiler diets on a natural *Eimeria* challenge in naïve and vaccinated birds. *Poultry Science* 90, 781–790.

Sheehan, N. (2010) Analysis of enzymes, principles and problems: developments in enzyme analysis. In: Bedford, M.R. and Partridge, G.G. (eds) *Enzymes in Farm Animal Nutrition*, 2nd edn. CAB International, Wallingford, UK, pp. 260–272.

Snow, J.L., Baker, D.H. and Parsons, C.M. (2004) Phytase, citric acid and 1α-hydroxycholecalciferol improve phytate phosphorus utilization in chicks fed a corn–soybean meal diet. *Poultry Science* 83, 1187–1192.

Sulabo, R.C., Jones, C.K., Tokach, M.D., Goodband, R.D., Dritz, S.S., *et al.* (2011) Factors affecting storage stability of various commercial phytase sources. *Journal of Animal Science* 89, 4262–4271.

Svihus, B. (2010) Effect of digestive tract conditions, feed processing and ingredients on response to NSP enzymes. In: Bedford, M.R. and Partridge, G.G. (eds) *Enzymes in Farm Animal Nutrition*, 2nd edn. CAB International, Wallingford, UK, pp. 129–159.

Svihus, B., Lund, V.B., Borjgen, B., Bedford, M.R. and Bakken, M. (2013) Effect of intermittent feeding, structural components and phytase on performance and behaviour of broiler chickens. *British Poultry Science* 54, 222–230.

Tancharoenrat, P., Ravindran, V., Molan, A.L. and Ravindran, G. (2014) Influence of fat source and xylanase supplementation on performance, utilisation of energy and fat, and caecal microbiota counts in broiler starters fed wheat-based diets. *Journal of Poultry Science* 51, 172–179.

Tiwari, U.P., Chen, H., Kim, S.W. and Jha, R. (2018) Supplemental effect of xylanase and mannanase on nutrient digestibility and gut health of nursery pigs studied using both *in vivo* and *in vitro* models. *Animal Feed Science and Technology* 245, 77–90.

Vieira, S.L., Freitas, D.M., Coneglian, J.L., Pena, J.E.M. and Berres, J. (2007) Live performance evaluation of broilers fed all vegetable corn–soy diets supplemented with an alpha amylase–beta glucanase blend. *Poultry Science Journal* 86, 399–400.

Waititu, S.M., Yin, F., Patterson, R., Rodriguez-Lecompte, J.C. and Nyachoti, C.M. (2016) Short-term effect of supplemental yeast extract without or with feed enzymes on growth performance, immune status and gut structure of weaned pigs challenged with *Escherichia coli* lipopolysaccharide. *Journal of Animal Science and Biotechnology* 7, 64–77.

Walk, C.L. and Rama Rao, S.V. (2020) Increasing dietary phytate has a significant anti-nutrient effect on apparent ileal amino acid digestibility and digestible amino acid intake requiring increasing doses of phytase as evidenced by prediction equations in broilers. *Poultry Science* 99, 290–330.

Walk, C.L., Wilcock, P. and Magowan, E. (2015) Evaluation of the effects of pharmacological zinc oxide and phosphorus source on weaned piglet growth performance, plasma minerals and mineral digestibility. *Animal* 9, 1145–1152.

Wang, T., Bedford, M.R. and Adeola, O. (2019) Investigation of xylanase, diet formulation method for energy, and choice of digestibility index marker on nutrient and energy utilization for broiler chickens and pigs. *Journal of Animal Science* 97, 279–290.

Wealleans, A.L., Walsh, M.C., Romero, L.F. and Ravindran, V. (2017) Comparative effects of two multi-enzyme combinations and a *Bacillus* probiotic on growth performance, digestibility of energy and nutrients, disappearance of non-starch polysaccharides, and gut microflora in broiler chickens. *Poultry Science* 96, 4287–4297.

Wu, Y.B. and Ravindran, V. (2004) Influence of whole wheat inclusion and xylanase supplementation on the performance, digestive tract measurements and carcass characteristics of broiler chickens. *Animal Feed Science and Technology* 116, 129–139.

Yan, F., Dibner, J.J., Knight, C.D. and Vazquez-Anon, M. (2017) Effect of carbohydrase and protease on growth performance and gut health of young broilers fed diets containing rye, wheat, and feather meal. *Poultry Science* 96, 817–828.

Yin, Y.-L., McEvoy, J.D.G., Schulze, H., Hennig, U., Souffrant, W.-B. and McCracken, K.J. (2000) Apparent digestibility (ileal and overall) of nutrients and endogenous nitrogen losses in growing pigs fed wheat (var. Soissons) or its by-products without or with xylanase supplementation. *Livestock Production Science* 62, 119–132.

Yin, Y.-L., McEvoy, J.D., Schulze, H. and McCracken, K.J. (2001a) Effects of xylanase and antibiotic addition on ileal and faecal apparent digestibilities of dietary nutrients and evaluating HCl-insoluble ash as a dietary marker in growing pigs. *Animal Science* 72, 95–103.

Yin, Y.-L., Baidoo, S.K., Jin, L.Z., Liu, Y.G., Schulze, H. and Simmins, P.H. (2001b) The effect of different carbohydrase and protease supplementation on apparent (ileal and overall) digestibility of nutrients of five hulless barley varieties in young pigs. *Livestock Production Science* 71, 109–120.

Zeller, E., Schollenberger, M., Witzig, M., Shastak, Y., Kühn, I., *et al.* (2015) Interactions between supplemented mineral phosphorus and phytase on phytate hydrolysis and inositol phosphates in the small intestine of broilers. *Poultry Science* 94, 1018–1029.

Zeng, Z.K., Li, Q.Y., Tian, Q.Y., Xu, Y.T. and Piao, X.S. (2018) The combination of carbohydrases and phytase to improve nutritional value and non-starch polysaccharides degradation for growing pigs fed diets with or without wheat bran. *Animal Feed Science and Technology* 235, 138–146.

Zuo, J., Ling, B., Long, L., Li, T., Lahaye, L., *et al.* (2015) Effect of dietary supplementation with protease on growth performance, nutrient digestibility, intestinal morphology, digestive enzymes and gene expression of weaned piglets. *Animal Nutrition* 1, 276–282.

17 Evolving Enzyme Applications

Michael R. Bedford[1], Carrie L. Walk[2] and Milan Hruby[3]

[1]AB Vista, Marlborough, UK; [2]DSM Nutritional Products, Heanor, UK; [3]ADM, Decatur, Illinois, USA

17.1 Doses

With the advancement of production strains or production capabilities to yield more enzyme activity per gram of protein, the use of super- or megadoses of enzymes may become more economical and commercially applicable in the future. Superdosing phytase has gained considerable traction in the market over the past 10 years, with benefits associated with feed efficiency, feed cost savings and sustainability. Diets containing superdoses of phytase now account for almost 15% of phytase sales by value and it is increasing in proportion with time.

The use of by-product feed ingredients, novel feed ingredients, or local cereals and legumes in production animal diets might result in greater concentrations of phytate and fibre and variable ingredient quality. To ensure optimal utilization of nutrients by the animal and mitigation of any antinutritional effects on growth performance or digestibility, the use of superdoses or megadoses of enzymes might be required to ensure rapid and efficient breakdown of phytate, fibre fractions or polysaccharides. However, care must be taken with increasing doses of some enzymes. For example, overdosing some carbohydrases may potentiate the depolymerization of beneficial oligosaccharides and overdosing some proteases may degrade non-target proteins and thus digestive efficiency. The stand-out anomaly here is phytases, where an optimum dose seems to be well above even current superdosed levels, particularly to target the lower phytate esters.

17.2 Animal Categories

The need and desire to produce animal protein in a more sustainable fashion and changing human meat consumption patterns will increase the use, adaptation and uptake of enzymes into the diets of ruminants and fish. The use of enzymes in sustainable animal nutrition is not new. Phytase was developed to improve P utilization by pigs and poultry and thereby reduce excretion of P and prevent eutrophication of rivers, lakes and streams. In the future, the use of enzymes in sustainable agriculture will include new categories of enzymes, endogenous enzyme inhibitors and the species to which they are applied. For example, the additives 3-nitrooxypropanol (3-NOP) and lubabegron are both endogenous enzyme inhibitors; 3-NOP has been shown to reduce emissions of the greenhouse gas methane from dairy cows by 30% and lubabegron to reduce ammonia in beef cattle manure and urine. Supplementation of carbohydrases into ruminant diets increases milk yield

DOI: 10.1079/9781789241563.0017

and improves fibre digestion. On the other hand, the use of phytase and xylanase in the diets of some species of fish allows for the use of more plant-based protein sources, thereby decreasing the use of animal-based protein meals while improving nutrient utilization and reducing waste runoff into water courses.

In addition, changing human consumption patterns towards less meat (beef, pork, chicken) might increase the consumption of fish and aquaculture to a greater extent than is currently forecast. If this were to occur, the development of enzymes (phytase, carbohydrases, protease or others) specific to the gastrointestinal properties of fish (pH, temperature, time) may take place. In turn, the use of plant-based ingredients in aquaculture could expand to include novel protein meals and alternatives to soybean meal, which contain a much greater content of fibre and phytate than found in fishmeal. The knowledge of endogenous enzymes and the use of enzyme inhibitors in combination with exogenous enzymes to improve nutrient utilization and reduce excretion will facilitate more sustainable animal production. In addition, wider categories of animals and animal products will benefit from exogenous enzymes in the future.

17.2.1   Pets

The global pet food market is worth over US$70 billion annually and expected to grow year on year. Although inclusion of enzymes in pet food is becoming an increasingly popular trend to aid digestion, there still appears to be relatively few brands that incorporate and advertise enzymes as part of their pet food and other pet products portfolio. Many brands, particularly premium brands, promote addition of enzymes together with other beneficial dietary components including prebiotics and probiotics, antioxidant-rich ingredients and natural ingredients. Heat-labile compounds like enzymes, but also vitamins, amino acids, probiotics, fatty acids and medicines, are not well suited to high-temperature and -pressure

processing such as extrusion used to manufacture pet food and treats. To maintain functionality of enzymes, some manufacturers add enzymes after the food has been heat-treated and there are also new technological trends gaining ground including cold extrusion, which could be particularly useful with ingredients known to be sensitive to heat. The main trends in the pet food market are related to humanization of pets and pet food quality. For example, humans are increasingly aware of their lifestyle and the impact nutrition has on their own health and longevity, as well as that of their pets. There is also a drive to focus on natural and minimally processed ingredients and nutrients to improve nutrient digestibility and reduce potential digestive disorders. Due to the trend to increase animal protein levels in pet food products, protease will likely be a key enzyme in the future. Interest to include other plant materials like vegetables, fruits and ancient grains will also allow for carbohydrase enzymes and amylase to find a growth opportunity space within the significantly growing pet food market.

17.2.2   Humans

Enzymes in human food preparation have a long history. They can be found in numerous applications within various food industries including starch and sugar, baking, brewing, dairy, meat, juice and wine. They are irreplaceable in many food-production processes not only to improve the quality of final products (bread, fruit juice, meat tenderness, cheese production and flavour, beer, wine, shelf life) but also to help individuals with specific disorders like lactose intolerance or are used to improve the digestion of complex carbohydrates (e.g. α-galactosidase-containing products).

Specific enzyme supplements are also available in the market to complement enzymes produced by the human body (protease, amylase, maltase, lipase) as well as to provide other activities such as xylanase, β-glucanase, α-galactosidase, cellulase, nattokinase and phytase. We see consumers taking greater control of their healthcare and looking to various supplements, including enzymes, in the future. Digestion of plant proteins including gluten, blood glucose control, cardiovascular support and even focus on diseases such as Alzheimer's are strong future opportunities for enzymes in this fast-evolving human nutrition and health area.

17.3   Minor or Novel Enzyme Classes

17.3.1   Antimicrobial enzymes

The major shift in animal production methods towards no antibiotics ever or no growth-promoting antibiotics has resulted in a plethora of research around antimicrobial mitigation. Numerous products are available, such as enzymes, yeast cell walls or oligosaccharides, organic acids, and immune activators or mitigators, with variable rates of success. The use of exogenous antimicrobial enzymes, such as lysozyme, might be a useful control of pathogenic bacteria and act to complement the animals' own antimicrobial enzyme secretions. For example, hen egg white lysozyme has been shown to decrease pathogenic bacteria in the gastrointestinal tract. Other functions of antimicrobial enzymes may be to break down dead bacterial cell walls (muramidase) or dephosphorylate lipopolysaccharides (alkaline phosphatase) and thereby reduce the pro-inflammatory response associated with the presence of these end products in the gut lumen. Bacteriophage lysins are enzymes which break open target cells and can be engineered to be produced and fed as a targeted antimicrobial approach. In this regard, the benefits of antimicrobial enzymes could be twofold: to decrease pathogenic bacteria and/or the immune response associated with the presence of the bacteria or bacterial products. Wider uptake of antimicrobial enzymes, specifically ones known to reduce pathogenic bacteria, in the market will require a re-evaluation of product registration criteria and categories, as they are not antibiotics but do have antimicrobial properties.

17.3.2   Lipases

Most fat sources in animal diets are highly digestible by the animal and once absorbed, the fat source retains a considerable amount of its original form and is only modified for transport across the enterocytes and into the tissues. In broilers, body fat is similar in structure and form as that in the diet. Therefore, the use of exogenous lipases to digest or aid in fat digestion might not be as widespread as that of phytase or carbohydrases. However, the use of lipases in young animals or geriatric pets, with inefficient digestive enzymes, may be a growth area in the future. In addition, the use of lipases to enable the use of poorly digested sources of fat or help to release other fatty acids and fat-based coatings could provide areas of growth for lipases.

17.3.3   Enzymes for by-products or novel feed ingredients (keratinases, targeted oligosaccharide producers, local cereals and legumes)

If carbon footprint develops as a significant factor in animal protein production, then use of local ingredients will become critical in the quest to minimize the effect of raising farm animals on climate change. Credible alternatives to corn, wheat and soya, which all have high input or transportation requirements, include rye and rapeseed. Development/adaptation of current enzyme strategies to take account of such changes in the diet, should they occur, will inevitably contribute to reducing the environmental impact of animal protein production. Other protein sources, such as algal, insect and yeast, are all potential targets for enzymatic improvements but the volumes available will probably limit their ability to replace the current annual usage of 330 million tonnes of soybean meal.

17.3.4   *In situ* enzyme expression

In-plant or in-animal expression of enzymes, particularly phytase and xylanase, has been tested over the past 40 years. Recently, corn-derived phytase has been shown to increase P digestibility and maintain growth performance of broilers and pigs fed low-P diets, whereas saliva-expressed phytase resulted in significant improvements in P digestibility of pigs. Therefore, the use of *in situ* enzymes is a possibility. However, consumer preference and concerns regarding genetically modified organisms as a source of food or in animal feeds may halt any further advancements towards in-plant or in-animal expression of enzymes. This phenomenon seems to be country specific and may mean the end of further advancements in the expression of exogenous or even overexpression of endogenous enzymes in animals.

In conclusion, the future of enzyme application in production animal diets will continue to grow and evolve. Current enzyme uses and recommendations will become more precise and targeted. Novel enzyme categories will enable the use of alternative feed ingredients or uptake of enzymes into new animal categories. Consumer preferences will continue to drive animal production guidelines, and this will facilitate enzyme development into new categories focused on gut health and functionality, improved nutrient utilization and digestibility, and of course sustainability.

Index

Note: Page numbers in *italics* denote tables and figures.

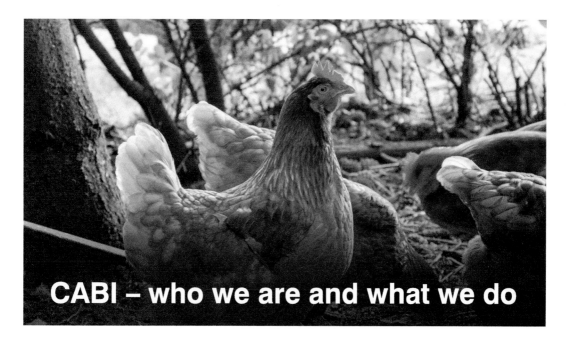

CABI – who we are and what we do

This book is published by **CABI**, an international not-for-profit organisation that improves people's lives worldwide by providing information and applying scientific expertise to solve problems in agriculture and the environment.

CABI is also a global publisher producing key scientific publications, including world renowned databases, as well as compendia, books, ebooks and full text electronic resources. We publish content in a wide range of subject areas including: agriculture and crop science / animal and veterinary sciences / ecology and conservation / environmental science / horticulture and plant sciences / human health, food science and nutrition / international development / leisure and tourism.

The profits from CABI's publishing activities enable us to work with farming communities around the world, supporting them as they battle with poor soil, invasive species and pests and diseases, to improve their livelihoods and help provide food for an ever growing population.

CABI is an international intergovernmental organisation, and we gratefully acknowledge the core financial support from our member countries (and lead agencies) including:

 Ministry of Agriculture People's Republic of China

 Australian Government Australian Centre for International Agricultural Research

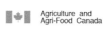 Agriculture and Agri-Food Canada

 Ministry of Foreign Affairs of the Netherlands

 Schweizerische Eidgenossenschaft Confédération suisse Confederazione Svizzera Confederaziun svizra
Swiss Agency for Development and Cooperation SDC

Discover more

To read more about CABI's work, please visit: **www.cabi.org**

Browse our books at: **www.cabi.org/bookshop**,
or explore our online products at: **www.cabi.org/publishing-products**

Interested in writing for CABI? Find our author guidelines here:
www.cabi.org/publishing-products/information-for-authors/